Medicine and Biomedical Sciences in Modern History

The aim of this series is to illuminate the development and impact of medicine and the biomedical sciences in the modern era.The series was founded by the late Professor John Pickstone, and its ambitions reflect his commitment to the integrated study of medicine, science and technology in their contexts. He repeatedly commented that it was a pity that the foundation discipline of the field, for which he popularized the acronym 'HSTM' (History of Science, Technology and Medicine) had been the history of science rather than the history of medicine. His point was that historians of science had too often focused just on scientific ideas and institutions, while historians of medicine always had to consider the understanding, management and meanings of diseases in their socioeconomic, cultural, technological and political contexts. In the event, most of the books in the series dealt with medicine and the biomedical sciences, and the changed series title reflects this. However, as the new editors we share Professor Pickstone's enthusiasm for the integrated study of medicine, science and technology, encouraging studies on biomedical science, translational medicine, clinical practice, disease histories, medical technologies, medical specialisms and health policies.

The books in this series will present medicine and biomedical science as crucial features of modern culture, analysing their economic, social and political aspects, while not neglecting their expert content and context. Our authors investigate the uses and consequences of technical knowledge, and how it shaped, and was shaped by, particular economic, social and political structures. In re-launching the series, we hope to build on its strengths but extend its geographical range beyond Western Europe and North America.

Medicine and Biomedical Sciences in Modern History is intended to supply analysis and stimulate debate. All books are based on searching historical study of topics which are important, not least because they cut across conventional academic boundaries. They should appeal not just to historians, nor just to medical practitioners, scientists and engineers, but to all who are interested in the place of medicine and biomedical sciences in modern history.

This series continues the Science, Technology and Medicine in Modern History series.

Suryakanthie Chetty

Reconstructive Surgery and Modernisation in Twentieth-Century South Africa

The Professional and Public Life of Jack Penn

palgrave
macmillan

Suryakanthie Chetty
Department of History
Stellenbosch University
Stellenbosch
Western Cape, South Africa

ISSN 2947-9142 ISSN 2947-9150 (electronic)
Medicine and Biomedical Sciences in Modern History
ISBN 978-3-031-38672-5 ISBN 978-3-031-38673-2 (eBook)
https://doi.org/10.1007/978-3-031-38673-2

Cover illustration: Jack Penn (left) and Albert Schweitzer" (mss_bc748_c01) reproduced with permission of Special Collections, University of Cape Town Libraries

This Palgrave Macmillan imprint is published by the registered company Springer Nature Switzerland AG
The registered company address is: Gewerbestrasse 11, 6330 Cham, Switzerland

Preface and Acknowledgements

This work has been a challenge to write as it morphed from what was envisioned as a simple biography of a surgical pioneer as a lens into the history of medicine and surgery, into a much broader engagement with twentieth-century South African history in relation to science, technology and the ideology of modernisation.

While my postgraduate research focused on the Second World War—as it related to gender—I subsequently turned to my other passion, the history of science. In 2019, reading about the work of Harold Gillies, I inadvertently stumbled upon Jack Penn, a plastic and reconstructive surgeon. Upon reading his autobiography, *The Right to Look Human*, I was enthralled. I had paid very little attention to plastic surgery—or the history of medicine itself—prior to this but Penn seemed the ideal figure to combine my research interests in the Second World War with the history of science. What followed, however, was a project that became far more ambitious—frequently testing my abilities—that would lead me on a figurative journey around the world.

During a time of tremendous upheaval, working on this project has been a means of highlighting what I believe to be the central role of the historian—an attempt to create meaning and bring a sense of order to the perceived chaos. Through the construction of a narrative from disparate sources, historians can trace the greater patterns of which an individual life forms part. Penn was not unaware of the importance of a human life and a belief in the sense of responsibility on the part of the individual to contribute to the greater good. And it was this belief that in many ways, made up for the various shortcomings that characterised some of his thinking which created much frustration as I sought to tie the various elements of his life together. That too, provided an important lesson in empathy and raised thought-provoking questions about the responsibility of the historian in recreating a life, especially one of a complex public and sometimes controversial figure.

While much of this journey has been necessarily undertaken during conditions of individual and social restriction, I have not been isolated and I wish to extend my heartfelt gratitude to various people who have given generously of their time to encourage me in numerous ways, from reading drafts to suggesting sources—and frequently providing a much-needed shoulder: first and foremost, Anne and John Samson for their unwavering support and kindness, Tilman Dedering, Saul Dubow, Johannes Du Bruyn, Anton Ehlers, Karen Jennings and Alex and Aline Mouton.

This work was also made possible through the dedication of the staff at the various archives around the country: Jennifer Kimble at the Brenthurst Library, Clive Kirkwood at the Jagger Library, the acting curator at the Adler Museum, Sepeke Sekgwele and Steve de Agrela at the Department of Defence Archives. I would also like to extend my thanks to Vivien Jandera at APRASSA and my colleagues at the History Department, Stellenbosch University.

Finally, this project is dedicated to my mother and to Nicholas Southey.

Stellenbosch, South Africa Suryakanthie Chetty

Contents

CHAPTER 1

Introduction

The history of modern plastic and reconstructive surgery during the first decades of the twentieth century is one that is marked by a struggle for acceptance. In contrast to other areas of surgery, it had greater associations with the aesthetic and was therefore not seen as essential as surgical specialisations directly related to the treatment of life-threatening injury. As the First World War demonstrated, however, the psychological effects of injuries—especially those related to the face—were as significant as the physical trauma itself.

While plastic surgery has a history dating back to ancient Egypt, in its modern form its development is intertwined with modern conflict and the First World War. As a specialisation in the twentieth century then, plastic surgery was bound to the ideology of modernisation. This is evident in the career of pioneering South African plastic surgeon, Jack Penn that was contextualised by the significant events of a tumultuous century—the Second World War, the Cold War, decolonisation and apartheid.

In the *Shock of the Old*, David Edgerton makes the claim that there is little that is "new" about technology. Rather than a simple association with linear progression and modernity, technological developments draw upon and are based on elements of the past which continue into

S. Chetty, *Reconstructive Surgery and Modernisation in Twentieth-Century South Africa*, Medicine and Biomedical Sciences in Modern History, https://doi.org/10.1007/978-3-031-38673-2_1

the present in diverse ways.[1] This is evident in plastic and reconstructive surgery. Throughout its history plastic surgery has been associated with conflict that precipitated the kinds of injuries requiring the intervention of a plastic surgeon. The techniques developed in the past were, however, refined during the First and Second World Wars with the former perceived as the birth of modern reconstructive surgery. The surgical treatment of the wounded was based on the adaptation of older techniques to address the injuries caused by the weapons of modern warfare—the artillery of the First World War and the burns incurred by pilots during the Second World War. There were also developments in the use of materials ranging from metals to plastics to aid reconstruction, the collaboration with other specialists such as dental surgeons, the availability of new technology such as X-rays that co-existed with the artistic impressions of injuries and the availability of new drugs such as penicillin to address infection. An important development during the First and Second World Wars, however, was the better organisation of medical services with the creation of reconstructive surgical units close to the front lines as well as surgical units at hospitals. Soldiers could thus receive early treatment, thereby reducing the chances of infection and complications, before being sent to surgical centres for long-term recuperation. Penn's development of the Brenthurst Splint provided immediate treatment for facial injuries without the need for medical personnel. War itself also contributed to the professionalisation of plastic surgery. While plastic and reconstructive surgery in the twentieth century is based on the use of increasingly sophisticated instrumentation and techniques to redress physical injury and deformity, it cannot simply be equated to technological development, retaining throughout elements of its past.

Yet it is the narrative of progress and modernity that underpinned Jack's Penn's work in plastic surgery and the history of the specialisation. Penn's story also highlights another aspect of Edgerton's argument—the ideological context of technology and the ways in which it may be considered conservative rather than simply progressive where "old power relations are transmitted through new technology".[2]

[1] *Cf* David Edgerton, *The Shock of the Old: Technology and Global History Since 1900* (London, Profile Books Ltd, 2008).

[2] Ibid., p159.

This is evident in the South African context in Bill Freund's overview of the developmental history of the country from the early twentieth century to the end of apartheid. Freund makes a noteworthy point by demonstrating that modernisation cannot simply be equated to "whiteness" with development occurring unevenly in Europe and, later in South Africa, and accompanied by resistance to the changes it wrought.[3] As Freund shows in the South African context—and this is further borne out in David Edgerton's work—modernisation and development do not exist in their idealised form within a state but engage with the socio-economic context as well as the state's unique history. In South Africa, modernisation was linked with race from the inception of the state in 1910 and the control over black labour. During the first stage of Penn's career, race was marked by paternalism coupled with segregation. Penn's work during the Second World War was part of a "modernist" bent by the state under Jan Smuts to take the lead in promoting science and technological development. As Freund shows, this continued from 1948. Within the context of decolonisation however, race becomes more explicit in Penn's writings with increasing black urbanisation requiring a balancing act on the part of the state to uphold the ideology of racial distinction while simultaneously addressing the changing needs of the economy. It also impelled the state to make overtures to possible allies on the African continent and elsewhere, due to increasing isolation. The economic success of the apartheid state came to an end with the crises of 1973, and it is here that Freund provides the context for Penn's views on racial distinction and difference. The economic crisis of 1973 coupled with the Soweto uprising of 1976 led to reform initiatives to the system of apartheid and this contextualised Penn's later role in the President's Council with its recommendations for limited reform during P.W. Botha's tenure. Freund's work therefore provides a narrative for the modernisation of the state that contextualises the work of Jack Penn as both surgeon and political figure.

Freund draws in part upon the work of Saul Dubow in showing the dominant political ideologies throughout southern African history from the late nineteenth century and the development of colonial nationalism, asserting itself against dominant British imperialism; the Anglo-centric attempts at reconstruction under Alfred Milner in the wake of the South

[3] Bill Freund, *Twentieth-Century South Africa: A Developmental History* (Cambridge, Cambridge University Press, 2019), p4.

African War (1899–1902) and South Africanism during the era of segregation that sought to reconcile English- and Afrikaans-speaking white South Africans while entrenching the exclusion of other groups. Even when the Second World War signalled the potential for a brief thawing in the system of segregation, the rise of the apartheid state in 1948 marked a return to uncompromising racially based policies.[4] The final phase then, is that of Afrikaner nationalism with the state privileging security over development.

Penn's career straddled both the worlds of segregation and apartheid with his early education and training taking place before the Second World War and his major exposure to the international trends in plastic surgery occurring during the War itself as he travelled to Britain and just immediately after the War, the United States. Yet, his career correlated even more closely with the narrative of development as promulgated by the apartheid state in the 1950s and 1960s that contextualised Penn's sharing of his medical expertise with countries such as Japan, Gabon and Israel. His later political involvement and philosophical writings suggested a man whose career engaged with the prevailing developmental ethos after 1948.

In the South African historiography, there are a number of figures who have focused on the history of medicine: Howard Phillips has addressed medicine from a social history perspective with a focus on epidemics[5]; Julie Parle has been prominent in focusing on the history of psychiatry.[6] As will be addressed in this book, medicine and race are intertwined within the South African context. Co-existing with health and healing is the role of medicine as part of the "civilising mission" dating from the nineteenth century. In the twentieth century, this also meant a significant role in modernisation—as is argued here. As a modern field, medicine is associated with the domination of the white male professional. In the South African context, it is deeply implicated in both racial domination and resistance. The work of Shula Marks and Simmone Horwitz addresses the racial inequalities in nursing, focusing on the unenviable position of

[4] Saul Dubow, *A Commonwealth of Knowledge: Science, Sensibility, and White South Africa, 1820–2000* (Oxford, Oxford University Press, 2007).

[5] *Cf* for instance Howard Phillips, *Plague, Pox and Epidemics: A Jacana Pocket History* (Johannesburg, Jacana, 2012).

[6] Julie Parle, *States of Mind: Searching for Mental Health in Natal & Zululand, 1868–1918* (Scottsville, UKZN Press, 2007).

black nurses. Marks demonstrates the position of black nurses from the nineteenth century as part of the "civilising mission" and their professionalisation as part of an elite, educated black middle class. Horwitz addresses the ways in which nursing was associated with both respectability as well as an idealised gendered role.[7] The ideology of the apartheid state however would reinforce inequality within the nursing profession. Vanessa Noble's *A School of Struggle* looks at the fraught environment of medical education under apartheid. With a focus on the Natal Medical School, Noble highlights the unequal and racialised system of medical education that would eventually lead to the political radicalisation of these medical students. She also addresses the unique position of black doctors in South Africa where their individual aspirations were often subsumed by their leadership and sense of responsibility to the communities from which they originated.[8] In *An Ambulance of the Wrong Colour*, Laurel Baldwin-Ragaven, Leslie London and Jeanelle De Gruchy discuss the uneasy positioning of the universality and ethics underlying medical treatment within the context of racial inequality and the oppression of the apartheid state. This was evident in both the unequal treatment afforded to black and white medical professionals but even more poignantly in significantly different mortality rates between black and white South Africans. An unequal health care system was coupled with segregation in hospitals, ambulances and even blood.[9] This study will incorporate these works to contextualise the career of Jack Penn.

Penn's work is also situated within the broader history of plastic and reconstructive surgery in the twentieth century, culminating in the professionalisation of the field. Plastic surgery had parallels with the earlier development of military medicine and *Between Flesh and Steel* by Richard Gabriel demonstrates the perennial problems faced in war conditions—infection and disease, the evacuation of the wounded, the setting up of

[7] Shula Marks, *Divided Sisterhood: Race, Class and Gender in the South African Nursing Profession* (Johannesburg, Witwatersrand University Press, 1994) and Simmone Horwitz, "'Black Nurses in White': Exploring Young Women's Entry into the Nursing Profession at Baragwanath Hospital, Soweto, 1948 –1980", *Social History of Medicine*, 20, 1, 131–164, 2007.

[8] Vanessa Noble, *A School of Struggle: Durban's Medical School and the Education of Black Doctors in South Africa* (Scottsville, University of KwaZulu-Natal Press, 2013).

[9] Laurel Baldwin-Ragaven, Jeanelle de Gruchy and Leslie London, *An Ambulance of the Wrong Colour: Health Professionals, Human Rights and Ethics in South Africa* (Cape Town, University of Cape Town Press, 1999).

hospitals, the provision of adequate medical care as well as the relationship between technology, injury and developments in medicine. Gabriel also addresses the role of the surgeon in military medicine, warfare providing the necessary conditions for the experience and expertise that would serve to distinguish the initially lowly barber surgeon from the educated medical professional with more theoretical approaches to medicine. It was also warfare that provided the impetus for the increased recognition and status of the surgeon.[10]

While Gabriel focuses on the development of military medicine via various conflicts across time, the edited collection by Thomas Scotland and Steven Heys, *War Surgery*, discusses the watershed moment of the First World War where nineteenth-century medicine met twentieth-century warfare and the sheer number of casualties drove dramatic change in military medicine. This ranged from the evacuation of the wounded, the role of casualty clearing stations and base hospitals that was dependent on the nature of the War, the use of anaesthesia as well as new understanding of the causes and effects of shock and with this, the use of blood transfusions. Benefiting from this was the emerging field of plastic and reconstructive surgery impelled by the profusion of projectile wounds to the face and jaw that characterised trench warfare.[11]

The history of plastic and reconstructive surgery is an understudied area. There have, however, been articles and dissertations that focus in particular on Harold Gillies' work during the First World War as well as the four major treatment centres in Britain during the Second World War. In addition, Emily Mayhew's work on the Guinea Pig Club has proved invaluable in understanding the challenges of plastic surgery during the Second World War.[12] Its focus is on the work of Archie McIndoe—arguably the most prominent plastic surgeon during the conflict and one who would exert a considerable influence on Penn. Mayhew's work has been complemented by Hugh McLeave's biography of McIndoe which is revealing in terms of its portrayal of the relationship between Gillies and

[10] Richard A. Gabriel, *Between Flesh and Steel: A History of Military Medicine from the Middle Ages to the War in Afghanistan* (Lincoln, Potomac Books, 2016).

[11] Thomas Scotland and Steven Heys (eds), *War Surgery, 1914–18* (Solihull, Helion and Company, 2012).

[12] Emily Mayhew, *Guinea Pig Club: Archibald McIndoe and the RAF in World War II* (Barnsley, Pen and Sword Books, 2018).

McIndoe.[13] Other published works that have been of value to this study are *Faces from the Front* by Andrew Bamji[14] as well as *Reconstructing Faces* by Murray Meikle.[15]

It is important to note however that the consideration of race is largely absent from these discussions of plastic surgery. The origin of Gillies' work on soldiers from the Western Front as well as McIndoe's later work on the airmen from the Battle of Britain suggested a norm in plastic surgery as it related to war: the white male. This mirrors in part of the history of medicine where the white male body was considered the standard by which other bodies were measured. Gillies' landmark work *Plastic Surgery of the Face* does not visually depict black patients as either soldiers or civilians.[16] Race is rendered invisible yet race seems essential to reconstruction and plastic surgery in terms of consideration of facial features as well as skin pigment. It is further reinforced in the relationship between art and plastic surgery—in the powerful drawings of Henry Tonks or in the sculptures of Jack Penn. In the case of the latter, black skin presented what he termed "The Problem of Pigment", the term "problem" highlighting its departure from the standard. While acknowledging that pigmented skin was just "the width of tissue paper", pigment cells ran deeper, presenting difficulties for the plastic surgeon. Skin grafts tended to be darker than regular skin; there was a greater likelihood of the formation of "thick scars"; darker skin could not easily permit the diagnosis of lack of blood flow as "European skin" did.[17] At the same time, prominent surgeons such as Archie McIndoe and Penn—as is discussed later—engaged in humanitarian work in Africa, for instance. McIndoe would work on those injured and scarred during the Mau Mau Rebellion in Kenya.[18] Plastic and reconstructive surgery therefore becomes the

[13] Hugh McLeave, *McIndoe: Plastic Surgeon* (London, Frederick Muller Limited, 1961).

[14] Andrew Bamji, *Faces from the Front: Harold Gillies, the Queen's Hospital, Sidcup and the Origins of Modern Plastic Surgery* (Solihull, Helion and Company, 2017).

[15] Murray C. Meikle, *Reconstructing Faces: The Art and Wartime Surgery of Gillies, Pickerill, McIndoe and Mowlem* (Otago University Press, 2015).

[16] *Cf.* H.D. Gillies, *Plastic Surgery of the Face* (London, Henry Frowde and Hodder and Stoughton, 1920).

[17] Jack Penn, *The Right to Look Human: An Autobiography* (Johannesburg, Hugh Keartland Publishers, 1976), p20. Penn's autobiography was also published by McGraw-Hill Book Company two years earlier. This book draws upon the later publication.

[18] McLeave, *McIndoe*, p152.

ideal illustration of the tension between a context of racial difference and the humanitarianism and universalism of medical treatment—that would be such a feature of Penn's career.

Apart from being an artist and surgeon, Jack Penn was a prolific writer and many of his writings underpin the arguments made in this book. Most significant is his autobiography *The Right to Look Human* focusing on his military and civilian career as well as his experiences in promoting the training of plastic surgery in Africa, Asia and the Middle East. Penn would later revise this autobiography with "A Surgeon's Story: It is the Divine Right of Man to Look Human", an unpublished manuscript. Penn also published work on his philosophical musings: his thinking on social, economic and political issues. These significant sources for analysis include *Reflections on Life* and *Letters to My Son*. He further contributed to an essay collection edited by Sarah Gertrude Millin and wrote another work that explicitly spelled out his idealised vision for society, "Towards a Modern Utopia". These works are housed at the Brenthurst Library.

His time in Lambarene is drawn largely from the correspondence between Penn and Albert Schweitzer as well as letters written to his family and friends detailing his views of and experiences in Schweitzer's hospital as well as his subsequent attempts to improve the hospital in light of modern medical practice. These form the core of the "Dr Jack Penn Collection" at the Jagger Library (University of Cape Town Libraries).

His political career has been drawn from the reports of the President's Council held in the Stellenbosch University Law Library and this has been contextualised and complemented by the detailed discussions of the workings and findings of the Council in the *Rand Daily Mail*.

The Department of Defence Archives contains documents relating to his military career—his trip to Britain on the outbreak of the Second World War to gain experience in reconstructive surgery under Gillies et al. as well as material relating to the establishment of the Tara hospital.

The Adler Museum at the University of the Witwatersrand Medical School contains several unpublished works by Penn including his Palestinian diary, collections of essays and a manuscript "Philosophy is Fun". In addition, there are newspaper and periodical clippings of interviews and features with Penn collected by him which focus largely on the latter part of his life. Further, there are copies of a regular column written by Penn for the *Washington Weekly* in the form of both the published articles as well as what appears to be typed drafts of articles that may or may not have been published.

The discussion of his surgical work is drawn partially from articles appearing in various medical journals and in the *Brenthurst Papers*, a journal established and edited by Penn during the Second World War and housed at the Brenthurst Library and Adler Museum. Other journal articles detail his work in medicine as well as research projects undertaken with Theodore Gillman. Additional primary material has also been incorporated into the narrative such as the use of newspaper articles.

The narrative has been divided into three parts, each dealing with a distinct element of Jack Penn's career. The first, "The Face of War", relates to his training as a surgeon and specialisation as a plastic surgeon. Here, a major component of Penn's experiences is the education and experience he received in Britain and the United States in both the interwar period and during the War itself. This underpinned the foundation for the Brenthurst Hospital established during the War and would later influence Penn's private practice.

Chapter 2 focuses on Penn's early life in Cape Town and Johannesburg as well as his secondary schooling and experiences at medical school where he first encountered the work of Harold Gillies. It briefly addresses the development of modern plastic surgery during the First World War. The subsequent chapter looks at Penn's formative experiences as a doctor with an emphasis on his specialisation as a surgeon in Britain and subsequent trip to the United States. It contextualises Penn's training abroad within the profound changes occurring in the field of medicine—and surgery—from the late nineteenth century, related to scientific research, education and professionalisation. Significant here—and marked by its absence in Penn's recollections—is the unavailability of medical training for black doctors in South Africa. As in the case of Penn, they were compelled to study abroad—particularly in Britain from the late nineteenth century and well into the twentieth and this would contribute to their political radicalisation. Medical training abroad then became both a necessity in a country that did not as yet have sufficient expertise for particular areas of specialisation but also one where societal racial discrimination was mirrored in the training and practice of medicine.

Upon the outbreak of the Second World War, Penn was given the opportunity to travel to Britain, one of a number of surgeons drawn from all over the Commonwealth and the Allied countries, to work under the pioneers of plastic surgery: Harold Gillies, Thomas Kilner, Archie McIndoe and Arthur Mowlem. Chapter 4 looks at Penn's impressions of these plastic surgeons and the impact of the War on the development of plastic surgery. Penn's experiences in Britain helped shape his vision for his own plastic surgery unit in Johannesburg, the Brenthurst Red Cross Military Hospital for Plastic Surgery, the focus of Chapter 5. Discussed here is the establishment of the hospital under the patronage of the wealthy and influential Oppenheimer family, the hiring of key members of staff and the efforts at surgical reconstruction. The hospital was also the site of an important technological development in the treatment of maxillo-facial injury—the Brenthurst Splint. Evident too is the segregation within the Union Defence Force. Although the exigencies of war meant that segregation on the front lines could not always be adhered to, boundaries were easier to maintain on the home front when treating those not faced with life-threatening injury such as soldiers undergoing reconstructive surgery. Simultaneously there was a recommendation to create a National Health Service providing equal access to health care. Penn's work at Brenthurst can therefore be contextualised by the constant tension between segregationist ideology and the idealised vision of medicine and the provision of universal health care. At the end of the War, Penn travelled to the United States, the new centre for the professionalisation of and innovation in plastic and reconstructive surgery. The sum of his experiences thus far also buttressed the establishment of his civilian practice, the Brenthurst Clinic, which is the focus on the final chapter in this part.

Chapter 6 looks at the establishment of the Brenthurst Clinic in Hillbrow and its subsequent relocation to its present location in Parktown, Johannesburg. It addresses the various aspects of Penn's vision of medical care from its architecture to the use of new technology and methods, the training of medical professionals and the creation of an idealised environment for treatment. The Clinic was also the site for the formalisation of plastic and reconstructive surgery when the Association of Plastic Surgeons of Southern Africa was founded in 1956. Further, Penn engaged in numerous research projects focusing on healing as well as hypnosis along with Theodore Gillman. Finally, while the Clinic was an important site for plastic and reconstructive surgery on the African continent, it did not fulfil Penn's vision of a "Medical City" and the chapter concludes with Penn's brief—but fruitless—attempt to convince the Iranian leadership to build such a city. The incident highlighted the complex relationship of non-Western states with modernisation, a complexity that applied in no small measure to South Africa.

Once Penn had acquired both the skills and experience necessary to his specialisation, he was able to, in turn, share those skills. The second part, "The Surgeon Ambassador" considers Penn's experiences in Africa, Japan and Israel. Occurring during the consolidation of apartheid, these trips can also be viewed as a means of creating and strengthening ties with potential allies of the South African state through the use of science and medicine. Joseph Nye's concept of "soft power" is particularly apt in contextualising Penn's travels here. Soft power can be defined as a form of diplomacy that is based on "attraction" rather than "coercion". One of the pillars of soft power is the exportation of culture which in this case, manifested as medicine—the impartation of the skills of plastic and reconstructive surgery as a means of fostering ties with potential allies of the apartheid state.[19]

Chapter 7 addresses Penn's encounter with Albert Schweitzer and his experiences at Schweitzer's hospital in Lambarene. The meeting of the two marked both convergence and clash of two perspectives on medicine and modernisation. While Penn was often critical of Schweitzer's methods, he was nevertheless influenced by Schweitzer's thinking which would have an impact on his own views of the value of imperialism as an agent of progress and modernity. These views included a sense of racial paternalism—evident in Schweitzer's humanitarian work and upon which Penn would draw in his own writings, marking again the dichotomy between the universalist discourse of medicine and its practical implementation in Africa. After Schweitzer's death, Penn—along with heart surgeon Christiaan Barnard—returned to newly independent Gabon to promote the benefits of South African science and medicine. Their visit represented the efforts by the South African state to use modernisation as a means of enhancing its relationship with newly independent African states.

Another potential ally was Japan and Penn's work on the victims of Hiroshima and Nagasaki as well as his treatment of sufferers of leprosy are the focus of the subsequent chapter. His trip to Japan presented Penn with the opportunity to promote plastic and reconstructive surgery and assist with its professionalisation in Japan. It also reflected, in part, the

[19] Joseph S. Nye Jr., "Public Diplomacy and Soft Power", *The Annals of the American Academy of Public and Social Science*, Vol 616, "Public Diplomacy in a Changing World", pp94–109, March 2008.

historical relationship between the Asian country and the apartheid state, with Japan a major trading and economic partner.

An additional alliance was that between South Africa and Israel. From the achievement of independence in 1948, Penn paid numerous visits to a country wracked by conflict, offering his services as a reconstructive surgeon. This is discussed in the final chapter of the part. While Gabon had presented the opportunity for the propagation of Penn's view of modern medicine and the same held true for Japan—which had had a different experience of modernisation—Israel was a country technologically on par with South Africa. Adding some complexity to this—and a theme that surfaces at various points in the narrative—is the nature of identity on the part of Jewish South Africans straddling the worlds of apartheid and Zionism. Penn's trips to Israel between 1948 and 1973 serve as a means of exploring the growing relationship between the apartheid state and Israel as well as the similar route to modernisation taken by both countries, a form of modernisation that would increasingly privilege state security. Penn's own role shifted from that of volunteer surgeon to advisor and his relations with figures like Moshe Dayan and David Ben-Gurion placed him on the periphery of the entente between the two countries that was based on a similar sense of identity, international isolation as well as the forging of scientific and technological ties. Also significant is the specifically South African context during Penn's later visits where an academic boycott had been implemented on the country, restricting the participation of South African intellectuals in the international arena. Penn's work in Israel was also a means of sharing knowledge and expertise in a climate that was increasingly restrictive. In this chapter, there is a clear indication that Penn moved beyond the simple sharing of medical expertise to the assessment of military capability and tactics during conflict that could potentially benefit South Africa. Simultaneously, his role as a reconstructive surgeon was also a means of strengthening these ties.

The final part, "Utopia?" discusses Penn's political career and ideological beliefs. Significant here are the ways in which he engaged with education, science and the "civilising mission" during a time when independence movements in Africa and anti-apartheid activism in South Africa threatened to undermine white minority rule. Penn's perspectives on education, genetic capability and the limits of self-rule are contextualised by the death throes of colonialism and cracks in the edifice of apartheid.

Central to Penn's understanding of the world was the value placed on education—it was the means by which he realised his own ambitions and at the heart of medicine, was the sharing of knowledge and skills. At the same time, while Penn believed in the power of education, it was this very power that needed to be limited. Education was the means of achieving equality but his own understanding of genetics and race led him to conclude that there were inherent limitations on intellectual ability. Penn's conservatism demonstrates a disregard for the struggles for equal access to medical training on the part of black doctors that had played out for much of the twentieth century as he privileged what he believed to be "nature" over environmental constraints. His views became a means of advocating racial paternalism—as evident in the following chapter. Penn's philosophy thus forms the basis for Chapter 10 and it is a philosophy that shaped his views on the burning political issues of the day—decolonisation, African nationalism and the criticism aimed at the apartheid state as discussed in Chapter 11. Attention is paid to Penn's perceptions of independence movements in Mozambique and South West Africa as well as South Africa's pariah-like status in the international community.

The final chapter looks at three disparate elements of Penn's life—his idealised vision for the world, his artistic endeavours and his foray into politics. Although very dissimilar, underlying these elements was Jack Penn's attempt to remake the world as he saw it through science, service and sculpture. Of significance was his role as a member of the Science Committee on the President's Council—an organisation attempting to introduce economic, social and political reform under President P.W. Botha. Penn's role on the Committee reflected his philosophy as evident in his earlier writings while demonstrating the changing political climate of South Africa in the 1980s, a climate that was characterised by tension and contradiction as Botha attempted to strike a balance between the conservative elements of his own party and the increasingly vociferous demands for change.

Throughout the narrative, plastic and reconstructive surgery—as embodied in the career of Jack Penn—is used as a lens through which can be viewed the complex ways in which medical knowledge was produced, disseminated and contextualised during the segregation era and under apartheid.

PART I

The Face of War

CHAPTER 2

Beginnings

The image in the photograph is almost in profile. Black and white, it depicts the face of a man past middle-age, grey hair combed back and a receding hairline. He has a neatly trimmed moustache and beneath generous eyebrows, are deep-set eyes, partly in shadow. His head rests on his raised left hand, the side farthest from the camera, the posture serving to give a pensive air to his expression. The face is that of plastic and reconstructive surgeon Jack Penn as it appears on the frontispiece of his autobiography, *The Right to Look Human*.[1] It seems apt to begin with a description of the face of a man whose professional life centred on the reconstruction of the human face in surgery and its portrayal in art.

Jack Penn was born in Cape Town on 14 August 1909. He was the youngest in a large family with three older sisters who were exuberant and musical and three older brothers with a passion for sport. From an account of his early childhood, there is a sense that Penn, due to his younger age and temperament, was slightly isolated from his older siblings. His father was described as kind yet with the occasional "flash of temper". For Penn, however, his mother was the true heart of the family with characteristics that would later be evident in her youngest son as

[1] Jack Penn, *The Right to Look Human: An Autobiography* (Johannesburg, Hugh Keartland Publishers, 1976).

S. Chetty, *Reconstructive Surgery and Modernisation in Twentieth-Century South Africa*, Medicine and Biomedical Sciences in Modern History, https://doi.org/10.1007/978-3-031-38673-2_2

well—"deep humanism and sympathy" as well as an all-important "sense of humour". Penn also inherited his father's talent—the older Penn was a man who worked with his hands.[2]

Penn's father was Solomon Penn[3]—who had changed his name from Penchansky—and had been born in Russia in 1867. His mother was Ann Penn nee Goldberg, born in Russian-controlled Lithuania in 1869.[4] Both parents, born in Eastern Europe, would have had some familiarity with the anti-Semitism and pogroms that drove ever increasing numbers of Jews to emigrate. The mineral revolution in South Africa, beginning with the discovery of diamonds and later, gold on the Witwatersrand, made the hitherto less than attractive tip of Africa a site of economic opportunity, especially as mining necessitated industrialisation and increasing urbanisation. Waves of Jewish immigrants arrived from Europe in the latter part of the nineteenth century, with some of the earliest figures—men like Barney Barnato and Sammy Marks—making an indelible impression on the country. Yet, although numbers increased, success stories were few and many Jews from the *shtetls* of Eastern Europe were incorporated into the working class—and subject to the same anti-Semitism they had sought to escape.[5]

As with Anne Penn, a greater majority of the Jewish immigrants making their way to South Africa from about 1880 came from Lithuania and the stark racial and ethnic divisions in South African society often meant that this immigrant population was able to retain a strong sense of cultural distinctiveness but one that also drew increasingly upon a British tradition. Eastern European Jewish immigration would continue for more than three decades, only coming to an end after the First World War when there was greater stability in Europe compounded by the implementation of policies designed to restrict immigration in South Africa and elsewhere.[6] Simultaneously, even as a certain sense of Jewish identity was maintained, over time there was less of an adherence to cultural and

[2] *Ibid*, p40.

[3] Death Notice—Solomon Penn, *Rand Daily Mail*, 2 June 1947.

[4] https://www.geni.com/people/Solomon-Penn/6000000084338103860, accessed 26 March 2021.

[5] Charles Van Onselen, *New Babylon New Nineveh: Everyday Life on the Witwatersrand, 1886–1914* (Johannesburg and Cape Town, Jonathan Ball Publishers, 2001), pp80–81.

[6] Samuel Shlomo Greenblatt, "'To a Golden Land': The Circle of Immigration of South African Jews" (Unpublished MA Thesis, University of the Witwatersrand, 2004), pp3–5.

religious practice which, as Greenblatt suggests, may have been related to a desire for "acculturation".[7] It is remarkable that in Jack Penn's published autobiography, there is little mention of his Jewish heritage and no indication of his parents' origins.

The anglicisation of Penchansky could be related to this sense of acculturation but just as easily be a response to the anti-Semitism experienced by South African Jewry over the ensuing decades. If Solomon and Anne Penn were one of the ten thousand Jews from Eastern Europe who settled in and around Cape Town between 1891 and 1904, they would have found themselves in an unenviable position—markedly different from the existing Jewish community who had long since assimilated—and thus singled out for racial discrimination. Largely poor, engaged in trading and forming part of a working class, they strained the famed liberal tolerance at the Cape and were subject to racial stereotyping. With the publication of the Public Health and Sanitation Report in 1897, they were viewed as a public health risk due to the overcrowded and unhealthy conditions in which they were forced to live. The situation worsened during the South African War when Jewish refugees streamed to the Cape from the Witwatersrand. By 1902, the Cape Immigration Restriction Act was implemented to limit unwanted immigration. Initially designed for Indians, it was as easily applied to Jews from Eastern Europe. At the same time, Jews at the Cape were still considered "white"[8] and whereas the more impoverished sectors of the population experienced anti-Semitism, the elite enjoyed the intellectual and economic benefits of the bourgeoisie.[9] By the time of Jack Penn's birth, it is likely that the family straddled the boundary between the working class and the petit bourgeoisie and was upwardly mobile.

[7] Ibid., pp4–5.

[8] Just as race is a fluid concept and has had a long and varied history, the same applies to the terms used to categorise race. These terms have been—and continue to be—contested. For the purposes of clarity, this project makes use of an adapted version of the racial categories used during apartheid that were subsequently adapted post-1994. "White" refers to people of European descent, whether English- or Afrikaans-speaking while "black" refers collectively to all groups which were not classified as white. Black is thus subdivided into "African" (indigenous origin), "Indian" (Asian and, particularly, South Asian origin) and "coloured" ("mixed" origin).

[9] Milton Shain, Richard Mendelsohn and Vivian Bickford-Smith, "Testing Cosmopolitan Tolerance: Port Jews in Cape Town During the Late Victorian and Edwardian Years", *Jewish Culture and History*, 7, 1–2, 235–246, May 2012.

Penn recalled two defining moments in his early childhood—the first was the outbreak of the First World War. Cape Town became a hub for soldiers from Australia and New Zealand, many of whom were hosted at the Penn home. His father enlisted and Penn remembered leaving school early to see his father off to war.[10] Solomon Penchansky enlisted in the Transport Regiment on 6 September 1914 and his occupation listed was that of a "wheelwright".[11]

The War was a significant moment in the young Union of South Africa, exposing tensions within Afrikaner society when several of Prime Minister Louis Botha's generals rebelled as a result of South African participation in support of Britain. This enmity towards the British was due partly to the still fresh memories of the South African War that had ended little more than a decade earlier. South African troops served in Africa and Europe with a significant event being the battle at Delville Wood in 1916 with high South African casualties. For black South Africans, already being marginalised in the new Union and prohibited from bearing arms, their sacrifices were recognised with the sinking of the Mendi, a troop-ship carrying members of the South African Native Labour Contingent (SANLC). The destruction wrought by the First World War was, however, not the only challenge the world would face in 1918.

A significant memory in young Penn's life—and one that may have made some contribution to his later decision to take up a career in medicine—was the Spanish influenza epidemic of 1918. Beginning as the First World War drew to a close, the epidemic did not receive as much historical attention as the conflict yet by the time it came to an end two years later, it is estimated that the flu killed between 2.5 and 5% of the world's population, with a conservative death toll of fifty million—almost three times the casualties of the First World War. Moreover, it was truly global in its scope, unlike the fairly restricted range of fighting that characterised the War.[12]

South Africa was especially vulnerable due to its railway links with the rest of the African continent and its large coastline with ports connecting it to the wider world. In September of 1918, two ships docked in Cape

[10] Penn, *The Right to Look Human*, p42.

[11] Solomon Penchansky service record, Department of Defence Archives (hereafter DOD).

[12] Laura Spinney, *Pale Rider: The Spanish Flu of 1918 and How It Changed the World* (New York, Public Affairs, 2017), pp4, 6.

Town from a flu hot zone in West Africa. The ships were transporting more than a thousand troops of the SANLC who were returning home from France. Suspected sufferers were quarantined but this was not foolproof and men returned to their homes, carrying the virus with them. From South Africa the virus spread north, wreaking havoc.[13]

The arrival of the second wave of the virus in Cape Town led to a death toll disproportionately higher than that of Natal and was particularly evident in the Transkei and Ciskei. It was also prevalent in areas distant from the Durban–Johannesburg rail network that had helped transmit the first phase.[14] Unsurprisingly, the largest toll was evident in urban areas due to concentrated populations allowing for the rapid transmission of the virus and Penn, residing in Cape Town, experienced its effects first-hand. Just nine years old in 1918, Penn's recollection of the waves of Australian and New Zealand soldiers who stopped at the city before travelling to France serves as a reminder of the importance of the port city—and its vulnerability to the virus. The influenza outbreak made a significant impression on the young Penn. He recalled deserted streets, carts collecting coffins and the sight of another cart piled haphazardly with the corpses of dead convicts, distinguished by their distinctive red and blue clothing and bearing the tell-tale physical signs of the flu. With the exception of himself and his mother, his entire family fell ill and Penn remembered his mother travelling across the city with him to attend to family members during the crisis: "When I look back, I cannot understand how she had the strength and tenacity to do it, nor can I imagine what would have happened to so many people if she had taken ill or broken down".[15] Penn's memories of his mother's actions during the epidemic may have also contributed to his later respect for female nurses who became integral to his medical work.

Penn's family was not immune to the upheaval of the preceding four years. A decision was taken to move north to Johannesburg in the hope of "better prospects for advancement".[16] In addition, two of Penn's older brothers left to study in Britain—one at the London School of Economics

[13] Ibid., p41.

[14] Ibid., p204.

[15] Penn, *The Right to Look Human*, pp43–44.

[16] Ibid., pp44, 46.

and the other, Hyman (Hymie), at Edinburgh and Glasgow where he qualified as a doctor, serving as a model for the young Penn.[17]

An article appearing in the *Rand Daily Mail* in 1928 entitled "Jewish Wedding: Penn—Cartoon", describes in great detail the wedding ceremony of Penn's older brother, Hymie, to Rose Cartoon at the Wolmarans Street Synagogue in Johannesburg.[18] The Great Synagogue had only been built fourteen years earlier by Theophile Schaerer who modelled it in part on the Hagia Sophia mosque in Istanbul with the inclusion of a large dome and arched windows and a capacity of fourteen hundred. Its location was, at the time, on the border of the largely Jewish neighbourhood of Doornfontein that had initially housed the early Randlords until their exodus to Parktown. At the time of the wedding—and until the 1960s—the heart of the area was Beit Street and the neighbourhood was a Jewish enclave with kosher butchers, various other trading stores and a number of schools, with Yiddish the dominant language spoken.[19] Penn and his brother, Benjamin, took an active role in the service as "canopy bearers", under which the young couple were betrothed.[20] At the time of the wedding, Hymie had completed his training in Edinburgh. After later serving in the South African Medical Corps (SAMC) during the Second World War, he would qualify as an ear, nose and throat specialist at the University of the Witwatersrand (Wits)—a career path that would be partly emulated by his younger sibling.[21]

"Better prospects" notwithstanding, Jack Penn experienced a trying period of adjustment in Johannesburg. The tone was set for his character as he became what he termed an "individualist", uneasy with a team ethos and focused on individual accomplishment. Later, this would be evident as he butted heads with military authority and bureaucracy, demanding to perform his work on his own terms. Yet, he still took part in sports while at school, demonstrating an aptitude for shooting. He also recalled a schooling system that privileged sport over intellectual achievement. His impression of his time at school was that it was a "mediocre existence",

[17] Ibid.

[18] "Jewish Wedding: Penn—Cartoon", *Rand Daily Mail*, 6 July 1928.

[19] Lucille Davie, "The Great Synagogue in Hillbrow", March 2020, http://www.theheritageportal.co.za/article/great-synagogue-hillbrow, accessed 26 March 2021.

[20] "Jewish Wedding: Penn—Cartoon".

[21] "Dr Hymie Penn Dies in Bus Accident", *Rand Daily Mail*, 19 September 1975.

bar the influence of some of his teachers who he considered to be exceptional men. One of those was his mathematics teacher, Clement Martyn Doke.[22]

Doke was born in England in 1893 and followed in the footsteps of his father and uncle by becoming a missionary. The family settled in South Africa in 1903. Clement accompanied his father, Joseph, as a Baptist missionary to Rhodesia, including present-day Ilamba. Joseph contracted and succumbed to typhoid in 1913 and Clement continued his father's mission, and was later joined by his sister, Olive.[23] It was in Ilamba that Clement developed his aptitude for African languages and an interest in linguistics, publishing a *Textbook of Lamba Grammar*. Doke eventually focused on isiZulu instead, joining the newly created Department of Bantu Studies at Wits. He went on to become head of the Department that also included Native Law and Administration and Anthropology and was thus very involved in thinking about ideas of race and policy at the time. It was during Doke's tenure at the Department that greater moves were made towards the hiring of black academic staff at the University, one of whom was B.W. Vilakazi. While Vilakazi was never accorded the official status of lecturer, he worked with Doke in the creation of the *Zulu–English Dictionary*, the first edition of which appeared in 1948. The year also saw the rise of the apartheid state and Doke soon condemned the racial inequalities that characterised apartheid policy. He held a strong belief in the importance of education as a means of fostering "development".[24] While expounding his own views of education for Africans, Penn would display a certain ambivalence—the importance of education and training in the name of progress and self-determination would sit uncomfortably with his views of the relationship between genetics and capability.

The mediocrity of Penn's schooling was temporarily alleviated by his school's proximity to a police barracks that became a site of violent conflict between police and strikers in 1922. The strike by white miners can also be attributed to the economic upheaval generated by the First

[22] Penn, *The Right to Look Human*, p45.

[23] Robert K. Herbert, "Contextualising a Missionary's Trek" in Clement M. Doke, *Trekking in South Central Africa, 1913–1919*, Robert K. Herbert (ed) (Johannesburg, University of the Witwatersrand Press, 1993), pp xi–xv, http://pzacad.pitzer.edu/NAM/newafrre/writers/dokec/17memoir/part1.pdf, accessed 31 August 2020.

[24] Ibid., pp xxiv–xxvi.

World War—that had led to the Penns' immigration inland. Falling gold prices and a move by mine owners to employ cheaper black labour in positions previously held by white workers precipitated the unrest. Jan Smuts, then Prime Minister, dealt harshly with the striking workers. Martial law was imposed, the Union Defence Force (UDF) was employed against strikers and air raids were carried out against the dissidents. Even though order was eventually restored, the incident led to growing working-class Afrikaner disillusionment with Smuts and strengthened the Afrikaner right wing. Smuts would eventually be toppled from power in the election two years later by an alliance of the National Party and the Labour Party who united to form the Pact Government. Penn's experience was a little more personal—a hail of gunfire, some of which inadvertently threatened his class and led to an early break from school.[25]

Penn was only sixteen when he completed his schooling and subsequently enrolled at the Wits Medical School to fulfil a lifelong ambition of becoming a doctor. It was also at this time that he became more heavily involved in his other passion—art. He took courses at the Technical College to learn the rudiments of sculpting.[26] His art teacher at the Johannesburg School of Arts and Crafts which was part of the Witwatersrand Technical College was Elizabeth Jane Macadam. Macadam was a graduate of the Regent Street Polytechnic School of Art in London and had returned to South Africa in 1920. She started lecturing at the Technical College that same year with a focus on woodcarving and sculpture. Like Penn, many of her sculptures were of notable contemporary public figures such as the boxer, Kid Lewis, and Colonel C.F. Stallard, military man and politician.[27]

Another influence at this point was Hymie who had returned to South Africa and set up his own medical practice after completing his studies. Penn accompanied him as he treated patients, observing his generosity towards those lacking the financial means to pay. His brother's generosity also extended to paying for Jack's education in its entirety and the latter

[25] Penn, *The Right to Look Human*, p45.

[26] Ibid., pp45–46, 51.

[27] H.E. Winder, "Tribute to the Late Elizabeth Macadam", *Rand Daily Mail*, 21 January 1976.

took great pride in his ability to repay the £1,280 once he had qualified and started working.[28]

Penn appeared to adjust more easily to student life at Wits than he had as a high school student. He joined the athletic team, becoming vice-captain. The captain was Lionel Melzer and a long association between the two men would ensue. Both studied together with Melzer going on to become an anaesthetist. Melzer would also be one of the South African doctors who travelled to Israel to offer their medical services during the various conflicts.

Penn found his medical teachers less than stimulating, with much of what they taught derived from textbooks and a belief that they produced little of great originality. He did however, find that he was more partial to the practical than the theoretical with an inclination towards "anatomy, pathology and surgery rather than physiology, psychiatry and medicine".[29] An exception in his assessment of the medical teaching staff was Raymond Dart, the prominent and controversial anatomist who had drawn the world's attention to the hominin discovery at Taung.[30] Penn's experiences at the Medical School—from which he graduated in 1932—also went some way to influencing his interest in education and the training of surgeons. While he acknowledged the validity of the degree, seeing it as on par with elsewhere in the country, he bemoaned the general lack of more widespread knowledge and a capacity for creative thinking. For Penn, this limited students, ill-preparing them to cope with changing times and improvements in technology.[31] Challenging certain forms of orthodoxy in the medical establishment and a willingness to use alternative forms of therapeutics such as music and hypnosis would later inform his career.

It was, however, a book in the Medical School Library that would set Penn on his lifelong path—albeit more than a decade in the future. It was here that he encountered *Plastic Surgery of the Face* written by reconstructive surgical pioneer Harold Gillies detailing his experiences of reconstructive surgery during the First World War. While Penn admitted to not entirely comprehending the material, he nevertheless devoured the

[28] Penn, *The Right to Look Human*, pp45–46, 51.

[29] Ibid., p46.

[30] Ibid., p47.

[31] Ibid.

book, reading it twice. The artist in him was just as taken with the illustrations by Henry Tonks, a poignant rendering of the damage to the face done by war. This was Penn's first introduction to reconstructive surgery and he resolved to be part of a similar assemblage of surgeons drawn from all over the Commonwealth, as had been the case at Sidcup during the First World War, should the opportunity present itself.[32]

Early Reconstructive Surgery

While Harold Gillies is popularly considered to be the originator of modern reconstructive surgery, the field drew upon earlier forms of treatment dating to antiquity. Just as the Renaissance drew upon the learning of ancient Greece, India, too, was considered to be the remnant of an ancient classical civilisation—albeit one that had declined in the contemporary era. Its medical knowledge had been accumulated through oral tradition, religious, spiritual and philosophical belief and its interaction with the Mediterranean and Islamic world. This helped shape the interaction between Indian "traditional" medicine and the "modern" medicine of British imperialism.[33]

Ayurveda is the collective term for Indian medical practice, some of which dates back more than two thousand years. A key text in Ayurvedic medicine is the *Sushruta Samhita* written in approximately the fourth century AD. This text is concerned with surgery as it relates to the treatment of injuries sustained during the war.[34] While Ayurvedic medicine had largely been marginalised under British imperialism, the Orientalists—through their fascination with classical civilisations—paid greater heed to Indian works in the eighteenth century including the *Sushruta Samhita*. These texts were translated and studied. In the nineteenth century, British medical practitioners made use of "traditional" medical knowledge in conjunction with modern medicine, to address the ailments with which they had little experience. Ayurvedic medicine, therefore, continued in

[32] Ibid.

[33] Pratik Chakrabarti, *Medicine and Empire, 1600–1960* (Basingstoke, Palgrave Macmillan, 2014), p185.

[34] Ibid.

various forms alongside Western medicine, eventually becoming a feature of Hindu "nationalist identity".[35]

Penn was familiar with the antecedents of modern reconstructive surgery such as the "Hindu rhinoplasty" as described in the *Sushruta Samhita*—a form of nasal construction to counter the punishment meted out during war or for female adultery. The nose was reconstructed with the use of a skin flap from the forehead which was grafted to the face until blood flow was restored to what became the new nose. This original operation would eventually be adapted by Harold Gillies and Penn himself who became adept at it, applying it to the facial injuries incurred in automobile and aeroplane crashes, as well as those resulting from the removal of tumours and due to disease such as syphilis.[36]

Reconstructive Surgery and War

It was the First World War that initiated modern plastic surgery. Reconstructive surgery is deeply intertwined with technology in two ways; the first is, as with other areas of surgery, the reliance on instruments to observe, diagnose and intervene. Simultaneously, the use of different forms of technology gave birth to new forms of injury and therefore developments in reconstructive surgery. War and plastic surgery have an intimate history, with each conflict bringing its own challenges—the facial injuries of the First World War due to trench warfare, the burns of pilots crashing during the Second World War as well as those inflicted on the casualties of Hiroshima and Nagasaki. It is no surprise then that modern reconstructive surgery had its origins in the first modern industrial war, a conflict defined by technology to wreak destruction—aeroplanes, tanks and chemical weapons.

The First World War raged on the Western Front in 1916 with trench warfare and the Battle of the Somme which took place over five months and became infamous for the horrific death toll. It was in 1916 then that the first plastic surgery unit was set up at Aldershot by Sir Arbuthnot

[35] Ibid., pp187–188.

[36] Ibid., pp80–81.

Lane.[37] Lane specialised in orthopaedic surgery, with a tendency to intervene internally in correcting fractures, using wires and metal screws. He took advantage of the developments in understanding of sepsis by Joseph Lister to reduce the rate of infection, creating a highly sterile operating environment to carry out treatment that his critics often found unnecessarily invasive.[38] This is likely to have predisposed him to the corrective procedures used in reconstructive surgery. Lane also took an interest in the cleft palate, writing a book that advocated the importance of early corrective surgery in childhood.[39] During the First World War, he was assigned to Aldershot Command and created the reconstructive surgery unit, choosing Gillies to lead it.[40]

Harold Delf Gillies was born in Dunedin, New Zealand in 1882 and studied medicine at Cambridge University before completing his internship at St Bartholomew's Hospital in London. While stationed in France during the First World War, he took special notice of the facial injuries incurred during the conflict as well as the work of French surgeons Charles Valadier and Hippolyte Morestin in treating them. Convinced of the need for a reconstructive surgery unit, Gillies—with the support of Lane—was allocated space at the Cambridge Hospital in Aldershot. This, however, was insufficient to deal with the influx of patients brought in from the Somme and Gillies eventually established another hospital in Sidcup which became known as the "The Queen's Hospital", to be later renamed "Queen Mary's Hospital". His unit encompassed medical staff from all over the Commonwealth as well as the United States, collaborating in treating the traumatic facial injury at a time when more effective methods of delivering anaesthesia had still to be developed and sepsis remained an omnipresent threat. The sheer range of injury led to developments in reconstructive surgery and Gillies is accredited with the

[37] Richard Battle, "Plastic Surgery in the Two World Wars and in the Years Between", *Journal of the Royal Society of Medicine*, 71, November 1978, p844.

[38] Richard A. Brand, "Sir William Arbuthnot Lane, 1856–1943", *Clinical Orthopaedics and Related Research*, 467, 8, August 2009, https://www.ncbi.nlm.nih.gov/pmc/articles/PMC2706364/, accessed 9 December 2020.

[39] Mackenzie Morris, Thea Price, Scott W. Cowan, Charles J. Yeo and Benjamin Phillips, "William Arbuthnot Lane (1856–1943): Surgical Innovator and His Theory of Autointoxication," Department of Surgery Gibbon Society Historical Profiles, Paper 48, 2017, https://jdc.jefferson.edu/gibbonsocietyprofiles/48, accessed 9 December 2020.

[40] Battle, "Plastic Surgery in the Two World Wars", p844.

development of the tube pedicle.[41] This involved the excising of a flap of skin and tissue from an undamaged area of the body which was sutured into the form of a tube. The tube retained blood flow and was eventually moved to the area of injury where it was attached. This reduced the possibility of infection and was used to treat large wounds with great efficacy.[42]

Gillies' experiences of plastic surgery during the First World War were recorded in the book that set Penn on his life's work, *Plastic Surgery of the Face*. Accompanying Gillies' descriptions of injury and treatment are powerful photographs depicting traumatic facial injuries which were rendered in even greater detail by the sketches made by Henry Tonks.[43] Like Penn, Tonks inhabited the two worlds of surgery and art—studying the former at the Royal Sussex County Hospital and the London Hospital where he trained under Frederick Treves, the surgeon who brought facial and other deformities to public attention with his treatment of Joseph Merrick, the "elephant man". Tonks also took night classes at the Westminster School of Art, eventually taking on a teaching position at the Slade School of Fine Art. During the First World War, he was assigned to the Cambridge Medical Hospital at Aldershot where he met Harold Gillies.[44] For Tonks, plastic surgery symbolised the unity between form and function, "Never is there a really fine architectural structure that is not functionally correct". The restoration of aesthetic facial structure thus accompanied the restoration of the patient's ability to speak, eat and express emotion.[45] The two men worked together, with Tonks visually depicting the injuries, surgical interventions and the outcomes that were recorded in *Plastic Surgery of the Face*.

[41] "Saints and Sinners: Sir Harold Gillies", *The Royal College of Surgeons of England Bulletin*, 2013, https://publishing.rcseng.ac.uk/doi/pdf/10.1308/003588413X13643054409063, accessed 9 December 2020.

[42] George Warren Pierce and Gerald B. O'Connor, "The Tubed Pedicle Flap in Reconstruction Surgery", *California and Western Medicine*, 35, 2, August 1931, p94, https://www.ncbi.nlm.nih.gov/pmc/articles/PMC1657906/?page=1, accessed 9 December 2020.

[43] *Cf.* H.D. Gillies, *Plastic Surgery of the Face* (London, Henry Frowde and Hodder and Stoughton, 1920).

[44] Suzannah Biernoff, "Flesh Poems: Henry Tonks and the Art of Surgery", *Visual Culture in Britain*, 11, 1, 25–47, 2010, pp25–26.

[45] Quoted in John D. Holmes, "Development of Plastic Surgery" in *War Surgery, 1914–1918*, Thomas Scotland and Steven Heys (eds) (Solihull, Helion and Company, 2012), p267.

In *Plastic Surgery of the Face*, Gillies discussed in detail the various facial injuries incurred during the war and the corrective procedures used. While the First World War marked the onset of modern reconstructive surgery, he was nevertheless aware of the antecedents which contextualised the work at Aldershot. This included the two forms of reconstructive surgery used in antiquity on the Indian subcontinent, one of which involved the use of skin drawn from the cheek to address nasal injury and the other using the forehead flap—as discussed above. The former method had also been employed in Europe, but it was the latter method that came to dominate and was adapted to modern requirements. Another method was developed by the Italians in the fifteenth century that involved the use of skin derived from the arms to be used on the face. Again, this was eventually discarded. For Gillies, modern reconstructive surgery methods had their roots in the past but had nevertheless been uniquely adapted to the contemporary era. It was ultimately through trial and error that the most effective treatment was determined at Aldershot.[46]

Plastic Surgery of the Face contains detailed descriptions of the various injuries pertaining to the face with chapters on eyes, lips, chin and cheeks. Photographs of injured faces are accompanied by Tonks' sketches, of both the injuries and often the surgical methods used. Gillies' observations and descriptions are recorded in the first person, lending a certain intimacy to the work. In addressing the injuries, however, there is a clear indication of their origins within the context of war. The "depressed scars" resulting from cheek injuries, for instance, were due to "the exit of a bullet, of the glancing blow of a fragment, or of the entrance of a small shell or bomb fragment". The resulting scar, especially due to an exit wound, "radiated" outwards from the central point of origin and proved more challenging to rectify with the "excision of each scar in addition to the central core".[47] Gillies' factual description, however, was belied by the images of the scarred soldier that bespoke physical and psychological suffering. In addition to the various wounds caused by gunshots, burns were a significant injury. Gillies specified five types of burns, the most prevalent of which were "cordite burns", resulting from proximity to weapons and explosives and often involving those in naval service. "Petrol burns" were those

[46] Gillies, *Plastic Surgery of the Face*, pp3–4.

[47] Ibid., p38.

specifically associated with aeroplanes and pilots trapped in the burning wreckage resulting in severe facial injury. "Acid burns" occurred usually when working in factories. Of greater rarity were burns incurred from flamethrowers and "electric burns". All resulted in different facial areas of injury but all tended to include adverse effects on the eyelids which were often largely burned off and had to be reconstructed.[48]

While plastic surgery had the potential to remedy much of the facial disfiguration resulting from injury, the conclusion was not always a happy one. Gillies related the tragic case of a pilot who had suffered severe facial burns and was sent to Aldershot fifteen months later, having all but lost his sight in his right eye with severe damage to the left. The recommended treatment was the use of a flap of skin from the chest to be applied to the entire face. After the initial procedures were performed, the patient had two and a half months to recover. He proved to be a slow healer and the possibility was raised for another year of recuperation before the resumption of treatment. The patient's condition had also been exacerbated by a growing dependence on "stimulants" and morphine in the wake of his injury. Clearly in a fragile mental state, it was decided that he would be unable to cope with another year and the major part of the operation was performed. After, the circulation to the flap slowed and then stopped, gangrene set in and the patient, a captain in the Royal Army Medical Corps (RAMC), succumbed just a day after the operation. Gillies considered the extensive nature of the surgery to be partially the cause, believing that he should have waited a year and performed the operation in separate stages, allowing for healing in-between.[49] What "Case 388" reveals, however, is the devastation—both psychological and physiological—wrought by facial injuries and the unenviable position of the medical personnel treating the wounded.

While the War enacted a vast human toll, it also provided the opportunity for the development and refinement of techniques in reconstructive surgery—especially rhinoplasty. Gillies paid homage to the work of Denis Francis Keegan, a plastic surgeon in India in the late nineteenth century who focused on rhinoplasty due to a customary Indian punishment of cutting off the tip of the nose for infidelity. Born in Ireland in 1840 and educated at Trinity College, Dublin, Keegan worked in the

[48] Ibid., pp347–349.

[49] Ibid., p364.

Indian Medical Service for almost twenty-five years, retiring in 1894. His long sojourn in India gave him new insight into rhinoplasty which was published in an article *The Lancet*, just three years prior to his retirement. The article, entitled simply "Rhinoplasty" was a landmark in nasal reconstruction. As Keegan pointed out, rhinoplasty in Europe was shaped by the prevalent cases of facial disfigurement due to syphilis or lupus. This was in contrast to the injuries evident in India resulting from deliberate mutilation. Also different was Keegan's operations on patients who tended to be young and in good health. Along with his Indian assistant, Gunput Singh, Keegan developed a method of using flaps to rectify the nasal mutilation. While this form of injury was novel in Europe, the advent of modern warfare and the facial injuries incurred by healthy, young men meant that Keegan's early work took on new significance. In his subsequent monograph, published at the turn of the century, *Rhinoplastic Operations with a Description of Recent Improvements in the Indian Method*, Keegan made use of what would become a standard in detailing the efficacy of reconstructive surgery—the use of "before" and "after" photographs.[50]

The innumerable cases of facial injury wrought by the War allowed the surgeons at Aldershot to try various methods of reconstruction until they had become proficient. The War provided "sufficient material" necessary "to elevate this branch of surgery", through the efforts of the formidable surgical team that had been assembled at Aldershot.[51] Procedures were attempted, discarded and refined and rhinoplasty became one of the areas of reconstructive surgery with which Gillies was most associated—and which Penn would later adapt.

While the War unleashed the power of technology with the aim of destruction, mechanical means also proved important in assisting reconstructive surgery. Key to the treatment of the various facial injuries that included severe deformation was the need to maintain alignment of the jaw, teeth and various facial features. This was done through metal apparatus such as splints and more elaborate head and facial gear. Also used

[50] M. Felix Freshwater, "Denis F. Keegan: Forgotten Pioneer of Plastic Surgery", *Journal of Plastic, Reconstructive and Aesthetic Surgery*, 65, 8, 1131–1136, March 2012, pp1131–1134.

[51] Gillies, *Plastic Surgery of the Face*, p211.

were prosthetics made of rubber or metal to replace bone and cartilage.[52] Again, the sheer number of casualties incurred by trench warfare furthered technological development and Gillies incorporated these in treatment, including one used to maintain dental alignment and developed by Major John Norman Rishworth of the New Zealand Dental Corps (NZDC).[53] The NZDC was formed in late 1915 as a branch distinct from the New Zealand Medical Corps with Colonel Thomas Hunter as its Director and Majors Pickerill and Rishworth serving as Assistant Directors. Initially, most of the treatment consisted of the conventional—fillings, extractions and dentures—yet necessary to maintain the fighting capability of soldiers. Dental units served in Egypt and at Gallipoli, learning to provide medical treatment under adverse conditions and while under fire. The Western front necessitated the formation of mobile units to treat soldiers on the front lines as soon as possible to the incurring of injury. Just a year after its formation, the experiences of the NZDC led to it serving in an advisory capacity with Henry Pickerill assigned to Britain and being instrumental in the formation of a hospital for the treatment of maxillo-facial injuries.[54] This was the No 2 New Zealand General Hospital which was subsequently moved to Sidcup where Pickerill worked alongside Gillies and acquired some renown for his publications on the treatment of facial and jaw injuries due to gunshot wounds.[55] The global experience of the First World War thus also provided the opportunity to draw together experts from various parts of the Dominion as well as the United States to foster the development of modern plastic surgery. As Gillies put it, "Our wounded had call upon surgical skill from the whole Anglo-Saxon race".[56]

The successful treatment of the wounded of the First World War could also prove a double-edged sword. Gillies related the case of an officer from one of the Dominion states admitted with a severe gash on his left cheek, cutting to the bone, fracturing his jaw and leaving his face partially

[52] Ibid., Chapter V.

[53] Ibid., p195.

[54] T.V. Anson, *The New Zealand Dental Services* (Wellington, Historical Publications Branch, 1960), pp5–9, http://nzetc.victoria.ac.nz/tm/scholarly/tei-WH2Dent-c1.html#name-023303-mention, accessed 10 February 2021.

[55] M.C. Meikle, "The Evolution of Plastic and Maxillofacial Surgery in the Twentieth Century: The Dunedin Connection", *The Surgeon*, 4, 5, 325–334, October 2006, p329.

[56] Quoted in John D. Holmes, "Development of Plastic Surgery", p265.

paralysed. The use of flaps containing fat from adjacent areas was "rolled" into the wound and the result was covered with skin. The patient was healed with little indication of the extreme trauma he had suffered and was pronounced fit for duty:

> The final history of this gallant officer from the Dominions is pathetic. Soon after being posted back to duty he volunteered for foreign service again, was shot through the knee-joint and died of wounds in the same Casualty Clearing Station as that which received him when his face was wounded.[57]

The dilemma faced by the Gillies would be the same faced by Archie McIndoe and Penn himself and related to the conflicting responsibilities of the military medical practitioner. On the one hand was the conventional and paramount role of saving the life of the individual soldier and alleviating his suffering—which was both physical and psychological. The other role was to ready the soldier to return to the field of combat so as "to ensure minimum wastage of manpower".[58] Even as the War had created the opportunities for innovation in reconstructive surgery, it was the destruction that retained dominance.

[57] Gillies, *Plastic Surgery of the Face*, p40.

[58] Thomas R. Scotland and Steven D. Heys, "Setting the Scene" in *War Surgery, 1914–1918*, Thomas Scotland and Steven Heys (eds) (Solihull, Helion and Company, 2012), p46.

CHAPTER 3

The Making of a Surgeon

Immediately upon Penn qualifying as a doctor in 1931, his first placement was at Greys Hospital in Pietermaritzburg. The staff had been struck down with enteritis and the novice doctor now found himself heading the entire hospital. The support of the nursing staff as he was placed in this unenviable position would make an impression on him and indicate that openness, i.e. his admission of the emergency situation that they faced, would garner trust and support. Penn's willingness to take on the position with absolutely no experience indicated not just an inclination to assist where needed but also a certain level of confidence in his abilities.[1]

His second placing was less of an ad hoc measure—he requested and was granted a position as the surgeon in the Children's Hospital in Johannesburg. This, too, furthered his training. The calming of injured children as he treated them not only helped him cultivate his bedside manner and sense of empathy, but also suggested to him the importance of the patient's state of mind in the experience of injury and pain. Penn would later develop this notion with the use of hypnosis as an alternative to anaesthesia.[2]

[1] Jack Penn, *The Right to Look Human: An Autobiography* (Johannesburg, Hugh Keartland Publishers, 1976), p48.

[2] Ibid.

S. Chetty, *Reconstructive Surgery and Modernisation in Twentieth-Century South Africa*, Medicine and Biomedical Sciences in Modern History, https://doi.org/10.1007/978-3-031-38673-2_3

He subsequently began work in his brother's general practice.[3] Even though Penn would come to prefer specialisation, he found that the early years he had spent in general practice were essential to the development of the ideal medical professional. They provided an understanding of the social, economic and cultural complexities that defined the lives of his patients and allowed the development of the relationship between doctor and patient. Unlike the specialist, the general practitioner had in-depth knowledge of his patients. This also perhaps marked the point when Penn adopted a more holistic view of medicine and expanded his philosophy so that it would eventually move beyond the confines of medical intervention:

> To become a specialist without ever having had the opportunity of working in people's homes and thus becoming an intimate friend of the families, poor and rich, coloured and white, is like becoming a general without ever having been on a battle field [sic].[4]

In this scenario it is also important to note that Penn likened the medical professional to the "general", a position of ultimate authority.

Penn's period of general practice equipped him with important skills and also allowed the attainment of a degree of financial independence. Significantly goal-orientated, he amassed sufficient savings to repay his brother for the latter's financial assistance. At the same time, realising that he had had sufficient experience in general practice, Penn wished to specialise, valuing the "responsibilities and intensity" that this would bring—and he wished to specialise as a surgeon.[5]

His financial independence also allowed him to further his personal ambitions. He met and was instantly drawn to Diana Malkin. The two married in December 1934 in what Penn's son would describe as "the best decision" of his father's life and the couple would remain together for more than sixty years until Penn's death in 1996. Their union produced two children—a daughter, Joan, and a son, John, who would eventually

[3] Ibid., pp48–49.

[4] Ibid., p50.

[5] Ibid., pp50–51.

become a plastic surgeon and work alongside his father.[6] Penn immortalised his wife in a sculpture that captured her attributes—a soft smile and her "gentility"—and his feelings towards her.[7]

The date of their marriage was related in part to Penn's professional plans as the couple left immediately after for Britain so that Penn could begin his surgical specialisation. Although his ultimate destination was Edinburgh, Diana and Penn first spent four months in the English capital. Initially planning on staying six months in London, Penn ended his visit prematurely due to a sense of disenchantment that he experienced with the medical profession in the city. England's historical pre-eminence in science and technology, its initiation of the Industrial Revolution and its reputation as the "birthplace of democracy" had created an idealised image of the country in his imagination—one that fell short of the reality. In Penn's view, "the true scientist" could no longer be found in the social class conscious, tradition-bound world of England where "To go to the right school, belong to the right clubs and have the right address is far more important on the march to success than having the right knowledge and being the right kind of human being".[8] He believed elitism and privilege had served to stifle English innovation—a perspective that can also be contextualised by his own modest beginnings. It was instead scientists such as himself—"the true scientists"—that were the "true representative of British endeavour".[9] It is a remarkable perspective on the relationship between Britain—the site of the origins of the scientific tradition as begun with Isaac Newton, Francis Bacon and medical pioneer William Harvey—and a member of a former British colony that was heir to this tradition.

Penn subsequently cut short his stay in London, bought an eccentric-looking used Morris Oxford for £35 and along with Diana, travelled to Edinburgh.[10] Described by Penn as "the city with the greatest surgical traditions in the world",[11] the Scottish capital had seen the development

[6] Ibid., p50 and John G. Penn, "Obituary: Jack Penn", *Plastic and Reconstructive Surgery*, 100, 4, September 1997, p1077.

[7] Penn, *The Right to Look Human*, pp49–50.

[8] Ibid., p52.

[9] Ibid., p52.

[10] Ibid., p53.

[11] Ibid., p55.

and professionalisation of surgery from the early sixteenth century when the condition for the guild of Barber Surgeons to practice surgery was literacy, a novel pre-requisite at the time. The guild was awarded the Seal of Cause that amongst other privileges, allowed one human dissection per year to further the study of anatomy and almost half a century later, members of the guild were exempt from combat during war while expected to provide treatment for the wounded, the first clearly defined role of the "army doctor". Over the next one hundred and fifty years, there was a growing distinction between surgeons and barbers, with the former engaging in formal medical training. Simultaneously, there was increasing association and blurring of the boundaries between surgeons and physicians, placing surgeons firmly in the world of medicine and leading to the professionalisation of surgery. Medical education was a significant factor throughout and the Faculty of Medicine at Edinburgh University came into existence in 1726. From the outset, students from the rest of the British Isles and as far afield as North America, came to Edinburgh to be trained as doctors. By the late nineteenth century, members of the Royal College of Surgeons could be found providing surgical services throughout the far-flung reaches of the British Empire, including South Africa and eventually, some of these settlers returned to Edinburgh to be trained in turn.[12]

At Edinburgh University, Penn was taught by two professors of surgery—David Wilkie and John Fraser, a study in contrasts who nevertheless "complemented and supplemented each other admirably".[13] Fraser was described in his obituary as a "born teacher"—an assessment with which Penn was in full agreement, emphasising Fraser's popularity.[14] Fraser was a graduate of Edinburgh University in 1907 and studied in Paris where he undertook research in tuberculosis, the product of which was *Tuberculosis of the Bones and Joints in Children* in 1914. The outbreak of the First World War saw him serving in the RAMC, which had been formed just sixteen years earlier and had already been involved in the South African War. The RAMC was established in light of the growing

[12] Iain MacLaren, "A Brief History of the Royal College of Surgeons of Edinburgh", *Res Medica*, 268, 2, 2005, pp55–56.

[13] Penn, *The Right to Look Human*, p54.

[14] "Obituary: Sir John Fraser", *British Medical Journal*, 2, 978, 1947, https://www.bmj.com/content/2/4536/978.1, accessed 1 September 2020; Penn, *The Right to Look Human*, p54.

realisation that medical personnel were essential to the maintenance of military manpower by providing ready treatment to troops on the battlefield. This became even more essential in the light of the enormous numbers of casualties arising from the conflicts of the twentieth century.[15] While not combatants, members of the RAMC also incurred the same risks as regular troops and Fraser was subsequently wounded and awarded the Military Cross. At the end of the war, he returned to Edinburgh, taking on surgical positions at the Royal Hospital for Sick Children and the Edinburgh Royal Infirmary. At the time of Penn's encounter with him, Fraser was the *regius* chair for clinical surgery at Edinburgh University. By 1944, he had become the Principal and Vice Chancellor of the university. Fraser also demonstrated the alliance between medical professionals with, not only his position as a Fellow of the Royal College of Surgeons of Edinburgh, but also honorary positions in the American College of Surgeons as well as the Australasian College of Surgeons. As a teacher, he was able to communicate clearly surgical principles and was "a master of the art of demonstration", making him "popular" with students and was also acknowledged for embodying the spirit of service that Penn so valued.[16]

It was however, David Wilkie with whom Penn appeared to have a closer affinity and Wilkie's example that Penn hoped to follow, "David Wilkie was quiet, efficient, modest, knowledgeable and a fine steady operator. I enjoyed and respected everything he did..."[17] Wilkie received his medical degree from Edinburgh University and travelled to the surgical centres in Austria, Germany and Switzerland to further his surgical knowledge. He had a desire to be a "surgical scientist", engaging in research as well as surgical practice. After serving as a surgeon during the First World War, he returned to Scotland where his aptitude for teaching was apparent and he became Chair of Systematic Surgery at Edinburgh in 1924. Like Penn, his idealised view of surgery and medical training was shaped by his travels in the United States and he sought to emulate what he viewed as American ideals of "discipline, criticism and forthrightness" at Edinburgh. Key to this was a rethinking of the way in which

[15] "Obituary: Sir John Fraser" and "The RAMC in War", http://www.ramc-ww1.com/ramc_in_war.php?osCsid=predohql7qef5j37ndf368ksi6, accessed 1 September 2020.

[16] "Obituary: Sir John Fraser".

[17] Penn, *The Right to Look Human*, p54.

surgical research and training was conducted. With funding provided by the Rockefeller Foundation, Wilkie departed from the convention that had surgeons derive their income largely from private practice while in the employ of Edinburgh University. He devoted his attention instead to teaching and research, radically redesigning the department and installing state-of-the-art equipment. While drawing inspiration from the American model, Wilkie's re-envisioned department was likely the first of its kind outside the United States. Officially opened in 1926, the new surgical research department had as one of its aims the availability of research and teaching facilities to novice surgeons from all over the world—one of whom was Jack Penn.[18]

Wilkie also engaged in numerous philanthropic activities ranging from a social centre to adult education and contributed to the expansion of his own research laboratory at Edinburgh. Moreover, the young surgeons he trained were in agreement with Penn regarding his personality which was as noteworthy as his surgical skill, "Like most of the others of my generation – Wilkie's young men as we were called – my admiration for him was nigh unto idolatory".[19] Wilkie's influence on Penn can be seen in both the emphasis on research and training, a willingness to innovate and a perception that the role of the surgeon extended beyond the operating theatre.

Penn complemented his lectures (which he did not attend all that frequently) with his preferred method of learning—hands-on training. He believed that he could acquire the fundamentals of surgery and the rest would resolve itself in due course. In contrast to his colleagues then, much of his time was spent observing the doctors at work in the wards. This also allowed him insight into their points of view and idiosyncratic approaches to surgery. This stood him in good stead during the exams where his answers tended to be tailored towards the inclination of the examiner, believing that he lacked sufficient experience to formulate his own views.[20] Penn was admitted as a Fellow of the Royal College of Surgeons in 1935.[21]

[18] Iain Macintyre, "Sir David Wilkie (1882–1938): Surgeon, Scientist and Philanthropist", *Journal of Medical Biography*, 5, 206–212, November 2007, pp206–209. My thanks to Dr Iain Macintyre for sending me this article.

[19] Macintyre, "Sir David Wilkie", p210.

[20] Penn, *The Right to Look Human*, pp54–55.

[21] Ibid., p56.

Edinburgh continued to hold a place in his affections and he would revisit his alma mater decades later, now an established surgeon and "as a guest Professor of Plastic Surgery". At this time, he left a lasting impression when he fulfilled a request to sculpt a bust of prominent surgeon Joseph Lister who had transformed the practice of surgery through the use of antiseptics for the sterilisation of surgical instruments and to prevent the infections that severely impacted healing and led to a high mortality rate amongst post-operative patients.[22]

Although he had achieved his ambition of being admitted to the Royal College of Surgeons, Penn still felt that his education lacked sufficient "practical experience" and returned to London to remedy this.[23] His first position was at the British Postgraduate Medical School which was part of the University of London and had just been established on the site of Hammersmith Hospital. The Postgraduate Medical School had been designed to fulfil both national and imperial needs. This was emphasised by King George V who opened the School in 1935 with the hope that it:

> ...would play an imperial role in the winning and dissemination of medical knowledge, in the relief of suffering among my peoples in this country and overseas, and in enabling the doctors of all lands to come together in a task where all must be allies and helpers.[24]

The monarch's vision was one of a collaboration between imperial power and the colonies, a noble image of benevolent paternalism, a joint effort that nonetheless privileged the medical leadership of the metropole.

While the British Postgraduate Medical School was designed to foster the ties of Empire, it was based on an American model accredited to the Rockefeller Foundation. The emphasis on scientific medical research originated in Germany and Austria in the 1870s and the influence of these European institutions on American medical practitioners was profound. This influence was felt in the establishment of the Johns Hopkins University Medical School in the late nineteenth century. It was the first

[22] Ibid., pp55–56.

[23] Ibid., p56.

[24] Mark E. Silverman, Arthur Hollman and Dennis M. Krikler, "The Hammersmith Hospital and the Royal Postgraduate Medical School" in *British Cardiology in the 20th Century*, Mark E. Silverman, Peter R. Fleming, Arthur Hollman, Desmond G. Julian and Dennis M. Krikler (eds) (London, Springer, 2000), p103.

American institution to dedicate itself to "full-time clinical teaching", incorporating a strong research element.[25] The trend evident at Johns Hopkins was given further impetus with the formation of the Rockefeller Institute of Medical Research in 1901. While John D. Rockefeller provided both the funding and the impetus for the establishment of the Institute, it was the brainchild of Frederick T. Gates. Envisaged as a ground-breaking "institute of biomedical research in the United States", Gates drew his inspiration from similar European institutes—the Koch Institute of Germany and the Pasteur Institute in France. The Rockefeller Institute was run by scientists for scientists—divided into particular laboratories, each led by a medical pioneer, the aim was to prevent funding and bureaucratic concerns impeding scientific medical progress. This soon bore fruit with breakthroughs such as the development of a cure for cerebrospinal meningitis in 1907. Five years later Rockefeller funded the Rockefeller Hospital as a site for putting laboratory findings into practice as well as gaining a practical understanding of disease.[26]

The First World War and the Influenza Epidemic of 1919 had an important influence on the development of scientific medicine. The emphasis on scientific thinking had infiltrated various areas of knowledge production from the nineteenth century and in the field of medicine, it was believed to be a panacea. Scientific medicine was envisioned as having a particularly "preventative" role in contrast to existing forms of medicine that focused on treatment. The First World War with periodic outbreaks of dysentery and enormous death toll and the global impact of the Influenza Epidemic stimulated the development of scientific medicine. The Rockefeller Foundation was a key player in the fostering of scientific knowledge and medicine and had formulated a plan for the introduction of scientific medical training at tertiary level with London identified as a site due to its centrality in the British Empire. By 1921 then, the Foundation had begun its collaboration with the University of London and the British Government to establish the London School of Hygiene and Tropical Medicine. The Foundation provided funding to the amount of

[25] Fisher, "The Rockefeller Foundation and the Development of Scientific Medicine in Great Britain", p21.

[26] Scott Kohler "Case 1: Rockefeller University (Formerly the Rockefeller Institute for Medical Research), 1901", Center for Strategic Philanthropy and Civil Society (Duke), 2007, https://cspcs.sanford.duke.edu/sites/default/files/descriptive/rockefeller_university.pdf, accessed 10 February 2021.

£461,000 for this venture that would be aimed at improving the health of the metropole, "the British Dominions and Possessions and other countries".[27]

Tropical medicine was itself intertwined with empire. By 1914, most of the world outside Europe was under colonial control with Britain the frontrunner, the culmination of a process that had been ongoing for centuries. This was also the point at which there was a greater scientific understanding of disease, particularly those associated with overseas possessions in Africa, Asia, the Caribbean and South and Central America. With high European mortality in these tropical regions, climate in various ways came to be associated with race and the tropics were viewed as the sites of disease—cholera, for instance, was largely associated with India. Understanding the spread of disease in the tropics was a means by which Europeans could survive and dominate these alien environments. By the late nineteenth century, great strides were made in the understanding of the origin of disease with the identification of the bacteria and parasites responsible. Yet, while scientific evidence suggested that these organisms could thrive in most environments, European preconceptions of the tropics—which were often seen as an unvarying environment across continents—meant that these spaces retained a reputation for disease. Tropical medicine therefore, as studied at the London School of Tropical Medicine, was marked by both colonial thinking and new developments in scientific medicine.[28]

Medical science, based in the laboratory and employing new technologies to seek and identify the origins of illness, became harnessed to the "civilising mission" characteristic of empire. As Chakrabarti points out, through increasing understanding and intervention, it represented "the colonisation of the body and the colonisation of the mind", marginalising indigenous knowledge systems and establishing medicine as "modern" and overwhelmingly "Western".[29] With the construction of the Panama Canal by the Americans in the early twentieth century—symbolic of American hegemony in Central America—the exposure of workers to yellow fever marked the onset of the contribution of the Rockefeller

[27] Fisher, "The Rockefeller Foundation and the Development of Scientific Medicine in Great Britain", pp25–27.

[28] Pratik Chakrabarti, *Medicine and Empire: 1600–1960* (Basingstoke, Palgrave Macmillan, 2014), pp141–146.

[29] Ibid., p178.

Foundation to public health in South America. It extended its role to Africa and Asia, sending a representative to India to decide on the funding and medical intervention required and working in tandem with the League of Nations Health Organisation.[30] The spirit of philanthropy, paternalism and context of empire that had led to the establishment of the London School of Hygiene and Tropical Medicine along with the avowal of scientific medicine saw the creation of the British Postgraduate Medical School soon thereafter.

The Medical School had been established to fill a perceived gap in postgraduate medical education. Most of the medical schools in London were centuries old, often predating the University of London itself. These medical schools were historically less associated with universities than they were with hospitals, with students undertaking a form of "apprenticeship" in hospitals. The tremendous development in the sciences in the nineteenth century, especially those associated with medicine—biology, physics and chemistry—exceeded the skills of the existing medical instructors at the hospitals. Beginning in the mid-nineteenth century, it therefore became necessary to hire instructors with the requisite knowledge. Medical teaching could no longer be haphazardly done and also needed to incorporate other fields of medical study to reflect developments in science such as anatomy and pathology.[31] While some medical schools subsequently became affiliated with the University of London in the late nineteenth and early twentieth centuries, it would only be in the wake of the First World War that a concerted effort was made to better incorporate both science and research into medical education—as well as greater professionalisation in teaching and training.[32]

The Rockefeller Foundation played a significant role here and the British Postgraduate Medical School was envisaged as a site of teaching and research with four departments: medicine, obstetrics and gynaecology, pathology and Penn's department, surgery. Research was a defining quality of the Medical School, marking a significant point of departure from earlier teaching hospitals that were funded by donors where work done was on a purely voluntary basis. While there had been

[30] Ibid., pp95–96, 115, 202.

[31] Donald Fisher, "The Rockefeller Foundation and the Development of Scientific Medicine in Great Britain", *Minerva*, 16, 1, 20–41, 1978, p23.

[32] Ibid., pp23–24.

some attempts at creating medical research institutions in the interwar period, the Medical School was the most ambitious with medical professionals hired by the University of London and paid to engage in research and to impart their wisdom to postgraduate students.[33]

The American influence on the British Postgraduate Medical School may account for the unique spirit of egalitarianism that permeated the relationship between student and teacher, leading to a ferment of discussion, debate, creativity and learning.[34] Penn was under the tutelage of Professor George Grey Turner, the head of surgery.[35] Turner had been based in the north of England for much of his career—receiving his medical degree from the University of Durham's Newcastle Medical School. He also established a renowned private practice with patients drawn from both the rural and industrial backgrounds that characterised the region. The medical tradition in Newcastle was considered to be as strong as that emanating from the great centres at Edinburgh and London, but Turner left this behind when he took on the position in Hammersmith. As a surgeon, he was involved in the treatment of cancer and as Penn recollected, many of his patients were terminal making the "experience" for the younger man, "valuable but harrowing" yet also demonstrating Turner's courage and commitment.[36]

While being exposed to Turner's teaching and the empathetic example he set as a surgeon was rewarding, there was little financial remuneration and Penn had to leave the Medical School for another position. He would subsequently work at two very different hospitals which would help shape his own vision for the ideal hospital—a vision that he hoped to realise.[37]

For a brief period, he served as an "acting senior surgeon" in a large County Council hospital based in London, filling in for a surgeon who had gone on leave.[38] While it presented the opportunity for Penn to have a sense of autonomy and gain important "practical experience", he

[33] Silverman et al., "The Hammersmith Hospital", p105.

[34] Ibid.

[35] Penn, *The Right to Look Human*, p56.

[36] "Obituary: George Grey Turner", *Plarr's Lives of the Fellows*, Royal College of Surgeons, https://livesonline.rcseng.ac.uk/client/en_GB/lives/search/detailnonmodal/ent:$002f$002fSD_ASSET$002f0$002fSD_ASSET:376907/one, accessed 7 September 2020; Penn, *The Right to Look Human*, p56.

[37] Penn, *The Right to Look Human*, p56.

[38] Ibid.

nonetheless preferred a more intimate atmosphere, equating the operation of the larger hospitals to an "impersonal conveyor belt". He therefore took the post of "resident surgical officer" at the Royal Salop Infirmary based in Shrewsbury, a town in the west of England.[39] The Infirmary had a long and noble history from its establishment in 1747 as a site for the treatment of the "Poor-Sick and Lame". It was administered and funded by the wealthy elite and a symbol of paternal benevolence in the eighteenth and nineteenth centuries with the key medical staff consisting of an Apothecary, Surgeon, Matron and Physician.[40] More than a century later, it was his experience at Shrewsbury that confirmed in Penn a desire to model his own hospital along the lines of a "cottage hospital", with distinctive units, each allowing for a more "personal" interaction between doctor and patient.[41]

It was while stationed at the Royal Salop Infirmary that Penn had his first encounter with Harold Gillies. Penn, still a relatively unknown young doctor, viewed the "father of modern plastic surgery" from afar, noting the delicate hands of an artist, the "moody and nervous [yet] charming" temperament with a "[brilliance]" that provoked ambivalence as it came with a strong sense of individuality. Gillies' visit was also marked by the demonstration of a nasal reconstruction that he had adapted from the Hindu rhinoplasty, a procedure that had become an important feature in his surgical repertoire. It was Penn's first direct experience of reconstructive surgery, provoking "exhilaration" and confirming in him a desire to pursue the specialisation further.[42]

The seeds of Penn's future career were sown during his time in Britain, but he remained ambivalent about the British class culture that couched elitism as good "taste". At the same time, he acknowledged the innovation and change that occurred in British society, despite the stifling traditionalism of the upper class. This was however, accredited to both the "quiet brilliance of the English intellectual" who, through international networks of knowledge, was partially immune to "snobbery and parochialism". In contrast to the more rarefied intellectual, credit was

[39] Ibid., pp56–58.

[40] W.B. Howie, "The Administration of an Eighteenth-Century Provincial Hospital: The Royal Salop Infirmary, 1747–1830", *Medical History*, 5, 1, 34–55, 1961.

[41] Penn, *The Right to Look Human*, p58.

[42] Ibid., pp58–59.

also given to the ordinary middle-class man on the street characterised by "common sense and innate decency" and able to keep in check the unruly "mobs" of the working class.[43] It can be deduced that Penn saw himself reflected in both—a "self-made man" who had acquired his position through ability and work rather than networks of patronage, an exemplar of the aspiring middle-class intellectual that had risen to prominence during the Enlightenment, the voice of reason as the bulwark against the elitism from above and rabble-rousing from below. It thus seemed a logical step that he would complete his training in the country that had been founded on the principles of the Enlightenment.

His imagination fired by a member of the Mayo Clinic visiting London, Penn completed his formative medical experiences across the Atlantic in the United States.[44]

It seemed to be almost an act of divine intervention that led to the formation of the Mayo Clinic in the town of Rochester less than 150 kilometres from the urban sprawl of Minneapolis in Minnesota. In the summer of 1883, a tornado devastated a part of the town, with numerous injuries in scattered locations that proved a challenge to treat by the town's doctor, William Worrall Mayo and his sons, Will and Charlie. The doctors were able to move some of the wounded to the students' quarters at a convent, the Sisters of Saint Francis. Eventually, Mother Alfred—who was a supervisor at the convent—confided to Mayo that she had received a message from God to build a hospital in Rochester that would be led by Mayo and would become "world renowned for its medical arts".[45] It was this unusual convergence between the secular and religious that led to the establishment of the Mayo Clinic.

An English immigrant to the United States in the mid-nineteenth century, William Mayo served as an "examining surgeon" in Rochester, a role that involved him deciding on the fitness level of recruits for the Union Army during the Civil War. The war itself proved to be a sharp learning curve for surgeons, exposing many to injuries they had never before seen such as bullet wounds.[46] There were also very early attempts

[43] Ibid., p60.

[44] Ibid., pp59–60.

[45] David Blistein and Ken Burns, *The Mayo Clinic: Faith, Hope, Science* (New York, RosettaBooks, 2018), pp22–23.

[46] Ibid., pp29, 37.

at plastic surgery due to the facial injuries sustained by increasingly accurate projectile weapons and Gordon Buck, a surgeon with the Union Army, became the first to carry out a complete facial reconstruction.[47] Upon the cessation of hostilities in 1865, Mayo remained in Rochester setting up his private practice. From the outset, he demonstrated a keen interest in medical developments, maintaining ties with an earlier place of employment, Bellevue Hospital in New York, reading the latest medical literature and in one memorable instance, mortgaging his house—with the consent of his long-suffering wife—to buy the latest in medical technology, a microscope developed in Germany that cost an astronomical $600.[48]

In the wake of the tornado and with the fund-raising efforts of Mother Alfred, the building of the Mayo Clinic began in 1888. The hospital, known as St Mary's, was completed a year later and its key figures were Will and Charlie Mayo who had been an integral part of their father's medical practice. Both men subscribed to the newly emergent germ theory proposed by Joseph Lister, maintaining high standards of sterilisation in their operating rooms leading to incredibly low mortality rates.[49] Their success meant increasing numbers of patients and more staff. The Mayo practice was where specialists diagnosed prospective patients who would subsequently be sent to the hospital for treatment.[50] What would become known as the Mayo Clinic, would eventually be a hallmark of collaboration between various medical specialists and as Will Mayo observed, "The people will demand, the medical profession must supply, adequate means for the proper care of patients, which means that individualism in medicine can no longer exist".[51] With a focus on cutting-edge medical techniques and technology, the Clinic expanded rapidly—eventually branching out into the rest of the country and influencing medical treatment internationally. At the time of Penn's visit, it had treated one million patients over its five-decade history and would soon send medical

[47] Richard A. Gabriel, *Between Flesh and Steel: A History of Military Medicine from the Middle Ages to the War in Afghanistan* (Lincoln, Potomac Books, 2016), p174.

[48] Blistein and Burns, *The Mayo Clinic*, pp29, 39.

[49] Ibid., pp51, 53–55.

[50] Ibid., p68.

[51] Ibid., p61.

professionals to the Pacific to treat both Allied and Japanese combatants.[52] Of particular interest to South African doctors in the ensuing decade in light of Christiaan Barnard's first heart transplant, the Clinic employed the first CT scanner in the United States as well as completed a number of surgeries using a heart–lung bypass machine.[53]

As Penn observed, the Mayo Clinic exceeded its British counterparts in terms of efficiency and quality of treatment. Decades before the use of computer technology, patient records were stored on "punch-cards", making them easily accessible for research purposes. There was a high degree of specialisation which culminated in effective treatment and in contrast to what Penn had been led to believe by his British counterparts, there was no indication of "exhibitionism" on the part of American surgeons but rather "modesty and knowledgeable efficiency".[54] Yet it was this very emphasis on rational efficiency as well as the scale of the Clinic that Penn found off-putting—patients were first examined in a single, large building and then referred to various specialists for treatment. The human body was perceived as a machine: "Patients came in on a conveyor belt principle, their organs were examined, cleaned and put back by a host of experts until the patient was in good running order…".[55] While the machine was returned to operating efficiency, the human element was reduced and there was little opportunity for the development of the "doctor-patient relationship" that Penn favoured.[56] Yet, as in Britain, the experience was invaluable in consolidating Penn's own vision for a hospital in his own country. In addition, it was from Will Mayo that Penn first heard the phrase, "the divine right of man to look human", which would become his credo.[57]

His funds exhausted and ready to begin his career and start a family, Jack and Diana Penn returned to Johannesburg in 1937. Upon his arrival in South Africa, Penn started at Wits, this time teaching clinical anatomy in the Department of Anatomy, a part-time position that had been

52 Ibid., pp121–122.

53 Ibid., p122.

54 Penn, *The Right to Look Human*, p61.

55 Ibid.

56 Ibid.

57 "Profile: Jack Penn", *S.A. Practice Management*, 9, 3, 1988, File: Biography—Jack Penn, Adler Museum, University of the Witwatersrand (hereafter AMUW).

extended to him by Raymond Dart.[58] Dart had become a figure of note—and controversy—more than a decade earlier with his discovery of the Taung skull which he classified as *Australopithecus africanus*, positing that Africa was the site of human evolution in contrast to prevailing doctrine that privileged Asia.

The making of facial masks was a significant part of the Department of Anatomy's—and Dart's—attempt to ascertain specific race types and to determine the connections between early hominins and the San. In 1930, Dart was part of an Italian expedition where he first encountered the use of facemasks by Lido Cipriani, a proponent of racial hierarchy. Dart was converted to the apparent efficacy of facemasks in delineating racial differences. Most of the subsequent expeditions by the Wits Department of Anatomy also included the making of facemasks, including the Witwatersrand Kalahari Bushmen Expedition in the winter of 1936. One of the academics accompanying Dart was Penn's former mathematics teacher, Clement Doke of the Department of Bantu Studies.[59]

The Expedition had been made at the behest of Donald Bain, great-grandson of prominent early geologist Andrew Geddes Bain. The younger Bain had been involved in obtaining skeletal specimens of "Bushmen" for scientific study. In 1936 he planned on taking a group of live "specimens" to the British Empire Exhibition to be held in Johannesburg. He therefore invited Dart to bring a contingent to study these "specimens". Bain's stated aim was the creation of a "Bushman" reserve to preserve the supposed cultural purity of this group.[60] Prior to Dart's arrival, Bain forwarded his photographs of the "specimens" considered to be ideal representatives of the "type" for the Exhibition, with photography another important means of recording physical "types" in the service of physical anthropology.[61]

On reaching Bain's camp at Tweerivieren, Dart and his assistant engaged in a mania of measurement. Facial and physical characteristics were recorded and the scientists subsequently categorised subjects based on their correlation to racial type. Following this, facial masks were

58 Penn, *The Right to Look Human*, p64.

59 Christa Kuljian, *Darwin's Hunch: Science, Race and the Search for Human Origins* (Johannesburg, Jacana Media, 2016), pp62–63.

60 Ibid., p61.

61 Ibid., p63.

created by Dart and another assistant, Eric Williams. The first to undergo the procedure was the leader of the group, a nonagenarian, !Gaurice. Called Abraham by the scientists, !Gaurice was also classified as "Kal 4 (Kalahari 4)". He was made to lie on a table, reeds were placed in his nostrils allowing him to breathe and his entire face was encased in Plaster of Paris. The plaster was removed after it dried. The superstitious awe and fear of the San encountering the masks was also noted. Almost seventy masks were produced during this exhibition and the making of facemasks became an integral part of subsequent expeditions for the next fifty years. More than a thousand masks are held in the Raymond Dart Collection of African Life and Death Masks.[62] Dart used the physical facial characteristics—as captured by the facemasks—to bolster his claim that the "Bushmen" were "living fossils", the "missing link" between ancient hominins and modern *Homo sapiens*. He would continue to employ physical characteristics to argue for specific "pure" racial types, even as this view becomes increasingly anachronistic.[63] And this privileging of racial typology would have real-world repercussions in a country fraught with racial tension and division.

During his brief sojourn at Wits, Penn was involved in analysing the "musculature of the Bantu face", noting differences with "European" faces. A detailed examination of 135 faces revealed the lack of the "Risorius muscle" as well as points of difference in terms of "the blood supply of the muscles and the cartilages of the nose".[64] Penn also related an incident where he was able to challenge existing understandings of the facial structure of indigenous Africans which had a practical and controversial application during a case in which Robert Broom was called to give testimony. As with Raymond Dart, Broom had by this time become a prominent figure in South African palaeoanthropology. Born in Scotland and qualifying as a medical doctor from Glasgow University, he demonstrated an interest in comparative anatomy which underpinned much of his later career. With the support of Jan Smuts and J.H. Hofmeyr, he was made Curator of Fossil Vertebrates and Anthropology at the Transvaal Museum. His discovery of the fossilised remains of Pleistocene mammals brought him to the attention of Dart's Department of Anatomy. This

[62] Ibid., pp63–66.

[63] Ibid., pp66–67.

[64] Penn, *The Right to Look Human*, p64.

would lead him to Sterkfontein and nearby Kromdraai where hominin finds came quickly, including remains that were later classified as *Australopithecus robustus*.[65] More than a decade before his own discoveries, Broom had also been an early supporter of Raymond Dart during the controversy over the Taung discovery.[66]

Robert Broom then was a figure not unused to controversy. While he is often recognised for his role in palaeoanthropology, he was also a medical doctor and from the 1930s, aired his concerns regarding the death rate of women in childbirth as well as the tendency of the medical profession to engage in what he believed to be superfluous procedures that did more harm than good such as the pre-emptive removal of tonsils and the appendix—the biological role of both not being fully understood. He believed that it was the unnecessary intervention of medical professionals that contributed to the high mortality rate. Unafraid of airing eyebrow-raising views—for the time—he also condemned the illegality of abortion comparing the number of women who died from abortion in South Africa to the much lower number in the Soviet Union where abortion was legal.[67] He continued in a similar vein during the Second World War, with a no-holds-barred attack on the medical profession which he believed needed to be reformed with a smaller number of more proficient doctors who could provide "expert" health care unlike the contemporary situation with large numbers of doctors who were "unregulated" and thus not necessarily capable of treating their patients, especially in the field of obstetrics.[68] In some ways, Broom's call for well-trained doctors and a regulated profession echoed that of Penn but in this case, the two men parted ways.

In the aforementioned court case—as related by Penn—a woman had given to a still-born baby who her husband claimed was actually fathered by an African servant. Initially basing his support of the husband's claim on earlier research on the Herero which posited that "the African had only one accessory cartilage between the upper and lower nasal cartilages", Broom subsequently had a change of mind when Penn revealed this to not

[65] D.M.S. Watson, "Robert Broom 1866–1951", *Biographical Memoirs of the Fellows of the Royal Society*, 37–41, November 1952.

[66] Kuljian, *Darwin's Hunch*, p47.

[67] "Famous Doctor Scourges His Own Profession", *Rand Daily Mail*, 10 May 1935.

[68] "Union Needs Fewer, Better Doctors", *Rand Daily Mail*, 24 November 1943.

be the case. Penn divulged his conclusions to Dart who informed Broom, leading to the latter "withdrawing his evidence", without which the case could not be pursued.[69] The case itself is revealing for the attempt to use scientific evidence to buttress racial difference at a time when the notion of the *swaart gevaar*[70] exerted a strong hold on the public imagination. During a period of increased African urbanisation and fears of social control and the loss of racial boundaries, *swaart gevaar* was the fear of the apparent threat posed by African men to the virtue of white women.

Penn's intervention saved the reputation of the woman and he appeared ambivalent about the potentially far-reaching consequences of minor biological differences, "So is the fate of men and women decided – by a small accessory cartilage".[71] This perception of the important yet constructed nature of racial difference would bear some similarity to a later experience when he was asked to operate on a woman in order to allow her to "pass" as white.

Penn's period at Wits was marked by the beginning of his academic contributions to plastic surgery. A global event would however prove the ultimate baptism of fire for the novice reconstructive surgeon.

[69] Penn, *The Right to Look Human*, pp64–65. While the only account of this case is evident in Penn's autobiography and it has proved a challenge to track it further, the case itself is relevant for the understanding of the biological conception of race and the use of experts in medicine and palaeoanthropology.

[70] Literally translated as "black danger".

[71] Penn, *The Right to Look Human*, p65.

CHAPTER 4

The Restoration of a Lost Soul: War

As Penn recalled in his memoirs more than thirty years later, he had begun to have misgivings about Nazi Germany during his residency in Britain. For Penn, the British seemed wilfully oblivious to the threat posed by Germany.[1] By 1937, Britain's view of Germany was ameliorated by an attitude of appeasement, as evident in its Prime Minister, Neville Chamberlain. There were also strong elements in society that held fascist views. Ian Kershaw has addressed the Nazi sympathies of a British aristocracy in decline, anxious about the rise of radical socialism and facing the challenges of nationalist movements within the British Empire.[2] In the wake of the Great Depression, Sir Oswald Mosley was convinced that liberal capitalism and Britain's parliamentary system were inadequate in dealing with the myriad crises that confronted Britain. Communism was not seen

[1] Jack Penn, *The Right to Look Human: An Autobiography* (Johannesburg, Hugh Keartland Publishers, 1976), p64.

[2] Ian Kershaw, *Making Friends with Hitler: Lord Londonderry, the Nazis and the Road to War* (Penguin Books, 2005).

Title paraphrased from Archie McIndoe quoted in Emily Mayhew, *Guinea Pig Club: Archibald McIndoe and the RAF in World War II* (Barnsley, Greenhill Books, 2018), p76.

S. Chetty, *Reconstructive Surgery and Modernisation in Twentieth-Century South Africa*, Medicine and Biomedical Sciences in Modern History, https://doi.org/10.1007/978-3-031-38673-2_4

as a viable solution. Mosley's conclusion was that fascism and its utility in protecting the economy of the British Empire was the answer. This contextualised the formation of the British Union of Fascists (BUF) in 1932. Presenting itself as a feasible alternative to communism and capitalism, Mosley's vision of fascism was based firmly on modernity, with an emphasis on science and technological progress, strong state intervention in the economy and a privileging of the collective over the individual with "discipline and collective service". The BUF also drew its inspiration from European fascist movements—espousing the economic policies of Italy and the organisational framework of the Nazi Party.[3]

In contrast to Mosley, was Robert Vansittart—who Penn considered a man to have bucked the trends of either appeasement or tacit support that characterised the British response to the Nazi threat. Vansittart had opposed German ambitions during the First World War, attended the peace talks that led to the implementation of the Treaty of Versailles and was convinced in the 1930s that Germany's expansionist policies would inevitably spell conflict in Europe. He was not enamoured with a diplomatic response or Neville Chamberlain's policy of appeasement, believing that Adolf Hitler was not amenable to reason. The solution was British rearmament in the hopes that this might, at best, serve as a deterrent to German aggression or, at worst, prepare Britain for eventual conflict.[4]

Penn was also uneasy by the anti-Semitism that characterised the Nazi state, as evident when prominent intellectuals and scientists such as Thomas Mann and Albert Einstein left Germany upon Hitler's rise to power in 1933. Like Vansittart, Penn was certain that German policies would inevitably lead to war. He was further convinced that South Africa would be drawn in on the side of the British—a decision that turned out to be more complex than he imagined—leading to a schism in the South African parliament, the resignation of Prime Minister Hertzog, Jan Smuts's installation as Prime Minister and South Africa's own version of fascism.[5]

[3] Matthew Worley, "Why Fascism? Sir Oswald Mosley and the Conception of the British Union of Fascists", *History*, 96, 1, 321, 68–83, January 2011.

[4] "Robert Vansittart", *Spartacus Educational*, https://spartacus-educational.com/Robert_Vansittart.htm, accessed 3 February 2021; Michael Lawrence Roi, "Sir Robert Vansittart, the Global Balance of Power and Nazi Germany, 1934–1937" (Unpublished PhD dissertation, University of Toronto, 1996), p183.

[5] Penn, *The Right to Look Human*, p64.

The argument can certainly be made that Penn was writing with hindsight in his implacable opposition to German fascism—by the time of the publication of his autobiography in 1976, the world was fully cognisant of the evils of fascism and the threat posed by Nazi Germany. However, upon returning to South Africa in 1937, Penn was convinced enough of the outbreak of war to enlist in the Union Defence Force. Upon enlistment, he also expressed his desire to engage in plastic surgery, "[The senior colonel] had never heard of it but, nevertheless, put it on my dossier – which was the main purpose of the exercise as far as I was concerned".[6] Enlisting as a lieutenant, Penn was a major attached to the 7th Field Ambulance when war was eventually declared in September 1939.[7] His service file records Penn's subsequent transfer to the No 2 Medical Officers Training Ambulance of the SAMC.[8]

The UDF officially came into being with the passing of the South Africa Defence Act (13 of 1912). Passed two years after the formation of the Union of South Africa in 1910, it was both an assertion of nascent nationhood as well as symbolic of the internal tensions that characterised the new nation. It was an uneasy amalgamation of Boer and British military systems that in its first decade of existence, was used to suppress rebellions by Boer generals as well as indigenous groups in southern Africa and unrest by white workers on the Rand.[9] The formation of the UDF reflected Jan Smuts's imperial ambitions in southern Africa, his alliance with Britain as well as a policy of reconciliation between English and Afrikaans-speakers—which aroused the ire of Afrikaner nationalists. It also reflected his partiality to science, technology and progress. This was apparent in the South African Air Force which was used to awesome effect in quelling insurrection and establishing South African dominance in southern Africa.[10] It therefore does not take a leap of imagination to consider the UDF a conducive environment for the relatively new field of reconstructive surgery.

[6] Ibid.

[7] Ibid.

[8] Jack Penn Service File, W.R. 12/6640, DOD.

[9] Ian van der Waag, *A Military History of Modern South Africa* (Johannesburg and Cape Town, Jonathan Ball Publishers, 2015), pp74, 76, 141.

[10] Ibid., pp148–149.

Yet the UDF was in a sorry state after the First World War and this was particularly evident in the Medical Services. The demobilisation at the end of the War had steadily diminished the number of medical staff, the Medical Training School was no longer in operation and the SAMC Units which formed part of the Active Citizen Force had been disbanded. With Smuts's ousting from power in 1924, the government—with Afrikaner nationalist leanings—did little to improve the UDF, adopting a more isolationist stance in contrast to the earlier use of the UDF to further imperial ambition. This was compounded by the Great Depression when the funding of the military was cut further. The situation began to change in the 1930s however, under the leadership of Oswald Pirow, the Minister of Defence. Structural changes were made to the UDF and the budget permitted its expansion, a trend that continued until 1939.[11]

The Field Ambulance as employed by British forces during the First World War was designed to address the early treatment and evacuation of the wounded during a time when there were challenges getting the wounded from the frontlines to the casualty clearing stations in the rear and any delay increased the chances of shock due to loss of blood and cold as well as the onset of infection. As an "independent mobile medical unit" a single field ambulance was allocated to a brigade of four thousand men and comprised medical supplies and equipment as well as 241 medical staff consisting of doctors, stretcher-bearers, nurses and cooks.[12] Within the Department of Defence Archives, there are reports on the Japanese medical services—which had achieved some renown during the Russo-Japanese War—as well as the organisation of the Field Ambulance system by the Canadian medical services during the Second World War.[13] This indicates South Africa's awareness of—and perhaps willingness to adapt to—the organisation of military medicine evident in other countries (both Axis and Allied). By 1940, the Field Ambulance system was being modified for the South African experience of war with a request for the units to be able to operate independently as each unit accompanied

[11] Ian van der Waag, "The Union Defence Force Between the Two World Wars, 1919–1940", *Scientia Militaria, South African Journal of Military Studies*, 30, 2, 2000, http://scientiamilitaria.journals.ac.za, accessed 26 November 2020, pp188, 202–204, 207.

[12] Thomas R. Scotland, "Evacuation Pathway for the Wounded" in *War Surgery, 1914–1918*, Thomas Scotland and Steven Heys (eds) (Solihull, Helion and Company, 2012), p59.

[13] Director General Medical Services, Box 26, File MD129/204, DOD.

a battalion on the frontlines of North Africa.[14] Penn, however, would not serve on the front lines and special provision was made, both for his training as a plastic surgeon during wartime and the establishment of a hospital for plastic surgery.

At the outbreak of the Second World War after some shuffling and organisation in the structure of the UDF, there were a number of Directorates under the command of the Chief of General Staff, one of these being the Director General Medical Services (DGMS).[15] The DGMS, Edward Thornton was amenable to Penn's desire to pursue reconstructive surgery during the War. Thornton—born and trained in England—had come to South Africa in 1903 as Plague Medical Officer at the Cape, later serving in the Cape Provincial Administration. He had been involved in the First World War, serving in South West Africa and later taking charge of the South African Military Hospital in Richmond, England.[16] Established for both the rehabilitation and vocational training of South African soldiers to prepare them for post-war life, the hospital at Richmond was based on the ethos of incorporating those seriously wounded such as amputees into the fold of civilian society.[17] Its aims were therefore little different to that of reconstructive surgeons and of relevance to Penn, Thornton was also involved in an administrative role at Sidcup, making him familiar with the use of plastic surgery in war. Upon Thornton's return to South Africa in 1920, he served as Director of Medical Services in the UDF.[18]

In a subsequent position as Secretary for the Department of Public Health, Thornton had been a significant figure in promoting contraception as part of the eugenicist orientation of a decade earlier. He believed birth control was less a means of empowering women but instead an

[14] Major M.S.O. for DGMS to G.O.C. 2 Div, 27 December 1940: Equipment Field Ambulances, Director General Medical Services, Box 92, File MD129/390: 17th Field Ambulance, DOD.

[15] W.A. Dorning, "A Concise History of the South African Defence Force (1912–1987)", *Scientia Militaria, South African Journal of Military Studies*, 17, 2, 1987, http://scientiamilitaria.journals.ac.za, accessed 26 November 2020, p10.

[16] "Death of Sir Edward Thornton; Long Service in Public Health", *Rand Daily Mail*, 28 October 1946.

[17] "Follow the Drum: South African Military Hospital", *The Library Blog*, 8 November 2017, https://libraryblog.lbrut.org.uk/2017/11/south-african-military-hospital/, accessed 25 November 2020.

[18] "Death of Sir Edward Thornton".

important aspect of public health related to mother and child mortality and more significantly, the control over the reproduction of "poor whites" as well as Indian, coloured and African women. The authority of the physician in determining how contraceptives were distributed would remain absolute.[19] Penn would later demonstrate a similar concern about overpopulation and the need for family planning. Two years after his retirement from the Department of Public Health, Thornton returned to military service as the Director General of Defence Medical Services in the UDF.[20] His prior experiences meant that he had little qualm in acquiescing to Penn's request to serve as a plastic surgeon in the event of war.[21]

Penn noted with approval that, "the Medical Corps was developed even in this faraway land. Among other innovations, plastic surgery found a place".[22] He had already begun the process of asserting himself in the field, publishing an article in 1938 on the surgical procedures to correct the cleft palate and lip and demonstrated his cognisance of the contemporary methods applied, ranging from the surgical procedure itself to antiseptic measures and the use of anaesthetic on very young patients. The article also engaged with the work of prominent surgeons in the field such as Vilray Blair, another figure who developed his techniques during the First World War.[23]

Penn was highly aware of the relationship between plastic surgery and war, publishing an article that referred to the antecedents of modern plastic surgery in India, Greece and Rome, all precipitated by wartime injury. The techniques developed in antiquity were also brought into use during the Napoleonic wars that ravaged Europe however, as discussed here, it was the First World War that gave birth to modern plastic surgery. These wartime developments had influenced plastic surgery on civilians during the interwar period, even as the specialisation adapted to different types of injuries as well as cosmetic surgery. Penn was therefore confident

[19] Susanne Klausen, "The Race Welfare Society: Eugenics and Birth Control in Johannesburg, 1930–1940", in *Science and Society in Southern Africa*, Saul Dubow (ed) (Manchester and New York, Manchester University Press, 2000), pp174–175.

[20] "Sir Edward Thornton's New Appointment", *Rand Daily Mail*, 10 August 1940.

[21] Penn, *The Right to Look Human*, p65.

[22] Ibid.

[23] Jack Penn, "Treatment of Hair-Lip and Cleft-Palate", *South African Medical Journal*, 25 June 1938, pp425–429.

that the Second World War would once again provide the impetus for further development in the field.[24]

It did however, seem to be the DGMS that made the first attempt to ascertain the relevance of plastic surgery as well as the feasibility of sending South Africans to Britain for further training.[25] The response made reference to a surgeon who had had some experience in Britain, "[studying] plastic surgery under the famous Dr. Gillies of England" and the decision was taken to send two South African representatives, in addition to a Dr. Becker who had already been sent abroad for training.[26] The first of the two candidates proposed was Norman Petersen who preceded Penn to Britain to begin a six-month stint of training.[27] For the remaining candidate, requests were sent out to surgeon Professor Innes Wares Brebner—who had served during the First World War and was subsequently part of the Department of Surgery at the Wits Medical School[28]—regarding Penn's suitability as a candidate.[29] A similar request was forwarded to Professor C.F.M. Saint at the University of Cape Town to ascertain the suitability of another potential candidate, R.L. Forsyth.[30] Brebner however, proved the speedier respondent:

> In reply to your letter of the 19th October, 1940, re Plastic Surgery, I think the man you mention will fit the bill for he is keen on this type of work and made a special study of the specialty overseas, both in England and the States. He has been doing the plastic surgery at the local Dental Hospital

[24] Jack Penn, "Aspects of Civilian Plastic Surgery", *South African Medical Journal*, 14 September 1940, pp335–338.

[25] Maj-Gen C.G.S. to D.G.M.S., 27 September 1940, Director General Medical Services, Box 92, File 129/376: Plastic Surgery: MOs Studying in England, DOD.

[26] Colonel, DGMS, 2 October 1940, Director General Medical Services, Box 92, File 129/376: Plastic Surgery: MOs Studying in England, DOD.

[27] Major, DGMS, 29 October 1940: Captain N. Petersen, SAMC, Director General Medical Services, Box 92, File 129/376: Plastic Surgery: MOs Studying in England, DOD.

[28] S2A3 Biographical Database of Southern African Science, http://www.s2a3.org.za/bio/Biograph_final.php?serial=344, accessed 14 August 2021.

[29] Lieut-Col, DGMS, to Prof I.W. Brebner, 19 October 1940, Director General Medical Services, Box 92, File 129/376: Plastic Surgery: MOs Studying in England, DOD.

[30] Lieut-Col, DGMS, to Prof C.F.M. Saint, 19 October 1940, Director General Medical Services, Box 92, File 129/376: Plastic Surgery: MOs Studying in England, DOD.

> and I have seen some of the results and these have been excellent. I have communicated with him and he is prepared to accept the appointment.[31]

Penn (like Petersen before him) was subsequently promoted to the rank of Acting Major due to take effect on the day of his departure—while paid the lower rate of a Captain—and the necessary paperwork was provided for his attendance at the "Post Graduate course". Upon his return to South Africa, he was to be posted to a yet undetermined military hospital.[32]

Serving as part of the RAMC,[33] Penn was sent to England aboard the *Athlone Castle*, leaving behind his wife and infant daughter, aware that "this was a great turning point in [his] life".[34] Arriving in wartime London was a stark contrast to Penn's earlier visit and without his wife, he seemed alone and alienated. A visit to South Africa House helped alleviate the anxiety when he was provided with a helmet, gas mask and that perennial signifier of home, *biltong*.[35]

He decided that he required as broad an experience as possible with exposure to a variety of injuries. He would spend time at four different centres of reconstructive surgery scattered over the country and largely under the aegis of the New Zealand pioneers of the First World War. The first was at East Grinstead under Archie McIndoe which focused on injuries incurred by Air Force personnel.[36] McIndoe's father, John, was one of the earliest settlers in Dunedin, New Zealand who emigrated from Glasgow in 1859 when John was just six months old. An earlier group of settlers who left Scotland included John's grandfather, John Gillies,

[31] James Brebner, 22 October 1940 to Lieut-Col, Egerton Brown, DGMS, 22 October 1940, Director General Medical Services, Box 92, File 129/376: Plastic Surgery: MOs Studying in England, DOD.

[32] Lieut-Col H. Egerton Brown, DGMS, to Adjutant General, 7 November 1940, Director General Medical Services, Box 92, File 129/376: Plastic Surgery: MOs Studying in England, DOD.

[33] Jack Penn, "A Surgeon's Story: It Is the Divine Right of Man to Look Human" (Unpublished manuscript), p205, Brn No 12057, 617.95 PEN, Brenthurst Library (hereafter BL).

[34] Penn, *The Right to Look Human*, p65.

[35] Ibid., p66.

[36] Ibid., p67.

who was a solicitor.[37] John Gillies had arrived with his teenage son, Robert, and the latter played a role in the discovery of gold in Otago—the province that encompassed Dunedin—which led to a tremendous expansion of the modest settlement. Robert also served in the House of Representatives for the Bruce district and, upon his early death from an aneurism, had eight children—one of whom was four-year-old Harold Gillies.[38] There were therefore strong familial—and geographical—links between the McIndoe and Gillies families.

Archie McIndoe was born in 1900 and while too young to take part in the First World War, served as Battalion Sergeant-Major of the New Zealand Cadet Force. It comprised six hundred boys, formed in reaction to fears of Japanese invasion. McIndoe had an early desire to study medicine, refusing to work in the garden as he would be "going to need [his] hands". He was also just as eager to avoid having to work in his father's printing business and on completing his education, enrolled in the Otago Medical School, graduating in 1923.[39] While serving as an intern at Waikato Hospital in Hamilton, he was informed that he was the candidate chosen by his university to apply for a scholarship to the Mayo Clinic, a scholarship he was subsequently awarded.[40] The Mayo Clinic and its founders were to have as huge an impact on McIndoe as they would on Jack Penn two decades later. McIndoe was particularly taken with Charles Mayo, admiring his diagnostic skill and sense of empathy and diplomacy. Mayo was also a proponent of plastic surgery.[41] The Mayo Clinic had a distinct vision of surgery, different from the "quick, cut-and-thrust surgery" that tended to characterise the profession. The testing and diagnosis processes were exhaustive but necessary before the decision to operate was taken.[42]

After six years at the Mayo Clinic, the ambitious McIndoe left for the Postgraduate Medical School at the University of London, in the hopes

[37] Hugh McLeave, *McIndoe: Plastic Surgeon* (London, Frederick Muller Limited, 1961), p19.

[38] "The Late Robert Gillies", *Bruce Herald*, 17, 1759, 18 June 1886, https://paperspast.natlib.govt.nz/newspapers/BH18860618.2.12, accessed 3 May 2021.

[39] McLeave, *McIndoe*, p22.

[40] Ibid., pp24–25.

[41] Ibid., p31.

[42] Ibid., p29.

of achieving a professorship, bolstered by the recommendation of a friend and mentor, Lord Moynihan, President of the Royal College of Surgeons in England—only to be deeply disappointed.[43] It was here however, that he first encountered Harold Gillies who had hitherto been oblivious to his cousin's existence. Gillies was instrumental in obtaining a post for McIndoe at the Hospital for Tropical Diseases. McIndoe was also exposed to Gillies' pioneering work in plastic surgery.[44] At the outbreak of the Second World War, McIndoe—now a proficient plastic surgeon in his own right and one of only four in England—was the Consultant in Plastic Surgery to the Royal Air Force (RAF). He was assigned East Grinstead.[45]

For a country that did not experience occupation, the efforts of the RAF were the most visible indicator of the fight against the Axis powers. When Prime Minister Winston Churchill uttered the stirring: "Never in the field of human conflict was so much owed by so many to so few", he was paying tribute to the heroism of the pilots of the Battle of Britain whose efforts to save Britain from German invasion were visible to the civilian population on the ground. Even prior to the outbreak of the War, there was an acknowledgement of the increasing importance of aerial warfare with a build-up of bases and aircraft. With the horrors of trench warfare still fresh in the memories of many, the war in the air, the despatch of bombers to distant targets and the role of fighter aircraft in defending the home front, were portrayed as a means of protecting British people from the ravages of bloody conflict. Yet once aerial warfare actually broke out and Allied pilots were confronted with the experience and might of the German Luftwaffe, they were forced to adapt and casualties were high.[46]

This was particularly the case for pilots of the smaller and more mobile fighter aircraft, the Spitfire, Hurricane and Defiant. Unlike the larger bombers, space was at a premium and a compromise had to be reached between the fuel-carrying capacity of these fighters and rendering the fuel tanks fireproof. Studies demonstrated that the sealant used on the fuel tanks to make them fireproof added additional weight which had an

[43] Ibid., pp35–36, 38.

[44] Ibid., pp39–40.

[45] Ibid., p69.

[46] Mayhew, *Guinea Pig Club*, pp18, 20–21.

adverse effect on range and manoeuvrability. The attempts to find a solution were hampered by the shortage of rubber as the war progressed. The best available form of protection for pilots then was the protective glass of the cockpit and the plane itself while the aerial tactics employed made them difficult targets. Casualties were nevertheless high—and the majority of injuries were extensive burns to the upper body and face.[47]

The "airman's burn" as these injuries were categorised was due largely to the explosion of the forward fuel tanks (and often, the wing tanks as well). The pilot's hands and face usually bore the full brunt of the explosion with the areas not protected by the helmet or oxygen mask particularly vulnerable, i.e. the nose, ears and cheeks. There were also "contact burns" due to the hot metal portions of the plane coming into contact with the human body. By 1940, 378 pilots were injured severely enough to warrant their hospitalisation at a time when pilots were most needed to fight the Luftwaffe. This made the treatment of pilots a priority and thrust East Grinstead to the forefront of attention.[48]

McIndoe's treatment for burns, prior to surgical reconstruction, centred on the daily immersion of patients in warm saline baths to reduce infection, moisten the area so that dressings could be easily removed and prevent stiffening of the joints. To carry out the treatment, there was a large contingent of nursing staff—more so than at most other hospitals—and both beds and baths were mobile with the former having specially designed headrests to allow for the application of facial dressings and the latter designed to withstand the corrosive nature of the saline as well as its conductivity, and equipped with instruments to monitor the saline solution.[49] An important aspect of the treatment of burn victims was their isolation from other injured patients. Burn patients were housed in Ward III as a means of preventing infection and to reduce the psychological trauma that could potentially be caused by the reaction of other patients to their disfiguring injuries.[50]

The common experience of pain, disfigurement, treatment and isolation fostered an *esprit de corps* amongst the burn patients. This was compounded by the lack of a traditional hierarchy—with the exception

[47] Ibid., pp29–33.

[48] Ibid., pp44–45.

[49] Ibid., pp62–63.

[50] Ibid., p64.

of McIndoe as the undisputed leader. Perhaps reflecting the "colonial" influence in contrast to the elitism that Penn had found so off-putting during his internship in Britain, there was a sense of egalitarianism in Ward III. No distinction was made between the ranks, meals were served as the patients requested them and to prevent the dehydration associated with their injuries, men were given watered-down beer as an inducement to help them maintain their fluid intake.[51] Also novel was the relationship between doctor and patient which was a collaborative effort. The process of rectifying disfigurement could take years with numerous surgeries, and trust and communication were key between the surgeon and patient regarding treatment, rehabilitation and expectations.[52] The common experiences led to the formation of the "Guinea Pig Club", considered "the most exclusive Club in the world [but with an] entrance fee…most men would not care to pay".[53]

As with the history of plastic surgery in general, nationality was not a mitigating factor. At the outbreak of the war, many individuals drawn from the dominions went to Britain to join the war effort. In his seminal account of his war experiences, Spitfire pilot and fellow patient, Richard Hillary wrote of a South African pilot, "Edmonds", who was brought to Ward III. The twenty-six-year-old, described by Hillary as being "the worst-burned pilot in the Air Force to live" had crashed his plane on the runway prior to his first solo flight and was trapped in the burning wreckage. He bore his disfigurement, the numerous reconstructive surgeries and even the onset of a *streptococcus* infection with an enviable equanimity, even demonstrating a sense of regret that he had not had the opportunity to play a more active role as a pilot.[54] Of prominence was the Royal Canadian Air Force with Canadian pilots working alongside their counterparts in the RAF—and also subject to the same level of injury. The Canadians made use of British medical services however the sheer number of injured Canadian airmen led to the arrival of Group Captain Ross Tilley, the Principal Medical Officer (Overseas), to East Grinstead. Tilley was initially part of McIndoe's coterie of trainees, learning the basics of treatment as implemented at East Grinstead before he set up

[51] Ibid., p78.

[52] Ibid., p76.

[53] Ibid., p78.

[54] Richard Hillary, *The Last Enemy* (London, Penguin Books, 2018).

a special Canadian unit at East Grinstead that was modelled closely on that of McIndoe.[55]

"I like the hounds at my heels",[56] was both a description and McIndoe's vision of the training of plastic surgeons at East Grinstead. In his recollection of his time at East Grinstead, Penn made passing reference to the conditions under which surgeons were trained. The hospital was inundated with patients and McIndoe and his team were constantly on call with little time for formal training sessions. As a result, younger surgeons gleaned what they could from following McIndoe from the ward to operating theatre and back again. The pace was frenetic and there was little published literature available as surgeons were confronted with the new and unprecedented. This did not mean that there was no value in training at East Grinstead. A former trainee recalled the punishing hours and constant exposure as an important means of learning from the more experienced surgeons.[57] Of no little significance was the common aim of these surgeons as articulated so eloquently by McIndoe: "...we can within a reasonable time create order out of chaos and make a face which does not excite pity or horror. By doing so we can restore a lost soul to normal living".[58]

His work at East Grinstead and the publicity accorded to the Guinea Pig Club meant that Archie McIndoe became the face of plastic surgery during the Second World War. Penn was unstinting in his admiration of the surgeon who stood out in British medical circles for his "colonialistic bluntness". For Penn, he was the ideal surgeon—highly skilled and confident in his ability with a popularity that was well-deserved:

> I consider that Archie was the best plastic surgical operator of all time. His hands were enormous, but gentle, decisive and strong. There was no unnecessary fuss in his surgery, no wasted movement or material, and everything he did had a purpose. He knew he was good and loved to have spectators round him. These he always had in good measure, not only doctors, but patients and laymen. It was sometimes difficult to get under

[55] Mayhew, *Guinea Pig Club*, pp124–126.

[56] Quoted in Mayhew, *Guinea Pig Club*, p123.

[57] Mayhew, *Guinea Pig Club*, p71.

[58] Quoted in Mayhew, *Guinea Pig Club*, p76.

> his elbow to see what he was doing, but it was sufficient for me to appreciate the general principles of his work, to admire it and try to emulate it.[59]

The setup of East Grinstead by McIndoe also impacted the ways in which Penn viewed his own practice. McIndoe emphasised the importance of nursing staff to provide the post-operative care essential to ensuring the success of skin grafts. Their presence was also a psychological balm to injured men, whose trauma extended beyond the physical. Like Penn at Brenthurst, McIndoe had little patience with military authority and was grateful that he remained a civilian during the War so that he could better confront the military bureaucratic challenges facing the patients in his care. He applied the same lack of military convention to his patients refusing to compel them to wear the "hospital blues"—uniforms that were assigned to the injured—as this would only single them out even further in the eyes of the civilian populace. The "hospital blues" were used instead as a form of chastisement for the very few men who exceeded the bounds of propriety. Finally, McIndoe attempted to give Ward III a homely atmosphere, using pastel paint on the walls and replacing the iron-framed hospital beds and cots with wooden ones. To complete the picture, chintz curtains were put up and flowers added extra colour to the garden.[60] In 1947, McIndoe also paid a visit to South Africa, operating on patients, and delivering a lecture, "Middle Third Facial Injuries" at Wits on 27 July.[61]

With McIndoe's death almost two decades later, Penn chose to create a bust of him based on his recollection of McIndoe during the War.[62] In contrast, Penn was more ambivalent in his assessment of Gillies who was portrayed as being less skilled than McIndoe with a more abrasive personality that alienated observers. His "excellent" skills as an instructor and "virile brain continuously probing for a breakthrough" compensated for his shortcomings. However, Penn observed that Gillies—unlike McIndoe—seemed content to leave the actual surgeries to his trainees. Moreover, the Park Prewett Hospital where Gillies was based, "lacked

[59] Penn, *The Right to Look Human*, p67.

[60] McLeave, *McIndoe*, pp72, 77, 79.

[61] Ibid., p145; Advertisement, *Rand Daily Mail*, 26 July 1947.

[62] Penn, *The Right to Look Human*, p70.

the personal cottage hospital atmosphere" to which the South African was partial, leading to him cutting short the time spent there.[63]

In a later article paying tribute to Gillies, just two years before the "founding father's" death, Penn acknowledged the indelible impact made by Gillies as one of many who had had the privilege to "[sit] at his feet" during the Second World War. Referring to him as the "maestro", Penn recognised the basic principles of plastic surgery invented by Gillies in the First World War and later, setting in place the foundational procedures on which succeeding generations of plastic surgeons would build—Penn included. Drawing upon his own experience in Hiroshima and Nagasaki, he discussed in detail the adaptation and use of the skin flaps and grafts employed by Gillies. Further variations were made to the use of the forehead flap when treating patients suffering deformation due to leprosy and syphilis. An important adaptation was the Brenthurst Splint—discussed in the following chapter. Penn had first observed the use of the "pin method" to hold the mandible in place at Basingstoke and was inspired to improve upon the model with the non-invasive Brenthurst Splint. It was therefore important for Penn to note that his own work did not "slavishly follow the methods used in the past" and that Gillies would himself appreciate the points of departure from his own methods. Simultaneously, it was just as significant to acknowledge Gillies' role in the development of modern plastic surgery.[64]

Penn's assessment should be viewed in light of Gillies' invaluable contribution to reconstructive surgery that made possible Penn's own training. In the years following the First World War when the other surgeons who had worked at Sidcup returned to their pre-war work, Gillies and Thomas Kilner continued their promotion of this new surgical field and Gillies was instrumental in laying the foundation for the four great centres of plastic surgery (and the many smaller centres) scattered across Britain. He kept alive reconstructive surgery in the collective mind of the military and was also influential in the careers of both McIndoe and Mowlem.[65]

[63] Ibid.

[64] Jack Penn, "In the Steps of the 'Maestro'", *American Journal of Surgery*, 95, 255–262, February 1958.

[65] Simon Robert Millar, "Rooksdown House and the Rooksdown Club: A Study into the Rehabilitation of Facially Disfigured Servicemen and Civilians Following the Second World War" (Unpublished PhD Dissertation, University of London, 2015), pp104–105.

Nine months prior to the outbreak of the War, Gillies and dental surgeon, Captain William Kelsey-Fry served as Consultant Advisors to the Ministry of Health and began preparing strategies to deal with the anticipated casualties that were likely to result from German air raids. For the first years of the War, Dr. John Hebb, who was the Director General of Emergency Medical Services, envisaged a system of transferring the wounded from casualty stations to advance bases and then to base hospitals. Gillies preferred a more streamlined system of moving the wounded from casualty stations—where they received initial treatment—to base hospitals. Only the seriously injured who could not easily be moved would remain at the advance bases. He suggested the creation of two base hospitals in London, each with a self-contained team consisting of a senior surgeon, an experienced assistant, four younger surgeons or trainees, two senior dental surgeons, two regular dental surgeons and two anaesthetists. Gillies also envisaged mobile surgical teams to move between the advanced bases and the base hospitals to address more serious cases. Finally, he advocated the creation of a plastic surgery unit in a similar vein to Sidcup that should ideally be located in the Midwest in proximity to the railway and which would be used to house patients requiring lengthy care. A proposed site was at Basingstoke and the Park Prewett Mental Hospital was converted for the purpose. The other plastic surgery units would be East Grinstead (McIndoe) and Hill End (Mowlem).[66] Gillies was also desirous that the various units which fell under the different branches of the military as well as Stoke Mandeville which was under the Ministry of Pensions, collaborate, with the movement of staff between them, as this would allow "for an elastic service for the common good".[67]

Gillies himself took charge of Rookdown House, the plastic surgery unit attached to the Park Prewett Mental Hospital. It became an important centre for the training of plastic surgeons for both the military and civilian practice. Plastic surgeons were trained for work abroad and the unit attracted "surgeons from the four corners of the earth" from as far afield as the Soviet Union to Canada and of course, South Africa. It also sent surgeons to treat the injured abroad with a team sent to Yugoslavia travelling under the aegis of the United Nations Relief and Rehabilitation

[66] Ibid., pp60, 115–120.

[67] Ibid., pp124–125.

Administration.[68] Yet Rookdown House did not achieve the level of fame of East Grinstead and this was in part due to Gillies' miscalculation. He failed to take into account the changing nature of warfare where airman's burns became the defining feature of plastic surgery during the Second World War in contrast to the projectile wounds associated with its predecessor.[69] Gillies was however a key figure in the organisation of the plastic surgery units to meet the demands of the Second World War as well as the training of surgeons so that the skills developed at these centres could be disseminated internationally.

Thomas Pomfret Kilner had worked with Gillies at Sidcup and was the surgeon in charge at Stoke Mandeville Hospital. In contrast to the other pioneering plastic surgeons, Kilner was born in Britain and studied medicine at Manchester University where he subsequently lectured until the outbreak of the First World War. At the War's end, he was assigned to "Queen Mary's Hospital for Face and Jaw Injuries" at Sidcup, working alongside Gillies.[70] Kilner and Gillies set up a private practice together and were strong yet harmonising personalities with Gillies revelling in his status as the standout while Kilner preferred a more collaborative approach. Both were intolerant of those who did not meet their high standards. And both eventually grew intolerant of each other. The Ministry of Pensions was in charge of Sidcup and wished to move the plastic surgery unit to Roehampton. Gillies refused and Kilner went to Roehampton instead, setting up his own unit. The rivalry between the two men manifested itself in long-standing tension.[71] In the decades preceding the Second World War, Kilner was associated with a number of hospitals in Britain where he also served as a plastic surgeon. His research interests ranged from skin transplants to facial and jaw injuries with a focus on congenital defects such as the cleft palate and lip. From Roehampton, Kilner was tasked with creating the plastic surgery unit at Stoke Mandeville Hospital in 1941—where Penn encountered him—and

[68] Ibid., pp109, 193.

[69] McLeave, *McIndoe*, p91.

[70] "Obituary Notices: T Pomfret Kilner", *British Medical Journal*, 2, 127, 11 July 1964, https://www.bmj.com/content/2/5401/127, accessed 10 December 2020.

[71] Richard Battle, "Plastic Surgery in the Two World Wars and in the Years Between", *Journal of the Royal Society of Medicine*, 71, November 1978, p844.

would eventually be made an honorary member of the Association of Plastic Surgeons of South Africa.[72]

The Ministry of Pensions in charge of Sidcup and Roehampton believed that the latter—which had been set up by Kilner in 1925—was insufficiently large enough to address the number of casualties expected. Stoke Mandeville was therefore constructed in 1941. With an initial focus on reconstructive surgery, it retained its association with Roehampton and Kilner was in charge of both institutions. Over time, Stoke Mandeville acquired a separate identity and also served the more general surgical needs of the local populace. The plastic surgery unit was actually run by Richard Battle with Kilner paying a supervisory visit every Monday. He was an exacting supervisor—referred to as "The Boss"—with inspections of the wards, discussion of the cases and various operations that ran well into the evening. Over the course of the rest of the week, surgery was undertaken by Battle and his trainees with operations carried out in the mornings and evenings and sometimes, two operations conducted concurrently. When confronted with an influx of air raid casualties, they worked into the night. Kilner also provided training sessions for the novice plastic surgeons at Stoke Mandeville—they would sit in on his consultations with outpatients at St Thomas's Hospital before assisting in various surgeries.[73] This provided them with invaluable practical experience and as Battle observed more than three decades later, Kilner and Gillies (and their trainees) had between them provided the basic training for all the plastic surgeons currently operating in Britain.[74] At the same time, there was a clear hierarchy of institutions with those focusing on injured servicemen—such as East Grinstead—paid greater attention. According to Penn, Kilner—"the man [whom he] liked best" as a person—was empathetic even if he lacked the strong personality traits of his peers. And, even though he was confined to "the backwater of plastic surgery", harboured little antipathy towards the younger surgeons such as McIndoe and Mowlem (both New Zealanders) who came later.[75]

[72] "Obituary Notices: T Pomfret Kilner".

[73] J.P. Reidy, "The Formation and Early History of the Stoke Mandeville Plastic Surgery Unit", *British Journal of Plastic Surgery*, 39, 85–95, 1986, pp85–86.

[74] Battle, "Plastic Surgery in the Two World Wars and in the Years Between", p844.

[75] Penn, *The Right to Look Human*, p71.

Unlike Kilner and Gillies, Arthur Rainsford Mowlem was too young to have cut his surgical teeth during the First World War. The son of a solicitor, Mowlem was born in Auckland, New Zealand, studied medicine at the University of Otago Medical School before leaving for Britain for further medical training. He was the Resident Surgical Officer at Hammersmith Hospital and was about to return home when he agreed to temporarily take the place of a medical officer who had fallen ill. The medical officer supervised a ward in which Harold Gillies treated reconstructive surgery cases. Mowlem's encounter with the pioneering reconstructive surgeon would shape the remainder of the younger man's career.[76] His relative youth notwithstanding, he acquired a similar reputation for intolerance towards those he considered ineffectual. His surgical unit was based at Hill End Hospital, St Albans, and focused on facial injuries incurred by Army personnel. In addition to the reconstructive surgical operations that characterised the other units, Mowlem's team was also involved in penicillin trials where penicillin in powdered form was dissolved in a saline solution and injected into patients suffering from injuries that had become infected. Penicillin was also administered orally. On the surgical front, Mowlem's contribution to orthopaedic surgery was the use of pins to position the jaw and bone grafts and it was in the latter where he made a significant impact. Traditional bone grafting techniques involved the use of cortical bone which is the heavier, external bone on the skeleton. Pieces of cortical bone were taken from the iliac crest or pelvic bone and grafted onto the injured bone to form a "scaffolding" on which new bone could grow. In contrast, Mowlem made use of the softer cancellous bone, with small pieces of bone used as grafts for damaged mandibles and maxillae, for instance. Also obtained from the iliac crest, Mowlem's method had the advantage of promoting quicker healing with greater imperviousness to infection.[77] Yet of the "Big Four" encountered and assessed by Jack Penn, Mowlem was paid the least attention, not indicative of great strength of feeling, "Mowlem was a deft operator with an honest surgical approach, and for this I respected him greatly.

[76] M.C. Meikle, "The Evolution of Plastic and Maxillofacial Surgery in the Twentieth Century: The Dunedin Connection", *The Surgeon*, 4, 5, 325–334, October 2006, p331.

[77] Ibid., p333.

My relationship with him was always friendly – but polite rather than warm".[78]

In addition to Penn's encounters with the doyens of plastic surgery, the experience proved invaluable for the relationships forged with reconstructive surgeons from all over the world—John Marquis Converse who was part of the American unit at Park Prewett Hospital and Stuart Gordon of Canada, attached to the Canadian unit at Park Prewett.[79] In addition to his work with Gillies, Converse—who received his medical degree from the Sorbonne and was attached to the French Army during the War—also served in North Africa and with Free French forces in Italy. He eventually became the head of the Department of Plastic Surgery at New York University.[80] Stuart Gordon followed in the footsteps of E. Fulton Risdon, a Canadian plastic surgeon who had worked with Gillies during the First World War and established the Canadian unit at Sidcup. He was the first Canadian surgeon to specialise in plastic surgery and was key in its formal professionalisation through the establishment of the American Association of Plastic Surgeons and the American Board of Plastic Surgery.[81] Gordon graduated with a degree in medicine from the University of Toronto before studying under Gillies during the interwar period. He returned to England as a member of the Royal Canadian Army Medical Corps and was stationed at Basingstoke where he worked in the Canadian unit. Described as having a similar temperament to Gillies as "a dynamic, driving sort of man", Gordon was instrumental in assuring the future of plastic surgery in Canada through his position as chief of plastic surgery at the Toronto General Hospital as well as initiating postgraduate training in plastic surgery at the University of Toronto.[82]

The relationships and international links forged by Penn were a hallmark of modern plastic surgery from its inception. From the early days

[78] Penn, *The Right to Look Human*, p71.

[79] Ibid., pp70–71.

[80] "Obituary: John Marquis Converse, Surgeon", *The New York Times*, 1 February 1981, New York Times Archive, https://www.nytimes.com/1981/02/01/obituaries/john-marquis-converse-surgeon.html, accessed 13 December 2020.

[81] Leith G. Douglas, *History of the Canadian Society of Plastic Surgeons* (The Canadian Society of Plastic Surgeons, 1983), p10, http://plasticsurgery.ca/wp-content-csps/uploads/2016/05/HISTORY.pdf, accessed 13 December 2020.

[82] Ibid., pp11–12.

of reconstructive surgery at the Queen's Hospital during the First World War, the field was based on collaboration. As Gillies observed:

> This was indeed an impressive array. Clinics were held for open discussion of immediate problems and for presentation of difficult cases. Out of many a heated meeting floated a symphony of accents, the Canadian North Irish brogue, the New Zealand Fiji twang, the Australian cockney, a Midwestern drawl, a Philadelphia bark and a New York Oxford accent.[83]

It is more than likely that the mix of cultures and backgrounds presented something of a shock to British norms regarding medical practitioners, with a nurse at Aldershot describing Gillies as having "the casual, free and easy manner of the Colonials".[84] Yet the first global war both required and drew together a global talent with Gillies as the epicentre. Varaztad Kazanjian, for instance, was born in Armenia and immigrated to the United States as a teenager where he earned a scholarship to Harvard Dental School and was part of the Harvard Surgical Unit during the First World War.[85] Described as the "miracle man of the Western Front", Kazanjian was one of the many surgeons who offered their expertise at Sidcup as the First World War presented injuries never before encountered.[86] The spirit of co-operation crossed specialties with Gillies cognisant of the importance of dental surgeons and initiating a working relationship between dental specialists and reconstructive surgeons that were emulated in later plastic surgery units.[87] Wounded troops from all corners of the Commonwealth were admitted for treatment and placed in units where they were treated by the medical specialists of their homelands—Australia, Canada, New Zealand and Britain, along with a contingent of American specialists who arrived in 1918.[88]

[83] Quoted in Millar, "Rooksdown House and the Rooksdown Club", p56.

[84] Meikle, "The Evolution of Plastic and Maxillofacial Surgery", p328.

[85] John Hedley-Whyte and Debra R. Milamed, "Severe Burns in World War II", *Ulster Medical Journal*, 86, 2, 114–118, 2017, pp115–116.

[86] Darryl Tong, Andrew Bamji, Tom Brooking and Robert Love, "Plastic Kiwis—New Zealanders and the Development of a Specialty", *Journal of Military and Veterans' Health*, 17, 1, 11–19, October 2008, p13.

[87] Meikle, "The Evolution of Plastic and Maxillofacial Surgery", p328.

[88] Ibid., p329.

Of the "Big Four" plastic surgeons based in Britain at the outbreak of the Second World, Gillies, McIndoe, Mowlem and Kilner, only the last was native to Britain. The other three hailed from the relatively small island nation of New Zealand, distant from Britain. Their careers followed a similar trajectory—an early education in New Zealand followed by further training in Britain. They remained in Britain, forming the core of reconstructive surgery expertise that would be drawn on for the Second World War, providing sites of training for prospective reconstructive surgeons drawn from other Allied countries and members of the Commonwealth, including Jack Penn.

Inspired by what he had seen, Penn returned to South Africa to establish his own reconstructive surgery unit—the Brenthurst Military Hospital for Plastic Surgery.

CHAPTER 5

A Divine Right to Look Human: Brenthurst and Beyond

In May 1941, an article appeared in the society pages of the *Rand Daily Mail* describing Sir Ernest Oppenheimer's generous donation of his home, "Brenthurst", as a Red Cross hospital during the War.[1] The Oppenheimers had moved to the Brenthurst Estate in 1922. Initially known as Marion's Court, it was renamed after their first home in nearby Parktown, an affluent leafy suburb of Johannesburg that housed the mining magnates who dominated the South African economy. Marion's Court had been designed by architect Herbert Baker and was situated in 45 acres of parkland, complete with a maze.[2] Born in Kent in the mid-nineteenth century, Baker had been trained in the architectural styles that typified the strength of the British Empire. In South Africa, he also incorporated the aesthetic tastes of the imperialist archetype, Cecil John

[1] "Vanity Fair", *Rand Daily Mail*, 1 May 1941.

[2] Anthony Hocking, *Oppenheimer and Son* (Johannesburg, McGraw-Hill Book Company, 1973), pp86, 106.

The title is paraphrased from Jack Penn's published autobiography, *The Right to Look Human*, as well as the quote appearing on the tapestry commissioned for the Brenthurst Clinic.

S. Chetty, *Reconstructive Surgery and Modernisation in Twentieth-Century South Africa*, Medicine and Biomedical Sciences in Modern History, https://doi.org/10.1007/978-3-031-38673-2_5

Rhodes, who had a particular fondness for Cape Dutch architecture.[3] Baker's first architectural success was his renovation of Rhodes's residence, "Groote Schuur". This was followed by iconic landmarks such as the Rhodes Monument with its classical Greek influence, and the Union Buildings in Pretoria, the centre of the government of the newly formed Union of South Africa in 1910.[4] Baker's work therefore included the sites of political and economic power and Brenthurst was no exception.

Born in Germany in 1880, Ernest Oppenheimer immigrated to England where he worked as a diamond sorter in London. He was just 22 when he first went to Kimberley and acquired some renown as an authority on diamonds, working for the firm Dunkelsbuhler, which was closely linked to De Beers. In 1916 he returned to South Africa to the gold mining centre of the Witwatersrand where he eventually created the Anglo-American Corporation of South Africa. At the end of the First World War, using his influential connections to men such as Smuts, Anglo-American bought a number of German mines in South West Africa, forming Consolidated Diamond Mines of South West Africa Limited. He eventually became a director of De Beers, rising to the position of chairman in 1929.[5] A philanthropist, he was at the height of his economic influence by the outbreak of the Second World War.

In addition to the donation of his home, Oppenheimer also supported the hospital financially. Moreover, while the drawing room remained as a social gathering place for patients, extensive reconstruction was undertaken on the rest of the house to transform it into a hospital capable of housing up to fifty patients.[6] Just two months later Brenthurst began to receive its first patients—twenty-five wounded soldiers from both South Africa and the rest of the Empire.[7] The actual opening of the hospital took place on 23 July and was attended by a number of luminaries, including the author Sarah Gertrude Millin, Bertha Solomon (the first female Member of Parliament), Lady Oppenheimer and the guest of

[3] J.M. Claassen, "'Yonder Lies Your Hinterland': Rhodes, Baker and the Twisted Strands of the South African Architectural Tradition", *Akroterion*, 54, 69–86, 2009, p69.

[4] Ibid., pp79, 80, 83.

[5] Jade Davenport, *Digging Deep: A History of Mining in South Africa* (Johannesburg, Jonathan Ball Publishers, 2013), pp249–253, 260–261, 263, 265, 270, 276.

[6] "Vanity Fair", 1 May 1941.

[7] "Vanity Fair", *Rand Daily Mail*, 5 July 1941.

honour, Prime Minister Jan Smuts. The image presented was of orderly yet vibrant colour:

> On the steps of the house itself stood some of the first patients, men in British battle-dress hospital blue and Union Defence Force uniform. On the winding paths up the kopje which leads to the house were the blue and red uniforms of the V.A.D.s and those allied with the Red Cross's clear colours of red and white made a vivid scene.[8]

Penn returned to Cape Town aboard a ship that was part of an enormous convoy carrying troops bound for the Middle and Far East. He disembarked at Cape Town with the remainder of the military passengers on board his ship *en route* to Singapore, destined for an appalling fate when Singapore fell to the Japanese in February 1942 and thousands were taken prisoners.[9] The convoy of which Penn was part also came under enemy attack with a ship sunk by a torpedo as it made its way south. Penn, however, was unaware of the incident and the remainder of his War would be relatively more sedate.[10] Upon reaching the South African coast, he boarded the train for Johannesburg and it was on this final part of his journey home that he claimed to come across an article detailing Oppenheimer's donation of Brenthurst to the war effort. The seed was sown and, when Penn was informed by the DGMS that he would not be permitted to go to North Africa as a plastic surgeon, he requested the use of Brenthurst to form his own plastic surgery unit. His focus on plastic surgery and his decision to remain in South Africa put paid to the chance of rising in the military ranks but his priority was clear. He met with Lady Oppenheimer to obtain permission to use Brenthurst as the plastic surgery unit. The Brenthurst Red Cross Military Hospital for Plastic Surgery would be unique in sub-Saharan Africa, drawing in the wounded from various parts of the Commonwealth. While Penn served as its Officer-in-Charge for the duration, his rank would remain that of major.[11] However, while it was an indication of Penn's prioritisation of reconstructive surgery, the lower rank would also prove a hindrance and source of frustration when dealing with the military chain of command.

8 "Vanity Fair", *Rand Daily Mail*, 24 July 1941.

9 Ibid., p73.

10 Ibid., pp73–74.

11 Penn, *The Right to Look Human*, pp73–74.

The house itself had to be adapted to the needs of a plastic surgery clinic with the provision of the necessary medical equipment. Just as important was the recruitment of staff. Janet Ford like Penn, just thirty years old, became Matron of the hospital and served as Penn's invaluable aide during the setting up and subsequent running of Brenthurst. Loquacious and enthusiastic, she was described by Penn as having "an instinctive sound common sense and a remarkable perspicacity of character", ultimately becoming a "loyal friend". The matron oversaw the nursing staff and obtained the required nurses to staff the hospital.[12] As was the case in Britain, plastic surgery units required a high contingent of nursing staff to assist patients during the lengthy period of rehabilitation and recuperation. The close working relationship between plastic surgeons and their nursing staff was exemplified by Penn who would employ nurses from various parts of the world when he established his own clinic, nurses who also went on to create their own journal, the *Brenthurst Phoenix*. More than two decades after the War ended, Penn was asked by the South African Nursing Association to sculpt a model of Henrietta Stockdale for the Kimberley Cathedral.[13] Stockdale symbolised modern nursing practice in South Africa and was instrumental in the professionalisation of the field in the late nineteenth century. Completed in 1969, Penn's sculpture of Stockdale—a life-sized rendering of the nurse—was "unveiled…by three student nurses—one white, one black and one coloured", symbolic of the universality of medical care and the profession itself.[14] At the unveiling, Penn was also awarded the South African Nursing Association Gold Medal in 1969, only the second man to be so distinguished. In the spirit of the universality of nursing care, he would later also sculpt the likeness of Cecilia Makiwane, the first black woman to qualify as a professional nurse in South Africa.[15] During his surgical work in the ensuing decades, Penn travelled with his own medical team, including a nurse, Marie Roux, who worked on a voluntary basis in Japan as well as the war zones in Israel.

[12] Ibid., pp74–75.

[13] Ibid., p118.

[14] Ibid., p120.

[15] "Nurses Pay Tribute to Specialist", *Rand Daily Mail*, 7 January 1969. The sculpture of Cecilia Makiwane is discussed in the final chapter.

An important aspect of surgery—and one almost as essential as the prevention of infection—was the use of anaesthesia. Diethyl ether was first used in the mid-nineteenth century at Massachusetts General Hospital to painlessly remove a tumour from the neck of patient Edward Abbott. Anaesthesia revolutionised the practice of surgery—surgeons had previously to contend with the pained agony of patients, loss of blood and shock. Surgeries had to be quick and thus lacked a level of finesse. The use of anaesthesia in the form of chloroform entered mainstream surgical practice soon after when it was administered to Queen Victoria during childbirth. By rendering the patient unconscious, surgeons were free to operate with greater care and accuracy, limiting blood loss. This was essential for the exacting demands of plastic surgery.[16] Significant strides had been made in the administering of anaesthesia during the First World War and this was necessitated by plastic surgery where it proved difficult to administer anaesthesia via facial mask. The use of endotracheal tubes was the innovative solution by Ivan Magill, working with Gillies at Sidcup.[17] By the mid-twentieth century, anaesthesia had progressed beyond the application of chloroform to a combination of narcotics to induce unconsciousness, painkillers and muscle relaxants. A ventilator is used and the anaesthetist is responsible for the close monitoring of heart rate and blood oxygen levels for the duration of the procedure.[18]

Another figure who would accompany Penn on his surgical travels and one who would prove to be vital to the medical team at Brenthurst was his anaesthetist, Hyman Bental—although first impressions did not augur particularly well for the lengthy and productive relationship that was to follow. The anaesthetist is a key part of the surgical team and Penn wanted "a first-class man". He was instead assigned a young lieutenant with no previous experience who was as "horrified" by his assignment as Penn was. With the nickname "Speedy" —hardly designed to inspire confidence—he proved more than willing to work towards developing the necessary skills, becoming an essential member of the medical staff at Brenthurst. Penn grew to value his role, so much so, that subsequent attempts to

[16] Arnold Van De Laar, *Under the Knife: Remarkable Stories from the History of Surgery*, Andy Brown (translator) (London, John Murray, 2018), pp100–105.

[17] E. Ann Robertson, "Anaesthesia, Shock and Resuscitation", in *War Surgery, 1914–1918*, Thomas Scotland and Steven Heys (eds) (Solihull, Helion and Company, 2012), pp112–113.

[18] Van De Laar, *Under the Knife*, pp100–105.

have him transferred by the military hierarchy were met with implacable resistance on the part of Penn. The two men would forge an important partnership, even co-authoring medical articles together. Through his love for music, Bental proved an important morale booster at Brenthurst, assembling patients into a music band with him playing a leading role as mandolin player and mediocre singer.[19]

Other members of staff included Sergeant Shrier, the administrative officer, who was a confidante to the men as well as a dentist, particularly necessary for facial and jaw injuries. In this, Penn followed the example set by Gillies during the First World War. In a similar vein was the employment of an artist, Cecile Ormerod.[20] Women were hired as physiotherapists and occupational therapists. Penn emulated the New Zealanders in Britain in another manner as well—the amelioration of strict military discipline as Penn was not inclined to "play soldiers". Soldiers were permitted to create their own disciplinary committee and not compelled to wear the blue uniforms that were the usual attire for military patients. Any privileges extended to them were based on an understanding that they would not act in any manner to bring the hospital into disrepute, especially when off the grounds. This atmosphere of mutual trust paid off and Penn noted that he had no cause "to take a single disciplinary action" against any of the men for the duration of the War.[21] Just as the British were nonplussed by Gillies's and McIndoe's attitudes to military discipline, the same applied to Brenthurst under Penn with a brigadier informing Janet Ford that it "was the most unmilitary establishment" he had ever seen yet "it seems to work".[22]

Looming large over the Brenthurst Hospital were its patrons, Ernest and Caroline Oppenheimer. Penn established a close relationship with Lady Oppenheimer who arguably played more of a hands-on role at the hospital than her husband, with Penn in later correspondence referring to her familiarly as "Ina".[23] Lady Oppenheimer was born into the British nobility, her father Thomas Harvey was a baronet, and she had

[19] Penn, *The Right to Look Human*, p76.

[20] Ibid., p77.

[21] Ibid.

[22] Anthony Hocking, *Oppenheimer and Son* (Johannesburg, McGraw-Hill Book Company, 1973), p195.

[23] Cf. Jack Penn, Letter to Lady Oppenheimer—5th April 1956, BC748 A1.10, Dr Jack Penn Collection A1.1—A1.81, Correspondence between Dr Jack Penn and Albert

grown up hobnobbing with royalty. She came to South Africa with her husband, Michael Oppenheimer, the nephew of Ernest, who was subsequently killed in a plane crash. Ernest soon contended with the loss of his son, Frank, and in their mutual grief, the two grew closer, eventually marrying.[24]

Like her husband, Lady Oppenheimer demonstrated a philanthropic bent and with the outbreak of the Second World War, created the Caledonian Market to raise funds to purchase "the little luxuries" that would boost the morale of the men on the frontlines. The Market was based in the basement of Paramount Stores, loaned to Lady Oppenheimer and her like-minded acquaintances and was an unqualified success. By then, the Oppenheimers had turned their attention to another project—a means of alleviating the strain on Johannesburg hospitals due to the returning wounded. This would lead to the conversion of the Brenthurst home into a hospital.[25]

Early patients were less injured than expected—soldiers who often had yet to serve on the frontlines and who were afflicted with ailments ranging from ingrown toenails to appendicitis. They were subsequently encouraged to present a suitably ill appearance for the colourful opening of the hospital. It was, however, with Penn's plan for a plastic surgery unit that Brenthurst would come into its own. He presented his ideas to Lady Oppenheimer who was initially reluctant due to his relative youth. During the interview, however, the enthusiastic surgeon told her to "hold on" while he brought her some photographs that would strengthen his case. Impressed by his "confidence"—indicated by his lack of adherence to social mores—she agreed to the use of the hospital for Penn's surgical work and persuaded her husband to do the same.[26]

In addition to providing medical equipment for the hospital as well as Lady Oppenheimer's fund-raising in the Caledonian Market, the Oppenheimers involved themselves in social and recreational activities such as those taking place over Christmas.[27] The interaction of young soldiers

Schweitzer and Others, Mainly at Lambarene, 1956–1957, University of Cape Town Libraries (hereafter UCTL).

[24] Hocking, *Oppenheimer and Son*, pp149, 161, 165–166.

[25] Ibid., p192.

[26] Ibid., p193.

[27] Ibid., p197.

and female nurses created the opportunities for wartime romance. A small excerpt appearing in the *Rand Daily Mail* in 1943 announced the wedding of Sister H.C. Hagemann to Lieutenant R.G. Van Eyssen, a patient at Brenthurst.[28] Nor was this an isolated incident. On learning of the engagement of a nurse, Ernest funded the wedding that took place at Brenthurst.[29] Concerts were held for the patients including one by the Liberty Club in 1942 that incorporated cabaret dancers. "Play-readings" were another example of the entertainment available to patients.[30] The Red Cross hospitals—of which Brenthurst was part—were portrayed in the press as idyllic oases for the recuperating soldier, based on community involvement in both creating a haven at the hospital itself and in incorporating the more mobile patient into mainstream society:

> There are often lazy, care-free days spent in the lovely surroundings of the convalescent hospitals into which some of Johannesburg's most lovely homes have been turned by the gift of private owners...There is generally a full-time doctor and diversions include daily visitors and pass-outs in the daytime for those men who are well enough to walk about freely. Most of the wards are supported by groups of people in the city, who make it their business to supply their own particular ward with every comfort. Libraries, games, concerts and drives all help to make the convalescent days pass with comfort and satisfaction.[31]

Ernest Oppenheimer highlighted both the national and international importance of the Red Cross that had worked across national and state boundaries to provide philanthropic aid and medical care with a rather diplomatic caveat that this sometimes gave governments the "excuse" not to bear their own burden of responsibility for doing the same.[32]

Penn's relationship with the Oppenheimers would continue after the end of the War. Not only was the family involved in the sending of medical personnel and equipment to Lambarene, but Penn also wrote letters to

[28] "Nurse and Patient Married", *Rand Daily Mail*, 22 November 1943.

[29] Hocking, *Oppenheimer and Son*, p196.

[30] "Women in War-Time", *Rand Daily Mail*, 28 February 1942.

[31] "Men Happy in City Military Hospitals", *Rand Daily Mail*, 10 November 1941.

[32] "Transvaal Raised £543 000", *Rand Daily Mail*, 17 May 1944.

Lady Oppenheimer, informing her of his experiences there and his impressions of Schweitzer. When Ernest took ill due to a misdiagnosis of his diabetes, Lady Oppenheimer turned to Penn who successfully treated the mogul.[33]

The patients who arrived at Brenthurst were determined by the course of the War. Initially, patients were those Allied troops who served in the Mediterranean, southern Europe and North Africa. These numbers would eventually decline as Allied advances allowed for the transport of the injured to Britain and after 1941, the United States.[34] With the influx of patients drawn from all over the world, Penn also established relationships with other plastic surgeons, one of whom was an Italian based in Milan who was treating South Africans, even as Penn treated Italians. The Red Cross served as a mediator allowing the exchange of patients and Penn found that the South Africans had received similar treatment to that which would have been afforded at Brenthurst as the Italian had also been trained in Britain.[35] Penn would later work alongside this doctor and, after both carried out reconstructive surgery on a young woman who had been injured in a bombing raid over Milan, he observed, "...if our leaders would talk the same language as we do, people such as this girl would never have needed our services".[36] For Penn, while plastic surgery could rectify the injury caused by war, the common practice of medicine had the potential to transcend the divisions that led to conflict.

The increasing number of soldiers sent to South Africa for treatment soon outstripped the capacity of Brenthurst. Eventually, an additional five private homes were placed at Penn's disposal allowing the treatment of up to two hundred patients. Brenthurst served as the hub where the medical procedures were carried out. One of these homes would also be converted into a fully-fledged hospital with a focus on jaw injuries.[37]

[33] Hocking, *Oppenheimer and Son*, p282.

[34] Penn, *The Right to Look Human*, pp94–95.

[35] Hocking, *Oppenheimer and Son*, p194.

[36] Jack Penn, "He Is My Younger Brother", in *White Africans are Also People*, Sarah Gertrude Millin (ed) (Howard Timmons, Cape Town, 1966), pp122–123, Brn. No: 14607, Call No: 323.1128 MIL, BL.

[37] Hocking, *Oppenheimer and Son*, p195.

The Brenthurst Splint and the Brenthurst Papers

As with the development of modern reconstructive surgery during the First World War, it was the exposure to war injuries at Brenthurst that was the mother of invention, and Penn and his team were able to make a significant contribution to the treatment of traumatic injury to the jaw. An important component in the treatment of the injury was the correct alignment of the jaw and the contribution was a mechanical means of doing so. A brief paper written by Major Jack Penn and Captain Lester Brown appeared in the *Brenthurst Papers*. Entitled "A New Conception in Extra-Oral Splintage", it was a collaborative effort between groups from various specialties in the creation of a technological innovation in reconstructive surgery that came to be known as the "Brenthurst Splint". The paper begins with "the background of the development and methods of jaw splintage" which considers the view of several reconstructive surgeons (including Harold Gillies) of the challenges and likely lack of success in producing such a device. It also addresses the various dangers associated with the existing technology which relied upon drilling into the jaw to position the devices. In contrast, the Brenthurst Splint was not invasive with "no chance of a bone burn, injury to tooth roots or to the inferior dental nerve" and would be suitable for a variety of patients ranging from wounded soldiers to young children—who had not yet developed permanent teeth. The article contained photographs of the steel device attached to the jawbone via clamps with screws used to adjust its positioning and grip.[38]

A press report hailed the Brenthurst Splint as a marvel of South African technological ingenuity that had overcome the shortcomings of the existing devices employed by the British and Americans with the former employing "steel screws" and the latter "steel pins", both directly drilled into the jaw. The South Africa model was both non-invasive and induced little discomfort with none of the side-effects associated with the more invasive methods.[39] The application of the splint to the outside of the jaw also allowed the patient to continue their normal diet as they

[38] Jack Penn and Lester Brown, "A New Conception in Extra-Oral Splintage", *Brenthurst Papers*, Jack Penn (ed) (Johannesburg, Witwatersrand University Press, 1944), Brn. No: 3297, Call No: 617.95 BRE, BL.

[39] "City Dentists Invent Revolutionary Surgical Appliance", *Rand Daily Mail*, 1 April 1943.

healed.[40] A great benefit was its simplicity, rendering it easy to use in frontline situations without the need for surgical specialists; this could thus lead to prompt treatment. The splint was the result of intensive collaboration—the result of eighteen months of painstaking research and testing and done in conjunction with engineers from the South African Air Force and the Railway Administration who had acted under the direction of the "three young South African dental surgeons" and the overall approval of the DGMS.[41]

Penn's own account of the invention was more detailed and began with his research at the Department of Anatomy at Witwatersrand University where he made a detailed examination of the various types of mandibles housed there, including those of early hominins. He accredited his earlier work with Dart in giving him some understanding of these fossilised mandibles. Across the variety of mandibles studied, Penn concluded that there was one constant point—regardless of age and individual differences—the "inferior border" to which a splint could be attached which held a fractured jaw in position. Penn and Lester Brown then began extensive research and testing, designing twenty-two different versions until they arrived at the ideal model which was subsequently put into production by the engineers of the South African Railways. Over the next two years, Penn treated more than two hundred patients, all of whom made a successful recovery.[42]

In an interesting addendum, Penn related the use of the Brenthurst Splint by Soviet surgeons who used it on wounded soldiers who were then returned to combat. The Soviet Union, however, accredited its invention to one of their own. Penn would experience some frustration with his Soviet counterpart at the Moscow Traumatological Institute due to, either the latter's lack of expertise in plastic surgery or his lack of transparency that hindered the free sharing of knowledge amongst the Allies.[43] This was in contrast to the opening pages of Penn's journal article on the splint that drew extensively upon the work and findings of other Allied reconstructive surgeons.

[40] Penn, *The Right to Look Human*, p83.

[41] "City Dentists Invent Revolutionary Surgical Appliance".

[42] Penn, *The Right to Look Human*, p83.

[43] Ibid.

The account of the development of the Brenthurst Splint had pride of place in the *Brenthurst Papers*, a journal of plastic surgery established by Penn that was an early step in the professionalisation of plastic surgery in South Africa. It also highlighted the unique contributions made by South Africans to the field. No longer simply the observer of the "fathers" of modern plastic surgery, Penn felt confident enough to assert his own expertise. From the establishment of the hospital as a plastic surgery unit until the first half of 1944, Penn had a high case load, a situation made more onerous by the lack of suitable assistants who did not meet his pre-requisites of both surgical skill and an artistic or aesthetic sensibility. The number of cases, however, provided the opportunity for the development of and improvements in surgical techniques. Not short of a sense of self-assurance, Penn published the *Brenthurst Papers* as:

> ...it became obvious that some of the techniques developed and established were of sufficient importance to be made known to surgeons elsewhere. The pressure of work, together with wider experience, created methods that were short cuts to better results, apart from various breakthroughs beyond the normal boundaries of knowledge.[44]

Penn had initially been hampered from making these developments known in the more established British and American journals due to the "normal backlog" (that was possibly extended by the War) and this led to the publication of the *Brenthurst Papers*, with the assistance of Lady Oppenheimer. Printed quarterly until after the end of the War and, as Penn believed, the first journal exclusively in English, it gives some insight into the injuries sustained during the War and the methods used to treat them.[45]

The articles are remarkable for following a similar format to Harold Gillies' *Plastic Surgery of the Face* with photographs of injuries, artistic renditions of the surgical procedures used, and photographs taken after treatment was completed. There is, however, a greater use of X-ray photographs. While X-rays had been discovered by Wilhelm Röntgen in 1895 and were already considered to have important medical uses just

[44] Ibid., pp93–94.

[45] Ibid., p93.

a year later, it would take decades before they became part of the established diagnostic practice.[46] During the First World War, the use of X-rays in war conditions was adversely affected, not just by technology that was in its infancy but also by a lack of a steady electricity supply close to the frontlines. It was scientist Marie Curie, who played a significant role in the adaptation of X-rays for the diagnosis of injuries incurred during wartime. As France's Director of the Red Cross Radiology Service, she had mobile trucks set up with the necessary X-ray equipment and electricity supplied from their engines to make more widespread use of X-rays as a diagnostic tool in combat areas. At the end of the War, she began training American soldiers.[47] The use of X-rays was certainly an important early component of plastic surgery as evident at Sidcup, but the quality was poor and required extensive input from radiologists, a field that was still in its infancy.[48]

The varying quality of X-rays during the First World War may account for Gillies's reliance on Henry Tonks to render the less visible aspects of injury, cementing the relationship between reconstructive surgery and art. In contrast, Penn's incorporation of X-rays suggests the more widespread use of and improvements in this technology in the latter conflict. X-ray images published in the *Brenthurst Papers* reveal the damage done to teeth, cartilage and bone as well as the use of corrective measures such as splints to position the bone.[49]

A range of cases were presented in the *Brenthurst Papers* ranging from burns to the trauma inflicted by projectiles such as bullets or shrapnel. There was an overall focus on facial injury—the jaw, cheeks, eyes and ears—although there were some exceptions. And a number of patients had already received some form of treatment at other sites before they were sent to Brenthurst. While the use of the pedicle was a key and

[46] Joel D. Howell, "Early Clinical Use of the X-Ray", *Transactions of the American Clinical and Climatological Association*, 127, 2016, pp341–349, https://www.ncbi.nlm.nih.gov/pmc/articles/PMC5216491/, accessed 21 December 2020.

[47] Norman L. Martin, "Radiology at Base Hospital #28 in France during WW1", University of Kansas Medical Center, http://www.kumc.edu/wwi/base-hospital-28/clinical-services/radiology.html, accessed 21 December 2020.

[48] Alexander MacDonald, "X-Rays During the Great War", in *War Surgery, 1914–1918*, Thomas Scotland and Steven Heys (eds) (Solihull, Helion and Company, 2012), pp143–144.

[49] Cf. *Brenthurst Papers*, Jack Penn (ed) (Johannesburg, Witwatersrand University Press, 1944), Brn. No: 3297, Call No: 617.95 BRE, BL.

very visible sign of reconstructive surgery in Britain, Penn preferred free grafts for the treatment of scarring resulting from facial burns. Consisting largely of skin with the accompanying fatty tissue, he believed the grafts to be more suitable in assisting with the replication of facial expression whereas pedicle grafts tended to create "a rather flabby and expressionless appearance". Penn employed the free graft method on a petty officer in the Royal Navy who suffered severe burns to the face and hands when his destroyer was sunk in the Mediterranean. The initial treatment he received further complicated his injuries. Tannic acid had been applied to the injuries which formed a stiff carapace over his wound and led to the development of infection beneath.[50] The use of tannic acid in the treatment of burns had been evident in the interwar period. The acid—used to "tan" hides in the preparation of leather—was supplemented with silver nitrate to enhance the speed at which it dried as well as a mixture of gentian violet to be applied to the more delicate areas that had been burned such as eyelids. By the outbreak of the Second World War, it was available in the form of a jelly-like substance, "Tannefax", in tubes and could be applied to patients immediately after injury. Archie McIndoe, through his treatment of airman burns, became aware of the deleterious effects of tannic acid as it led to a stiffening of the injured joints, further affecting circulation and thus contributing to sepsis. The stiffening of the eyelids not only prevented further treatment but also reduced the patient's ability to blink, in some cases culminating in blindness. McIndoe was most influential in ensuring that tannic acid was withdrawn from use in the treatment of burns.[51]

The petty officer admitted to Brenthurst in June 1941 then, was in a pitiful state—scarred and weak yet with a sense of optimism that was essential for a process that could take months, if not years, with frequent surgeries interspersed with bouts of rehabilitation. The facial scarring was particularly evident on the nose with loss of cartilage. There was further loss of skin on the cheeks and upper eyelids, making it a challenge for the patient to sleep. Additional loss of skin and scarring on the lips had left this feature immobile, making both facial expression and eating difficult. Free grafts were used to treat the injuries with priority given to the eyelids

[50] "Case No 2: The Use of Free Grafts for Facial Reconstruction in Burns", *Brenthurst Papers*.

[51] Emily Mayhew, *Guinea Pig Club: Archibald McIndoe and the RAF in World War II* (Barnsley, Greenhill Books, 2018), pp58–61.

(to preserve the cornea), lips and hands that would allow the patient some degree of independence. Later procedures were largely aesthetic—the replacement of the missing left eyebrow as well as the reconstruction of the cheeks, nose and ears. Grafts were obtained from undamaged areas of the body such as the abdomen with the graft for the eyebrow taken from behind the ear as it contained hair follicles. Throughout Penn's account of the process, there is a strong aesthetic sense with the texture of the eyebrow not being as "bushy as normal", concerns about maintaining a consistent skin tone to prevent a "patchwork quilt appearance" and surgery on the lips for "a mobile mouth with a pleasing natural expression at the corners". The accompanying images ranged from a photograph taken ten years before the injury, the scarred face upon admission, a sketch detailing the areas where the grafts were applied and a final photograph of the petty officer on his release from Brenthurst, a slight smile on his face. The last showed the extent to which reconstructive surgery was able to restore his initial appearance.[52]

Another account addressed the injuries to the hands of a sapper—involved in explosives work such as mine detection. Severe damage had been caused by a trench mortar, leaving him with a right hand to which function could not be restored and without the use of his left thumb. Penn's treatment involved the transplant of a part of the index finger bone from the left hand which was grafted onto the thumb. At the conclusion of the operation, the patient had full use of sensation in the thumb, allowing him some degree of functionality. In this case, Penn acknowledged the possibility that another mode of treatment may have improved the outcome however this was not attempted "as the functional result was considered adequate".[53]

The case of a young corporal in the Polish Army provided Penn and his surgical team with the opportunity to make use of the Brenthurst splint. It also highlights the nature of some of the cases where Penn had to redress earlier unsuccessful attempts at treatment. The corporal—just twenty-three at the time—was serving in the Western Desert campaign when he was shot in the face, the bullet entering his right check and exiting through his left. Preliminary treatment was carried out in the units on the frontlines before he was transferred to a "Maxillo-Facial Unit"

[52] "Case No 2: The Use of Free Grafts for Facial Reconstruction in Burns".

[53] "Case No 4: Thumb Reconstruction by Transplantation of Digit", *Brenthurst Papers*.

a week later. A number of surgical interventions were then undertaken, including the removal of bone and tooth fragments, the insertion of soft tissue grafts, and almost a year later, a bone graft on the jaw. The latter, however, was largely unsuccessful and the patient was sent to Brenthurst in early 1944. The core of the treatment was therefore to insert a bone graft on the mandible. An approximately 13-centimetre piece of bone was taken from the iliac crest and shaped to fit the mandible. Holes were made in the bone and the mandible and wire was threaded through to attach the bone graft to the mandible. The Brenthurst clamp was employed to keep the mandible in position and the result was an unqualified success, "The post-operative course was uneventful, there being no pain, sepsis or discomfort".[54]

During reconstructive procedures, Penn used tissue, skin, bone and cartilage—with a preference for implant material obtained from the body of the patient undergoing surgery to minimise rejection. The First World War had begun the process of using synthetic material as well as other natural materials such as ivory—all with limited success.[55] This would change during the Second World War, especially as there was a premium on natural resources such as rubber. While the first form of plastic in the form of celluloid was invented in 1869 and the first fully synthetic plastic, Bakelite was ubiquitous by the 1920s, the major developments in thermoplastics—or plastics that could be moulded—were evident in the 1930s and initially the prerogative of the military during the Second World War where they were used in everything from the manufacture of combs to parachutes and even the anti-corrosive gas containers required during the development of the atomic bomb.[56] The use of plastics became an increasingly common feature in plastic surgery. Penn, however, was circumspect about their use due to their novelty yet they also proved indispensable in some cases such as that of an airman who had suffered severe head trauma during a crash. The injury necessitated the removal of his left frontal lobe as well as the overlying skull. There was insufficient

[54] Case No 16: "Free Bone Graft Replacement of Both Horizontal Rami. Immobilization by Combined Intra and Extra-Oral Splintage", *Brenthurst Papers*.

[55] Penn, *The Right to Look Human*, p91.

[56] Susan Freinkel, "A Brief History of Plastic's Conquest of the World: Cheap Plastic has Unleashed a Flood of Consumer Goods", *Scientific American*, 29 May 2011, https://www.scientificamerican.com/article/a-brief-history-of-plastic-world-conquest/, accessed 1 February 2021.

bone available to graft onto the exposed area so Penn used a large acrylic "graft". The plastic shield contained perforations to allow the tissue to join with it. No infection resulted and the patient went on to become a lawyer with only the rare epileptic seizure a reminder of the injury.[57]

Ultimately, between two to three thousand wounded men passed through the doors of Brenthurst with Penn personally accounting for six thousand surgical procedures.[58] By early January 1944, however, Penn was granted an "indefinite release from whole-time military service to resume civil occupation".[59] Yet he would continue his work at Brenthurst. The hospital was a sterling example of a plastic surgery unit that had drawn its inspiration from similar models in Britain but had nevertheless been the site of medical and technological innovation that was purely South African. With an integral role in treating the wounded of the Second World War, a steady decline in patients as the War drew to a close meant that plans were afoot to return the house to its original condition preparatory to the Oppenheimers reoccupying it. On 28 August 1944, however, a fire broke out. Believed to be due to a fault in the electrical wiring, the conflagration took hours to extinguish, consumed a wing of the house and resulted in injury to a number of firefighters.[60] The patients resident at the hospital evacuated to the gardens in an orderly fashion and no further injuries occurred.[61] In the interim Penn continued treating patients at the convalescent home that had already been converted into a hospital. The fire had, however, hastened the process of the closure of the Brenthurst Red Cross Military Hospital for Plastic Surgery. This would in turn be followed by the closure of the associated convalescent homes with the DGMS resolving to consolidate all plastic surgical work in one location. This was a former estate occupied by the UDF which had also, ironically, been damaged by fire. The estate—whimsically called "Tara"—was given to Penn to convert into a hospital for plastic surgery.[62]

[57] Penn, *The Right to Look Human*, pp91–92.

[58] Hocking, *Oppenheimer and Son*, p212.

[59] Jack Penn Service File, W.R. 12/6640, DOD.

[60] "Part of Brenthurst Destroyed by Fire: Four Firemen Hurt", *Rand Daily Mail*, 29 August 1944.

[61] Hocking, *Oppenheimer and Son*, p212.

[62] Penn, *The Right to Look Human*, p95.

Tara

With the understanding that private homes could not be used indefinitely as hospitals, Thornton's replacement as Director General of Medical Services, Alexander Jeremiah Orenstein turned his attention to the site of Tara or Hurlingham. A UDF site, Orenstein saw it as a white elephant, requiring resources to be guarded while remaining in a dilapidated state. The solution was to renovate it and transform it into a hospital for plastic surgery as well as one that could promote occupational therapy for recuperating military personnel. Penn consulted with Orenstein and the feasibility of the project was touted to Prime Minister Smuts—it would cost approximately £18 250 to convert Tara into a hospital with a capacity of 185 beds. In response to Smuts's expressed reservations about the potential hospital's isolated location, Orenstein's response was that this was a strength, given the disfigurement of the proposed patients: "Distance from town is an advantage rather than a disadvantage because most such cases are shy of casual contacts with the public whilst deformed and also for other reasons concerning long-term hospitalization cases".[63]

Penn and Lester Brown's inspection of the site resulted in a report that highlighted the potential of Tara as a hospital with specific consideration made for the requirements of the Dental section to promote efficient treatment. Penn also requested the construction of three surgeries and a laboratory near the entrance of the hospital. His proposed plan was made in light of his own experience at Brenthurst as well as his observations of the main British plastic surgical centres under the "Big Four". In his report, he further requested permission for himself and Brown to inspect surgical units in North Africa and the Middle East to familiarise themselves with new developments that would shape the ongoing vision for Tara and allow the fostering of ties with other plastic surgeons to enhance their "clinical knowledge".[64]

[63] A.J. Orenstein, DGMS, to Brigadier Blaine, Cape Town, Repeat General Mitchell Baker Cape Town, 22 January 1944, and Secretary of Defence, Cape Town to Director General of Medical Services (for Brigadier Orenstein personally from Brigadier Blaine), 21 January 1944, Surgeon General, Group 2, Box 1138, File MD 580/2/1 (Vol 1): Red Cross Hospital for Plastic Surgery (Tara): Buildings and Accommodation, DOD.

[64] Letter to the DGMS by Penn, Major, SAMC, Surgeon in Charge, for Tara suitability, 25 February 1944, Surgeon General, Group 2, Box 1138, File MD 580/2/1 (Vol 1): Red Cross Hospital for Plastic Surgery (Tara): Buildings and Accommodation, DOD.

The hospital continued its association with the Red Cross with Orenstein proposing the retention of the name, the Brenthurst Hospital for Plastic Surgery, as an homage to the Oppenheimers. The proposal was politely rebuffed by the Red Cross—and the Oppenheimers—as it would likely "cause confusion".[65] The alliance between the UDF and the Red Cross in their running of the hospital was to be one of negotiation. The Red Cross made use of the premises as a hospital free of charge but was tasked with the provision of transport, including ambulances, as well as furniture, food and the payment of utilities as well as the staffing related to nursing, administration and maintenance of the building and the grounds. The UDF was to pay a daily allowance per patient, provided medical and surgical equipment, undertook the maintenance of the hospital and provided the medical staff including three medical officers, two dental officers and two dental mechanics. The payment and discipline of the UDF personnel also fell under the ambit of the military.[66]

For Penn, the hospital's potential could last beyond the War itself. As a military hospital, it could serve as a centre for reconstructive surgery that would extend beyond plastic surgery and could include specialists from various fields ranging from orthopaedics to neurosurgery and opthalmic surgery. It could ideally make use of specialists from beyond the confines of the UDF that would serve on a consultative basis.[67] Penn was also wary of what he saw as arbitrary military intervention in the movement of personnel at Brenthurst, creating disruption in the running of the hospital and was anxious to not have the situation repeat itself at Tara.[68] It spoke

[65] DGMS to Red Cross, 15 August 1994, and response of Red Cross, 29 August 1944, Surgeon General, Group 2, Box 1136, File MD 580/2: Tara: Red Cross Hospital for Plastic Surgery—General, DOD. The Oppenheimers would have no such qualms when Penn used the name for his civilian practice.

[66] DGMS Orenstein, 2 February 1945, Aide Memoire on Conference Held at Red Cross Plastic Surgery Hospital, Hurlingham, on 1st February 1945, Surgeon General, Group 2, Box 1136, File MD 580/2: Tara: Red Cross Hospital for Plastic Surgery—General, DOD.

[67] Memorandum on Tara Hall: Suggestions by Major Jack Penn, 13 July 1944, Surgeon General, Group 2, Box 1136, File MD 580/2: Tara: Red Cross Hospital for Plastic Surgery—General, DOD.

[68] Dental Officers and Mechanics – Tara Hall, Excerpt from Statement by Penn, 15 September 1944, Surgeon General, Group 2, Box 1137, File MD 580/2/5: Red Cross Hospital for Plastic Surgery (Tara): Establishment and Staff Matters, DOD.

to his own desire for control and an abhorrence of what he believed to be unnecessary and arbitrary bureaucratic intervention.

The UDF also clearly spelt out the patients that were eligible for admittance to Tara for treatment. Patients were restricted to male and female "Europeans" only requiring treatment in the form of plastic surgery for "mutilation", the implementation of skin grafts and those with complex fractures of the jaw. Cases falling outside these categories would be transferred instead to the military hospitals at Wynberg, Springfield and Voortrekkerhoogte—and all "non-European" cases that fell into the three categories could only be treated at the No 110 Military Hospital Voortrekkerhoogte.[69] The segregation evident in military hospitals mirrored that in the Union Defence Force. Since the onset of the War in 1939, a major point of contention for black nationalists and white conservatives was the extent to which blacks could participate in the war. Appeasing white unease over the arming of black men, these soldiers were auxiliary and fell under the Non-European Army Services. Combat became the hallmark of citizenship and was officially only the prerogative of white soldiers—although the exigencies of war may have belied official policy. To compensate for a shortage of manpower, a "dilution" policy was put into effect in 1942 permitting black auxiliaries to serve in previously all-white units, thus freeing white men for combat. Facing similar experiences to that of their white counterparts, black soldiers were nevertheless paid less, were often subject to greater restrictions and enjoyed fewer privileges. Yet dilution also presented the opportunity for men from various cultural, ethnic and racial backgrounds to work together for a common cause.[70] On the home front, however, and as evident in medical treatment, distinctions were retained.

Yet this period was key in the development of social medicine in South Africa. In contrast to the language of discrimination, social medicine related to a holistic view of health care contextualised by social conditions. In South Africa, these conditions were a result of racial policies that adversely affected the health of black South Africans. As discussed in Chapter Nine, Sidney Kark—a contemporary and acquaintance of

[69] A.J. Orenstein, DGMS: D.G.M.S., U.D.F. Medical Administrative Instruction, No. 137, 9 February 1945, Surgeon General, Group 2, Box 1136, File MD 580/2: Tara: Red Cross Hospital for Plastic Surgery—General, DOD.

[70] Cf. Suryakanthie Chetty, "'Subjects or Citizens?' Black Soldiers and the Dilemma of the Second World War", *Journal of Natal and Zulu History*, 30, 1, 53–79, 2012.

Jack Penn—became synonymous with social medicine. During the War, however, the National Health Services Commission was established under Henry Gluckman in 1942. The Commission sat for two years, eventually recommending the creation of a National Health Service to meet the health needs of the entire South African population, regardless of racial categorisation. While the recommendation was spurned by Jan Smuts, Shula Marks argues that the Commission report, while relatively circumspect, nevertheless stood in opposition to the segregationist ideals of the 1940s in its recommendation of universal basic health care.[71] The Gluckman Commission and the military segregation as implemented at Tara are thus an ideal illustration of the key tension in the history of medicine in the South African context: the easing of human suffering and the oppression of racial discrimination.

Extending beyond racial distinctions to that between soldier and civilian, the instructions at Tara were so unequivocal that the Red Cross—and Ernest Oppenheimer who served as the chairman of the Transvaal Branch—had to obtain special—albeit retroactive—permission when a seven-year-old girl with severe burns was admitted to the hospital, requiring extensive skin grafting. While Orenstein gave permission for the treatment of the patient, he made clear that the financial cost would fall solely on the Red Cross:

> ...it being understood, however, that no cost whatsoever to the public funds is to be incurred in connection with the treatment, i.e. that there be not capitation fee in respect of this patient, and that all drugs, dressings, etc., the property of the Union Government, will be paid for to your Society and credited against the accounts submitted to the Defence Department for the care of patients in the Plastic Hospital.[72]

The complicated relationship between the UDF and the Red Cross notwithstanding, Tara also provided the opportunity to draw attention to both the work of the Red Cross as well as the role of plastic surgery during the War. It served as the perfect fund-raising opportunity for the

[71] Shula Marks, "Reflections on the 1944 National Health Services Commission: A Response to Bill Freund and Anne Digby on the Gluckman Commission", *South African Historical Journal*, 66, 1, 169–187, 2014, p171.

[72] SA Red Cross Society (Transvaal Branch) to DGMS, 30 December 1944, and Orenstein response to Red Cross, 2 January 1945, Surgeon General, Group 2, Box 1136, File MD 580/2: Tara: Red Cross Hospital for Plastic Surgery—General, DOD.

organisation and Orenstein was again approached for permission to use Tara to make a "filmet" in collaboration with Penn. The storyboard put before the DGMS was as follows:

Action	*Voice*
1. Shot of burning plane on ground	The searing horror that is total war!
2. Shot of burning tank	Miraculous escapes are recorded—men dragged from burning wreckage without a scratch
3. Shot of casualties coming off hospital ship (stretcher cases)	But many thousands more are not so fortunate
4. Shot of patients at Hurlingham (with faces heavily bandaged)	Escaping with their lives but tragically disfigured
5. Shot of walking cases coming off troopship	These injuries would be a lifelong affliction
6. Operating theatre at Hurlingham during an operation	But for that miracle of modern medicine— plastic surgery
7. Long shot of Hurlingham, panning if possible to include hutments	This work is done in Johannesburg at the special Red Cross hospital, Hurlingham
8. Line of patients walking towards the camera with a view of Hurlingham in the background	Support this generously with your contributions so that these men may have a new start
9. Title. Send your donations to Red Cross, 77 De Villiers Street, Johannesburg (Drawn up with Red Cross badge as in Special "E")	In the free world for which they have fought

While Orenstein gave permission for images to be used of Tara, his response was characteristically judicious, pointing out that the word "thousands" at Shot 3 was an "exaggeration" and that "such" replace "this" in Shot 7 as Tara was not the sole site for plastic surgery in the country.[73]

Penn's first view of Tara "with its bedraggled out-buildings" had not inspired confidence but rather "an outsize migraine attack" and his autobiography offers far less detail about Tara than it does Brenthurst. Yet setting up Tara permitted Penn to initiate some of the design plans that he would later bring to fruition with his own clinic. Part of this

[73] Request by Red Cross to DGMS to make "Filmlet" in order to raise funds, focus on Hurlingham, 16 January 1945 and Reply from Orenstein to permission for film, 20 January 1945, Surgeon General, Group 2, Box 1136, File MD 580/2: Tara: Red Cross Hospital for Plastic Surgery—General, DOD.

stemmed from Tara's perceived shortcomings such as north-facing operating theatres when the contemporary trend was that they should be south-facing. In consultation with engineers and architects, Penn carried out several renovations and innovations including the installation of blinds in operating theatres. In his own clinic, he would later exclude windows altogether to prevent the influx of natural light that rendered artificial light less effective under operating conditions.[74] Tara also had a capacity more than three times that of Brenthurst.[75] At the same time, however, the War was nearing its end and Penn was able to move beyond war surgery. He continued to consult at Tara daily for which he was paid £40 a month and began his private practice, operating out of rooms that he rented in a nursing home.[76]

While Penn played less of a role in war-related reconstructive surgery, he nevertheless chafed under the military bureaucracy. The active role played by the Oppenheimers at Brenthurst as well as Brenthurst falling under the auspices of the Red Cross meant that Penn was, to some extent, shielded from the military hierarchy—yet their presence was keenly felt and often less than welcome. It was upon Penn's return from Britain and the establishment of the Brenthurst Hospital that he found himself subject to the full force of the military establishment. While the DGMS Edward Thornton was a notable exception, Penn was critical of the high-ranking officers, believing that they lacked sufficient understanding of medicine and only held their positions by virtue of "old age and seniority". This generation gap was reinforced by his view of these men as representing "conservative mediocrity" designed to clash with the young and confident "non-conformist".[77] In a book on his philosophical beliefs, *Reflections of Life*, published four decades later, Penn aired his views on evolution where "every now and then certain chromosomes spill over which are exceptions to the rule" and the result of these exceptions was either the "genius" or its opposite.[78] It was clear in which category Penn placed himself and he was unequivocal in his display of irritation towards

[74] Penn, *The Right to Look Human*, p95.

[75] "Red Cross Will Care for Soldiers Long After the War", *Rand Daily Mail*, 19 July 1944.

[76] Penn, *The Right to Look Human*, p96.

[77] Ibid., p74.

[78] Jack Penn, *Reflections on Life* (Johannesburg, Ernest Stanton Publishers, 1980), p33.

the military establishment that did not recognise this as well as similar personality types at Wits as well as the Medical Council "which should know that evolution depends on the chromosome that is different".[79] Unsurprisingly, Penn's perception of himself as a "non-conformist", his pioneering work in an unfamiliar medical field and the bureaucratic and hierarchical military establishment created conditions that were fraught. From the outset, Penn insisted on being in sole command of Brenthurst and met directly with the DGMS to be assured that he would have a free hand in running the hospital as he saw fit, regardless of his rank. He also requested—and was granted—direct access to the DGMS, bypassing the usual chain of command.[80] By March 1943, Penn's new commanding officer was Brigadier A.J. Orenstein who had served in the SAMC during the First World War and had been responsible for attempts to contain the influenza outbreak in 1919.[81] But Penn's reluctance to follow the chain of command remained and direct access to the DGMS was a condition he would repeat at the end of the War when asked to remain in the UDF as a consulting surgeon.

Penn's clash with the military bureaucracy continued while he was based at Tara. The hospital, with its large numbers of injured, particularly those with jaw and facial injuries, offered the perfect opportunity for training and Penn began offering courses for both surgeons and dentists. The first course was a "Mastership of Dental Surgery" and attracted dentists drawn from the greater Johannesburg area. Its success meant that Penn was eager to do the same for surgeons. First, however, he wanted to observe training institutions—both military and civilian—in the United States and also wanted to interact with practising plastic surgeons. Unsurprisingly for a man not enamoured with the chain of command and blessed with a strong sense of bravado, Penn went directly to Jan Smuts, the Commander in Chief of the UDF and Prime Minister of South Africa, to obtain permission.[82]

While Penn would later achieve some fame for his bust of Smuts that graced the Jan Smuts International Airport in Johannesburg—until

[79] Penn, *The Right to Look Human*, p75.

[80] Ibid.

[81] "New Posts for Brigadiers Orenstein and Thornton", *Rand Daily Mail*, 2 March 1943.

[82] Penn, *The Right to Look Human*, p98.

the renaming of the airport in the wake of the democratic transition in 1994—his impressions of Smuts were marked by a critical analysis of the General's physical and mental attributes. Smuts's personality was described as "electric", his voice as "surprisingly high-pitched", his demeanour "decisive and birdlike" and the overall impression "of a cultured man of high intelligence and courage, who knew his own mind and would brook no nonsense". Smuts also proved to be a tactful man—complimenting Penn on his work at Brenthurst but concluding that he would refer Penn's request to a colonel with whom Penn had already clashed. Penn had clearly made an enemy for life in the colonel who subsequently turned down his request. Undeterred and irrepressible, he would find his own way to the United States, bypassing the Union Defence Force entirely.[83]

An American Visit

Likely disappointed but unsurprised by Smuts's response, Penn met with Alexander Hood, the Director General of the RAMC who set the wheels in motion for his visit to the United States.[84] Behind the more distinctive features of the War—the firepower, offensives, military tactics, devastating defeats and larger-than-life heroes and villains—were the formidable logistical operations that underlay the provision of medical and surgical services. In 1938, while Prime Minister Neville Chamberlain professed that his meeting with Adolf Hitler would lead to "peace in our time", plans were already underfoot at the Royal College of Surgeons and the Surgical Travellers Club to prepare for war, including the creation of the Army Blood Transfusion Service. With the outbreak of war, medical developments such as penicillin were tested on wounded troops on the frontlines—as discussed in the previous chapter, this was also done at the surgical units in Britain. Prior to the invasion of Normandy in June 1944—the Allied offensive that would sound the death knell of Nazi ambitions—preparations were put in place for the evacuation of the wounded by their branches of service (both American and British), the provision of drinkable water and milk for troops as well as blood supplies and penicillin and the prospective handling of gangrene and tuberculosis.

[83] Ibid., pp98–99.

[84] Ibid., p99.

Medical personnel even determined the maximum amount of weight that individual troops could carry as they landed on the beaches of Normandy. Medical doctors allocated to the invasion numbered six thousand with additional tonnes of medical drugs and equipment. Overseeing this in Britain was General Hood who, for much of the war, met frequently with his officers to co-ordinate the medical side of the war effort.[85] Penn's approach to Hood was symptomatic of his unconventionality in bypassing regular channels and disdain for red tape—and it bore results.

Hood arranged for Penn's visit to the United States with his counterpart, Norman T. Kirk. In his capacity as Surgeon General, Kirk had been responsible for a dramatic overhauling and restructuring of the Army Medical Department and under his leadership, the mortality rate amongst troops had dropped dramatically from the First World War, even as military engagement in the second conflict was far more wide-ranging and occurred over different terrain. His medical policy was predicated on the greater use of civilians serving as consultants who would oversee military medical care as well as the standards of sanitation and hygiene designed to prevent the outbreak of illness. There was a restructuring of the various branches of medicine ranging from rehabilitation to surgery and even attention to the health and treatment within the women's auxiliary branches. The separate branches were given greater autonomy in advising on the requirements of their sections. With regards to surgery, a clear plan of action had been put in place—the initial treatment of the wound and measures taken to stabilise the patient close to the front lines, further treatment at general hospitals to reduce long-term effects of injury, and finally, corrective surgery such as plastic and reconstructive surgery if required. From 1944, there was a greater deployment of plastic and dental surgeons to frontline areas. The two were essential components of "maxillo-facial surgical teams", collaborating in treating facial injuries to minimise disfigurement as well as preserving tissue from the injured that could be used in their later treatment in plastic surgery hospitals.[86] Kirk had therefore demonstrated a progressive spirit in medicine,

[85] Cf. John Hedley-Whyte and Debra R. Milamed, "Surgical Travellers: Tapestry to Bayeux", *Ulster Medical Journal*, 83, 3, 171–177, 2014.

[86] Cf. Historical Division, Army Medical Library, "Developments in Military Medicine During the Administration of Surgeon General Norman T. Kirk", *Army Medical Bulletin*, 7, 7, July 1947, pp594–626, United States Army Academy of Health Sciences, Stimson Library Collections.

with an emphasis on organisation and an acknowledgement of the expertise of the specialists that fell under his ambit. He was thus warmly supportive of Penn's efforts.

Penn was feted by the military elite as he travelled through the country and demonstrated fond feelings towards them, highlighting their greater informality. In contrast to the devastation of war-torn Europe, the Americans were emerging from the War a military and economic powerhouse and Penn was allocated a staff car as an itinerary was drawn up scheduling his visits to various military hospitals. He was even offered a flight on a military plane, and he contrasted this ruefully with his experience in South Africa when he could only aspire to "[getting] a lift in a five-ton truck".[87]

Although Penn would travel throughout the United States, he was mainly based at the Valley Forge Hospital in Pennsylvania.[88] The medical history of Valley Forge and its association with war dated back to the late eighteenth century when George Washington's men were positioned in the area and the surrounding villages were used for the treatment and convalescence of injured soldiers.[89] Valley Forge's contemporary history began with the Second World War. The hospital was built during the War and accepted its first patients in 1943, one of the sixty-five Army General Hospitals operating in the United States. Capable of housing approximately three thousand patients, the hospital had a staffing component of more than half that was drawn from both the civilian and military spheres. It would remain in operation for a further three decades, overseeing the treatment of soldiers in the Korean and Vietnam Wars.[90]In May 1943, Valley Forge was one of the only two hospitals that was especially devoted to the treatment of soldiers blinded during the War with, as was Kirk's inclination, a strong component of rehabilitation involved in the treatment that would later be continued by other organisations once the patient had left the hospital.[91] By 1945, the hospital had become

[87] Penn, *The Right to Look Human*, pp99–100.

[88] Ibid., p103.

[89] Cf. Richard L. Blanco, "American Army Hospitals in Pennsylvania during the Revolutionary War", *Pennsylvania History: A Journal of Mid-Atlantic Studies*, 48, 4, 347–368, October 1981.

[90] "A Brief History of Valley Forge General Hospital, http://www.hspa-pa.org/History%20of%20Valley%20Forge%20Army%20Hospital.pdf, accessed 25 January 2021.

[91] Historical Division, Army Medical Library, "Developments in Military Medicine During the Administration of Surgeon General Norman T. Kirk", p634.

a major site for the development of prosthetic eyes under the guidance of dental surgeons Stanley Erpf, Milton Wirtz and Victor Dietz who had been assembled by Kirk. Pioneering the use of plastic due to its durability, the prosthetic eyes were designed to mimic as natural an appearance as possible and inserted into the socket to allow for normal movement.[92] In Penn's biography, however, he accredits Brenthurst with the first development of the plastic eye as early as 1941. Eye injuries amongst Allied troops were particularly evident during the early years of the War due in part to "booby traps" such as exploding fountain pens that were used to great effect by the Italians. The common treatment used in Britain was the insertion of a skin graft with a spherical gutta-percha mould that would remain in place for three months before an artificial eye could be inserted. This was, however, prone to inflammation and as Penn described it, "was mucky". Working with his dental technicians, he developed a new procedure called "The Gun Turret Operation" where an artificial mould was constructed out of plastic containing tubes through which fluid could be passed to cleanse the eye socket. The mould was covered with a skin graft. After just a week, the mould could then be removed and the artificial eye inserted. Although initially made of glass, wartime conditions meant that Brenthurst soon ran out of their imported supply of glass artificial eyes and there were no means in South Africa to make more. The solution was plastic, with the creation of artificial eyes painted by artists to resemble the real thing, complete with the use of silk thread to emulate blood vessels. In a dramatic demonstration of their efficacy and superiority to their glass counterparts, Penn tossed one at a wall. Once it had bounced around the room, the ignominious treatment was found to have had no effect.[93] Penn also adapted a technique from the United States, using dermal grafts to help flesh out the upper eyelid in order to give as natural an appearance as possible. As an homage to its inventors, he called it "The American Method". On his visit to Valley Forge, however, he served to introduce it to the hospital which had never employed it previously.[94]

[92] "Army Develops Superior Artificial Eyes", *Army Medical Bulletin*, Issue 86, March 1945, p12, United States Army Academy of Health Sciences, Stimson Library Collections.

[93] Penn, *The Right to Look Human*, pp88–89.

[94] Ibid., pp89–90.

During the War, nine general hospitals were involved in the very specialised field of hand surgery; Valley Forge would be one of the four remaining after 1945.[95] The hospital was therefore a significant site for the development of techniques in plastic and reconstructive surgery—a field that was coming into its own in the United States.

Penn's American trip was not happenstance. Just as the War had hastened the shift in the balance of power across the Atlantic, the same could be said for the development of plastic surgery. While modern plastic surgery had had its nascence in Britain, with the pioneering work of Harold Gillies and Thomas Kilner, their success in maintaining interest in the field was limited in the interwar period—despite both men and Gillies, in particular, working tirelessly to promote the specialisation. With an insufficient number of cases necessitating a focus on cosmetic surgery in this period as well as the obliviousness of the British public and medical profession, Gillies despaired that plastic surgery in Britain was being relegated to the "hospital scrap-basket".[96] The situation across the pond, however, was very different with expansion in the field and the United States had sixty fully-trained plastic surgeons to draw upon at the outbreak of the Second World War; Britain had four. The disparity may be explained counterintuitively by more stringent training requirements with prospective American surgeons having to undergo a further five years of surgical training after finishing medical school as well as the completion of fifty operations "under supervision". In contrast, British doctors could take up surgery as soon as they had completed their medical schooling. In addition, more stringent measures in the United States highlighted gaps in existing medical training, leading to the creation of "well-funded" training institutions that embraced new developments in surgery. Finally, cosmetic surgery—once safely in the hands of surgical professionals—did not bring with it the same sense of disdain that Gillies experienced in Britain.[97]

95 Historical Division, Army Medical Library, "Developments in Military Medicine during the Administration of Surgeon General Norman T. Kirk", p624.

96 James F. Fraser and Charles Scott Hultman, "America's Fertile Frontier: How America Surpassed Britain in the Development and Growth of Plastic Surgery During the Interwar Years of 1920–1940", *Annals of Plastic Surgery*, 64, 5, 610–613, May 2010, p611.

97 Ibid., pp610, 612.

As was the case in Britain and despite the greater number of full-time plastic surgeons at the outbreak of the War, the United States also had its own version of the "Big Four" —and Penn encountered all of them. The first was Robert Ivy, one of Kirk's "civilian consultants" who was born in England and had begun his career as a dentist before taking up plastic and reconstructive surgery and who, at the time of meeting Penn, was the Professor of Maxillo-facial and Oral Surgery at the University of Pennsylvania. Ivy was responsible for training officers in reconstructive surgery and Penn was also taken with the Ivy Plan. This entailed the provision of reconstructive surgery on children born with congenital defects in the hopes that it would prevent the ostracisation of a child with a facial deformity. Penn also attempted a similar plan in South Africa, with far less success, but it spoke to his belief in the importance of removing the stigma associated with facial deformity.[98]

During the First World War, Ivy had served as an assistant to Vilray Blair, a significant figure in the establishment of plastic surgery as a distinct field of specialisation. In 1897 Blair travelled to Britain to focus on surgery of the neck, head and mouth which, in 1912, led to the publication of a seminal work *Surgery and Diseases of the Mouth and Jaws*. This stood him in good stead with America's entry into the War in 1917 when he was tasked with leading Head and Neck Trauma—to which Ivy was also attached as his assistant. During the War, Blair went to Basingstoke to acquaint himself with the techniques pioneered by Gillies and dental surgeon, Major Kelsey-Fry. His return to the United States was marked by the creation of a multidisciplinary model for the treatment of facial and jaw injuries at the Walter Reed Hospital that would serve as an inspiration for similar models established elsewhere. Blair's espousal of collaboration inspired Ivy who developed his own pioneering American team focused on the treatment of the cleft palate and lip.[99] Also attached to Blair's

[98] Penn, *The Right to Look Human*, p101; Mansher Singh, R. Barrett Noone, Halimat Afolabi and Edward J. Caterson, "A Tribute to the Founding Figures of the American Board of Plastic Surgery", *Plastic and Reconstructive Surgery*, 135, 6, 1047–1054, June 2015, pp1049–1050.

[99] Cf. Eric J. Stelnicki, V. Leroy Young, Tom Francel and Peter Randall, "Vilray P. Blair, His Surgical Descendants, and Their Roles in Plastic Surgical Development", *Plastic and Reconstructive Surgery*, 103, 7, 1990–2009, June 1999.

team during the First World War was Armenian emigre, Varaztad Kazanjian, "the miracle man of the Western Front"[100] who despite the lack of verbal dexterity evident in his peers, was described by Penn as a figure of "tremendous charm" whose unconventional beginnings had resulted in both "tenacity and intelligence".[101] Arguably, Blair's greatest contribution to the field was in his role as a founder of the American Board of Plastic Surgery in late 1937. While Gillies struggled to gain recognition for the specialisation in Britain, Blair had worked to overcome the widely held perception of plastic surgery as the domain of "quacks" and "charlatans", figures with little or no qualification who operated on unwitting victims in "beauty shops" that had mushroomed across the United States. Before the establishment of the Board, Blair gave lectures across the United States, emphasising the need for an organisation that would ensure strict surgical standards and qualification criteria. He also persuaded the American Board of Surgery to recognise the specialisation. His efforts paid off when the American Board of Plastic Surgery was established with its motto "*Ad Formam, Functionem, Felicitatemque, Restituendam*", or "For restoring contour, function, and happiness", signifying the fundamental importance of a "normal" physical appearance to a fulfilled life.[102] The use of "happiness" is reminiscent of the founding document of the fledgling United States, the Declaration of Independence, with its right to "the pursuit of happiness". It would be echoed in Penn's civilian practice at the Brenthurst Clinic and the tapestry that proclaimed "It is the divine right of man to look human".

The final figure making up the "Big Four" and the "grand old man" of plastic surgery in the United States was John Staige Davis.[103] Born in January 1872, Staige Davis came from an illustrious line of medical practitioners—his grandfather was a Professor of Medicine at the University of Virginia and his father an Assistant Surgeon, first in the US Navy and then the Army. After graduating from Yale University, Staige Davis enrolled at the Johns Hopkins Medical School. Although the medical school had lecturers who were pioneers in their fields, their teaching left him uninspired, and he was contemptuous of their reliance on medical

[100] Cf. previous chapter.

[101] Penn, *The Right to Look Human*, p102.

[102] Singh et al., "A Tribute to the Founding Figures", pp1048–1049.

[103] Penn, *The Right to Look Human*, pp102–103.

research largely originating in Germany—seen as the centre of science. Specialising in surgery, Staige Davis developed a growing fascination with plastic surgery from as early as 1901 and with American entry into the First World War in 1917, the Surgeon General suggested that he would be the perfect candidate to teach medical officers the rudimentary aspects of plastic surgery at Johns Hopkins. However, the head of surgery at Johns Hopkins, William Halstead, had little interest in plastic surgery as a unique area of specialisation and vetoed the idea. Undeterred, Staige Davis produced one of the earliest texts on modern plastic surgery, *Plastic Surgery, Its Principles and Practice*, marking him out as a pioneer in the field. He would go on to write research papers on skin grafts—the "Davis grafts" —congenital defects, scarring and, ahead of his time, radiation burns. Even before the United States entered the Second World War, Staige Davis was already involved in organisations ensuring medical preparedness for the conflict and was a member of the Subcommittee on Plastic and Maxillo-Facial Surgery of the National Research Council. By 1946—the year of his death—he also served as president of the American Association of Plastic Surgeons.[104]

Staige Davis's career as a plastic surgeon echoed the frustrations felt by Gillies and later, Jack Penn. He was the first American to specialise wholly in the field of plastic surgery but received little recognition or support in the way of resources from his colleagues and supervisors at Johns Hopkins. Plastic surgery was initially seen as little other than an addendum to mainstream surgery, requiring skills that were not all that different. As a result, Staige Davis believed that there was insufficient development and innovation in the field, with a focus largely on maxillofacial surgery at the expense of limbs and the torso. His textbook was an attempt to highlight the specialised skills required of a plastic surgeon, making them an indispensable component of a surgical team. In contrast to Gillies, however, who had support from the RAMC and an exhaustive number of war wounded on which to base his research, Staige Davis was far more limited in what he was able to achieve.[105] He was nevertheless a pioneer in American plastic surgery—which swiftly caught up with its

[104] Cf. W. Bowdoin Davis, "The Life of John Staige Davis, M.D.", *Plastic and Reconstructive Surgery*, 62, 3, 368–378, September 1978.

[105] M. Felix Freshwater, "A Critical Comparison of Davis' *Principles of Plastic Surgery* with Gillies' *Plastic Surgery of the Face*", *Journal of Plastic, Reconstructive and Aesthetic Surgery*, 64, 17–26, 2011.

British counterpart—and saw his efforts reach fruition with the formation of the American Board of Plastic Surgery. It was the professionalisation of plastic surgery and its recognition as a distinct discipline that Penn would seek to emulate in South Africa.

The culmination of Penn's visit to North America was his attendance at the conference of the American Association of Plastic Surgeons held in Toronto, Canada on 3 June 1946 where he was more than gratified to be mentioned by Staige Davis in his presidential address in the same breath as Harold Gillies.[106] Staige Davis's speech was entitled "Plastic Surgery in World War I and in World War II". He detailed the birth of plastic surgery under Gillies during the First World War and its expansion in the Second, addressing its growth in the United States, emphasising the importance of plastic surgery, the need for collaboration across surgical specialisations and the path towards the recognition of the specialisation with the inaugural publication of the Association's journal, *Plastic and Reconstructive Surgery*. In his account of international developments in plastic surgery amongst the Allied countries—excepting the Soviet Union—Penn was given special mention for his contribution:

> In South Africa, Major Jack Penn and his staff have done fine military plastic surgery at 'Brenthurst' and later at the Witwatersrand University Hospital. Some of us have been fortunate in receiving 'Brenthurst Papers' edited by Major Penn.[107]

For the South African dealing with the perceived lack of support in his own country, it would have been an incredibly proud moment.

Penn both presented and wrote up his observations made in the United States during the War. Of note was the process of the professionalisation and specialisation of plastic surgery—which Penn would promote in South Africa. The certification of plastic surgeons in the United States was a rigorous process of years of training before an examination by the Board that was both practical and theoretical. It is only then that plastic surgeons were admitted to the Board of Plastic Surgeons. Penn highlighted the importance of the Board in ensuring that the highest

[106] Penn, *The Right to Look Human*, p102.

[107] John Staige Davis, "Plastic Surgery in World War I and in World War II", *Plastic and Reconstructive Surgery*, 1, 3, 255–264, November 1946.

standards were maintained in the surgical specialisation, instilling confidence in patients.[108] This spoke to Penn's beliefs regarding the specific requirements for the plastic surgeon that could be distinguished from the practice of surgery in general, including a willingness to be innovative and a strong sense of the aesthetic, combining both science and art.

Penn also saw the expansion of plastic surgery in the United States as a result of the wartime experiences of surgeons. In a similar structure to that in Britain, there were fourteen centres for plastic and reconstructive surgery distributed throughout the United States—nine attached to the Army and five to the Navy. With the diminishing need for these centres as the War drew to a close and the subsequent return of surgeons to civilian life, there would eventually be five permanent plastic surgical units.[109] Underlying Penn's description of the various reconstructive surgical procedures that were undertaken in the United States was both their similarity to those developed in the previous War as well as their advancement due to new technologies. Penn demonstrated differences in approach between American and British methods as well as differences in his own approach. In his discussion of jaw fractures, he pointed out the decreased use of extra-oral splintage due to the existing methods available, shortcomings that he hoped the Brenthurst clamp would address. Penn's report also addressed cosmetic surgery, particularly as carried out on women, such as face and breast lifts. He concluded with the importance of the American experience for South African surgeons who could adopt successful American techniques while avoiding the pitfalls. The key was the establishment of adequate teaching and training to ensure the highest "standards" of quality were maintained in the specialisation.[110]

With the end of the War in 1945, Penn was ready to resume his civilian practice but was persuaded by the Surgeon General to retain his military ties and remain as the Consultant Plastic Surgeon to the UDF. Initially hesitant due to his experiences with the chain of command during the War, he was promoted to the rank of Brigadier and guaranteed direct communication with the Surgeon General, thereby avoiding the bureaucratic red tape that he felt had hampered his efforts during the War—as

[108] Jack Penn, "Plastic Surgery in the USA", *S.A. Medical Journal*, 9 November 1946, p666.

[109] Ibid.

[110] Ibid., pp666–669.

well as allowing him to retain his sense of autonomy.[111] Despite continuing his military association, Penn's focus was now on civilian practice, but one that was based on his wartime experience.

[111] Jack Penn "A Surgeon's Story: It Is the Divine Right of Man to Look Human" (Unpublished manuscript), p205, Brn. No: 12057, 617.95 PEN, BL.

CHAPTER 6

The Post-war Years: Going Solo

Penn's time at Tara was characterised by a greatly reduced caseload. Sans the frenetic pace that had defined the early years at Brenthurst, he was able to devote more time to his academic and teaching roles at Wits as the "Oppenheimer Chair in Plastic, Maxillo-Facial and Oral Surgery" which was funded by Oppenheimer.[1] The latter donated £25,000 to expanding the floor space of the University's Dental and Oral Hospital to house the new department, with the state matching his donation. With space for 39 patients, the aim was to continue the work Penn had initiated at Brenthurst, treating injuries sustained in civilian accidents as well as congenital defects. Before construction began, two wards were set aside at the Hospital as the "Brenthurst section". With space for just six patients, it was funded by the Transvaal section of the Red Cross.[2]

Penn's six-year tenure at the Dental School was, however, marked by some tension due to strong and competing personalities. Disagreement over the disciplinary measures taken against a student added to a growing

[1] Jack Penn, *The Right to Look Human: An Autobiography* (Johannesburg, Hugh Keartland Publishers, 1976), p96.

[2] "Rand University to Have Chair of Plastic Surgery", *Rand Daily Mail*, 16 September 1944.

S. Chetty, *Reconstructive Surgery and Modernisation in Twentieth-Century South Africa*, Medicine and Biomedical Sciences in Modern History, https://doi.org/10.1007/978-3-031-38673-2_6

distance between Penn and the Dean of the Medical School, A.S. Strachan.[3] Archibald Sutherland Strachan was born in Glasgow, studying at the university there where he specialised in pathology. He came to South Africa in 1919, joining the Department of Pathology and Bacteriology before starting at Wits in 1943 where he was appointed Dean a year later—when the new plastic surgery unit was created. Held in some esteem in medical departments for his teaching skills as well as his expertise in silicosis—a lung disease that took a toll on the miners on the Witwatersrand—the middle-aged Strachan was at the height of his career in 1944.[4] Penn was already clearly a headstrong and independent figure with strong views and felt his authority increasingly undermined. This came to a head when he was not consulted in the establishment of a department specifically dedicated to plastic surgery and facial and jaw injuries. To add insult to injury, his assistant was asked to join this new department. While Penn did not challenge the decision, he clearly felt marginalised in the "unhealthy atmosphere just short of animosity".[5]

Another factor that possibly contributed to his disenchantment with the teaching position at Wits was that his appointment was in the Dental rather than Medical faculty, meaning that he had little access to surgical students. He was also influenced by the American teaching model that permitted training in private hospitals and not just state or tertiary institutions. Any training that took place at his private practice was however not acknowledged by the South African Medical and Dental Council.[6]

Penn believed that he had a great deal to offer as both teacher and researcher but what he described as the "bogged-down conservatism" of the Department contributed to him eventually resigning from the University. With hindsight, he would have wanted to remain had he known that the tenure of the individuals with whom he most clashed would be relatively short-lived. And he regretted the lost opportunities for training new generations of plastic surgeons.[7] Upon his decision to

[3] Penn, *The Right to Look Human*, pp106–107.

[4] Cedric Bremner and Rochelle Keene, "Archibald Sutherland Strachan (23 November 1891, Glasgow–20 February 1949, Johannesburg)", *Pioneers in African Occupational Health*, 26, 2, March/April 2020, p96.

[5] Penn, *The Right to Look Human*, p107.

[6] Warwick Morris, "The Plastic Surgeons of Southern Africa and the History of APRASSA", APRASSA, p5.

[7] Penn, *The Right to Look Human*, pp107–108.

resign from Wits in 1950, the Oppenheimers withdrew the £30,000 grant used to fund the Oppenheimer Chair in Plastic, Maxillo-Facial and Oral Surgery[8]—indicative of their strong support for him.

Acknowledging that his temperament prevented him from tolerating the "group relationships" that he had experienced in the military and at Wits, Penn was now ready to express his individualism with his own clinic.[9]

The Civilian Brenthurst Clinic/s

Jack Penn had been stationed in England in 1940, acquiring the skills and expertise necessary to set up the Brenthurst Hospital. This was during the Blitz when Britain faced nightly bombing raids over eight months from 1940 until 1941 that took a significant toll on London—and other metropolitan areas. Unwilling to join those taking refuge in the bomb shelters, Penn walked the city, and it was on one of these occasions where looking at a vast empty tract of land along the Thames, he envisioned a "Medical City" that would be an amalgamation of his various experiences in Britain and the United States. It would be an international centre of learning and treatment, the professional home of specialists in their fields and a beacon of modern medicine that stood in stark contrast to the elitism of "the crummy waiting rooms and 'antique' examination rooms of Harley and Wimpole Streets".[10] He would attempt to implement this vision over the course of his career, making overtures to various philanthropists and advocating its construction in places as distant from London as Israel and Iran, yet it did not come to fruition. Penn would, however, create on a less ambitious scale his own clinic in Johannesburg.

While plastic surgery had its origins in war, these developments were adapted and applied to the civilian sphere. In turn, the civilian practice of plastic surgery added a further level of refinement. The focus of the injuries shifted in civilian practice. There were congenital defects such as the cleft lip and palate as well as deformities due to illness such as mastectomies used to treat breast cancer. A further component

[8] Rochelle Keene, "Our Graduates: 1924–2012" (Johannesburg, Faculty of Health Sciences, University of the Witwatersrand, 2013), p10.

[9] Penn, *The Right to Look Human*, p108.

[10] Ibid., p72.

of civilian plastic surgery was its cosmetic aspect. There is, of course, an aesthetic element incorporated within plastic surgery evident in the artistic sensibilities of surgeons ranging from Gillies to Penn yet, now, elective surgeries were emphasised—ear tucks, facelifts, breast lifts and reductions. Penn, however, in 1940 was less than enamoured with the facelift procedure, which he believed to affect adversely a natural expression and, moreover, its effects were temporary. Aimed largely at women, he acknowledged its needs, however, for those whose professional lives were linked to their aesthetic appeal such as actresses.[11] In Penn's civilian practice therefore—begun before the Second World War but the subject of his focus in its aftermath—there was a significant change in emphasis in the specialisation.

Permitted to use the name by the Oppenheimers, the first civilian Brenthurst Clinic occupied three storeys in a building in Hillbrow and from the outset, reflected Penn's individualism, his desire for control and the lessons learnt from working within the military establishment as well as Wits:

> ...a clinic of my own, where I could teach and do research, limited though it may be, with my own staff trained by me, where the standard would be as high as I could make it, and where our future would depend entirely on good quality and integrity, and not on the whims and ambitions of other people.[12]

Today, an area in central Johannesburg that has acquired notoriety for high levels of crime and is emblematic of social ills such as poverty, unemployment and vice, Hillbrow had initially been envisaged as the "healthiest and most fashionable residential suburb" in the late nineteenth century, distant from the urban sprawl that characterised the rapid growth of Johannesburg in the wake of the mineral revolution. Contemporary ideas of health and the "importance of clean air" also influenced its location as a suitable site for early medical facilities such as the first hospital in the city in 1889 and within a decade, the first operating theatre. From the 1920s and, particularly after the Second World War, the area was marked by the erection of skyscrapers that served as apartment housing

[11] Jack Penn, "Aspects of Civilian Plastic Surgery", *South African Medical Journal*, 335–338, 14 September 1940.

[12] Penn, *The Right to Look Human*, p108.

and office space.[13] Penn rented space at the top of one of these newly erected edifices to house the Brenthurst Clinic.[14]

It was a prime location. Hillbrow became the focus of an expanding medical complex that included the adjacent "Hospital Hill", the site of a hospital for "non-Europeans", a training college for nurses, the Transvaal Memorial Hospital, the Queen Victoria Maternity Hospital and the Florence Nightingale Hospital. Further private and public medical practices were established, including the Rand Clinic, the Parklane Clinic and Penn's Brenthurst Clinic.[15] Penn occupied the site for the next six years with his clinic comprised two operating theatres, a capacity of thirty beds and a research laboratory.[16] The initial staff was modest—in addition to Penn, there was Dorothy Gallagher who served as his secretary and did the accounts, Audrey Benedict, the matron who worked alongside Penn in Israel, as did Marie Roux, the theatre nurse. The modest staff notwithstanding, the Brenthurst Clinic offered Penn the opportunity to forge his own path in medicine as a "lone rider".[17]

Civilian plastic surgery involved both cosmetic surgery as well as the removal of scars resulting from trauma ranging from mild scarification to deformity due to car accidents or burns. A relatively minor but problematic form of scarring was the common "cross-hatch" scar that was exacerbated by the initial method of suturing the wound and the length of time the stitches remained in place. Penn's solution was the use of "diamond-shaped" incisions to remove the scar and the resulting edges were made to fit together. This decreased the tension due to lateral incisions and the subsequent scarring arising from them.[18]

For severe burns, Penn advocated the "simple" solution proposed by a Belgian doctor which the former thought particularly suited to the South African context, especially in areas distant from the major metropolitan areas that lacked a burns unit. In this scenario, the burnt tissue was

[13] Jonathan Stadler and Charles Dugmore, "'Honey, Milk and Bile': A Social History of Hillbrow", *BMC Public Health*, 17, (Suppl 3), 444, 9–15, 2017, p9.

[14] Penn, *The Right to Look Human*, p108.

[15] Stadler and Dugmore, "'Honey, Milk and Bile'", p9.

[16] Penn, *The Right to Look Human*, p109.

[17] Ibid., p110.

[18] Jack Penn, "The Removal of 'Cross-Hatch' Scars", *Plastic and Reconstructive Surgery*, 25, 1, 73–76, January 1960.

"brushed" off the body, the patient was placed in an oxygen chamber and no dressings were used. This permitted an improvement in the monitoring of fluid intake—as loss of fluid and its associations with dehydration, shock and infection were an omnipresent concern in the case of serious injury. The grafting of skin to cover the burned areas could then be undertaken sooner than was the case with conventional burn treatments that made use of dressings.[19]

And decades after the First World War, its presence was still felt when a former lieutenant-colonel, wounded in the face in 1917 by shell fragments, was first treated by Penn in 1951. Part of the fragment had remained lodged in his face, between the nose and left eye and he was subject to rodent ulcers and carcinomas, the last forming over the shrapnel fragment and likely exacerbated by the South African climate. The major surgery required to remove the tumours and the fragment as well as procedures to rectify the resultant scarring was successful, with no resurgence of the carcinoma.[20]

Penn felt strongly about cases involving congenital defects in children—the cleft lip and palate—that led to the stigmatisation of such children and could result in delinquency. Rudimentary treatment provided to these children often exacerbated the problem, especially when families were unable to afford the "expert" treatment required. Drawing upon the Ivy Plan in the United States, where the government paid for such surgeries, Penn advocated the same in South Africa as a "humanitarian act" on the part of the state and one that would result in the creation of a "useful citizen" if provision was made for the surgery as well as the speech therapy and other forms of post-surgical rehabilitation.[21] As a private practitioner, he also initiated the Brenthurst Clinic Trust Fund that provided financial means to carry out these life-changing operations.[22]

Penn was also involved in cosmetic surgery that emphasised the aesthetic appearance of the patient such as the pinning back of protruding ears to reduce "embarrassment", to reconstructive nasal surgery where he

[19] Jack Penn, "Advances in Plastic and Reconstructive Surgery", *S.A. Medical Journal*, 259–263, 26 March 1966.

[20] Jack Penn and Edward Epstein, "Notes on a Case of Carcinoma Following Shell-Wound of the Face", *Plastic and Reconstructive Surgery*, 12, 2, 148–151, August 1953.

[21] Penn, "Advances in Plastic and Reconstructive Surgery", pp261–262.

[22] "Profile: Jack Penn", *S.A. Practice Management*, 9, 3, 1988, File: Biography—Jack Penn, AMUW.

advocated the deft touch of the artist in creating a nose that was perfectly proportioned to facial shape. There was also his view of "Women's breasts [which] are like army uniforms—with certain exceptions they are either too large or too small". At the time of his writing, advances had been made to reduce the dangers associated with breast reduction surgery while breast enhancement was still in development. Both were necessary for the psychological desire of the patient to have a "normal" appearance. Finally, there was the facelift to reduce the effect of ageing when appearance could potentially disadvantage people "if they are to compete in the world of economics".[23]

As a site for plastic and reconstructive surgery, the Brenthurst Clinic soon became prominent in sub-Saharan Africa and Penn was also called on to perform surgeries beyond the country's borders in present-day Zimbabwe as well as Mozambique. He would later venture even further afield to the Belgian Congo.[24] And within the confines of the Clinic itself, Penn engaged in research.

One research project was the use of hypnosis to alleviate pain without the need for anaesthetic. Penn had already proved keen on adopting new methods of anaesthetic collaborating closely with his anaesthetist, Speedy Bental. Hypnosis, however, presented a new prospect. During his early days as a doctor at the Children's Hospital in Johannesburg, he discovered that injured children (particularly those with broken bones) responded well to him speaking to them and "massaging" the afflicted site. Their responses were physiological—the "relaxation" of the muscles that allowed him to set the bone, often without "full anaesthesia". He later discovered that this was "a form of hypnotic suggestion".[25] The placebo effect is a significant one in medical research and hypnosis—as unconventional as it may seem in a field that relies heavily on pharmaceutical interventions—is another means of harnessing the power of suggestion. Archie McIndoe had also investigated the potential of the technique at East Grinstead in the 1950s. As Vice-President of the Dental and Medical Society for the Study of Hypnosis, he permitted the demonstration of the removal of a mole from the face of a patient without the use of anaesthesia, showing the efficacy of hypnosis to a contingent of

[23] Jack Penn, "Plastic Surgery in Perspective", *The Lancet*, 774–775, 13 October 1962.

[24] Penn, *The Right to Look Human*, p110.

[25] Ibid., p48.

foreign doctors who had assembled for an anaesthesiology conference. McIndoe did not, however, employ the technique in his own surgeries.[26]

With his research partner, Theodore Gillman, Penn desired to trace the healing process of an "incised wound" i.e., one caused by surgery, observing the changes microscopically. This necessitated the taking of daily samples from the wound for 36 days. The dilemmas faced by the researchers were the discomfort to the volunteer and the possibility that daily doses of anaesthetic would affect the findings. Penn turned to hypnotic suggestion as a solution and Marie Roux volunteered for the procedure. The hypnotic suggestion was that her "abdominal wall would be numb until such time as [Penn] restored normal sensation". Penn then made an incision across her abdomen that was about 25 centimetres in length and proceeded to suture it. Each day—with her active involvement throughout the process—he obtained a biopsy of the wound. Once this phase was complete, he removed the scar entirely. The total experiment lasted six weeks. At no point was anaesthetic used. When the post-hypnotic suggestion was removed, Roux immediately felt pain as the wound had not yet completely healed. Another week of post-hypnotic suggestion to numb the area was implemented with great success.[27]

Penn's use of hypnotic suggestion suggested his willingness to consider alternative forms of therapy. The use of hypnosis was not new to the surgical profession—it had been used in the nineteenth century with some success. However, with the advent of anaesthetic and the increasing use of chloroform, it was marginalised as a viable form of pain management from the mid-nineteenth century. Yet, a century later, as Penn was carrying out his experiment, its potential efficacy was flagged by the British Medical Association and three years later in 1958, by the American Medical Association.[28] Two decades later, David Scott highlighted the dearth of publications on the use of hypnosis in plastic surgery while simultaneously, promoting its use in plastic and reconstructive surgery. It could be especially useful for pedicle grafts, some of which required placing patients in awkward positions for lengthy periods. Hypnosis could

[26] Hugh McLeave, *McIndoe: Plastic Surgeon* (London, Frederick Muller Limited, 1961), p168.

[27] Penn, *The Right to Look Human*, p111.

[28] Albrecht W.K. Wobst, "Hypnosis and Surgery: Past, Present and Future", *Anesthesia and Analgesia*, (International Anesthesia Research Society) 104, 5, 1199–1208, May 2007, pp1199–1200.

also reduce the anxiety levels of patients. The process by which a person is hypnotised and made amenable to the power of suggestion can be considered the means by which the patient comes to place implicit trust in the surgeon:

> The induction of hypnosis should be considered as a learning process, in which the doctor/patient relationship is replaced by a teacher/pupil relationship. It usually involves a series of predictions by the therapist; as each proves true, the subject places more and more weight on what the therapist is saying. Finally, as hypnosis deepens and the critical faculty of the conscious mind had become suppressed and the subconscious mind has come to the surface, he accepts without query what is being said.[29]

And as Penn observed decades previously, research had also demonstrated the use of hypnosis in children as a form of pain management, with children particularly acquiescent to the power of suggestion. The role of hypnosis in pain management also stems from a more in-depth understanding of the concept of "pain" that addresses not just the physical sensation, but the sense of "threat" and the "negative emotions" associated with it.[30] Penn's research here is an early foray into an area that has been given increasing credence in pain management. It demonstrates his eagerness to consider new methods as soon as they were available. His research ambitions were also a source of frustration—as an individual, he had greater autonomy in pursuing new avenues of research but he also had less access to the funding available to larger and more established research institutions.

Penn's patron Ernest Oppenheimer initially provided funding for Theodore Gillman and this was later supplemented by real estate tycoon, John Schlesinger, who funded Gillman for another five years until Gillman left for England.[31] Like Penn, Gillman was a graduate of Wits where he was a member of the Department of Anatomy; his brother, Joseph Gillman was the chair of the Department of Physiology, an expert on childhood nutrition who would establish a "Medical Research

[29] David L. Scott, "Hypnosis in Pedicle Graft Surgery", *British Journal of Plastic Surgery*, 29, 8–13, 1976, pp8–9.

[30] Chantal Wood and Antoine Bioy, "Hypnosis and Pain in Children", *Journal of Pain and Symptom Management*, 35, 4, 437–446, April 2008, pp437–439.

[31] Penn, *The Right to Look Human*, pp110–111.

Unit" in Ghana.[32] Joseph was a contemporary of Raymond Dart and Robert Broom and both brothers had undertaken research with later Nobel Prize-winning biologist Sydney Brenner, publishing three papers together.[33] Joseph also served as mentor to leading palaeoanthropologist, Phillip Tobias.

Theodore, then, was part of an intellectual world with which Penn was well acquainted. He was younger than Penn, graduating with his Bachelor of Medicine degree from Wits in 1941 and his doctorate in 1958. As a researcher, he and his brother had focused on human pathology, addressing disease and malnutrition. He is also accredited with the invention of the "Gillman needle", used in liver biopsy. On a personal level, he was an avid lover of art and a sculptor in his own right which undoubtedly gave him much in common with Penn.[34]

At Brenthurst, the two men worked together on a number of research projects: "the nature of skin grafts, cross transplantation, the effect of the ageing of skin on cancer formation, and the physiology of wound healing"—the latter with Marie Roux's participation.[35] Of interest to Penn was the effects of the sun on South Africans of European descent that often led to skin cancer. As Penn treated a significant number of these cases, he was able to obtain samples for Gillman to study. Another group investigated were lepers—cured of the disease but with facial deformity requiring Penn's intervention. The skin samples obtained by Penn demonstrated—to the surprise of both men—"that the skin of lepers was astonishingly youthful", and this applied to those who were more advanced in age as well.[36] They presented their findings at a conference in Rome in April 1956. The paper addressed the stigmatisation and loss of confidence on the part of people who had suffered the facial deformities associated with Hansen's disease, even after being cured. It highlighted the most common deformities, all of which could be addressed via plastic

[32] "Famous Medical Alumni", https://www.wits.ac.za/media/wits-university/alumni..., accessed 15 April 2021.

[33] "Citation delivered by Deputy Vice-Chancellor, Professor S.P. Jackson, on the Occasion of the Conferment of the Degree of Doctor of Science, Honoris Causa, on Sydney Brenner", https://www.wits.ac.za/media/wits-university/alumni/documents/honorary-degree-citations, accessed 15 April 2021.

[34] "Obituary: Theodore Gillman", *The Lancet*, 271–272, 31 July 1971.

[35] Penn, *The Right to Look Human*, p111.

[36] Ibid., p112.

and reconstructive surgery via the use of pedicle grafts obtained from the forehead and arm as well as the use of skin grafts. Also discussed was the "youthful" skin of patients which was "thinner" than that usually found in adults without the disease and was described as "foetal or infant-like skin" with corresponding "foetal-like hair follicles". They believed that their experience of the treatment of leprosy sufferers should be brought to the attention of the World Health Organisation (WHO) as well as to nations particularly afflicted with the disease with the aim of providing standardised care and surgical treatment.[37]

Another paper related to the use of closing wounds. Although acknowledging that their study did not deal with wounds that were necessarily as deep as many surgical incisions, they were able to conclude that the use of tape to seal wounds was advantageous when compared to suturing, leading to less scarring and infection.[38] A more detailed analysis of the process of healing and scarification in relation to different types of skin grafts was also made and published in an extensive article in the *British Journal of Plastic Surgery*.[39]

Penn's work with Gillman lasted for seven years—the first two spent at the Clinic. In 1951, Gillman was appointed to a professorship in physiology at the University of Natal and was attached to the King Edward VIII Hospital in Durban, continuing his research into the healing process of wounds.[40] Despite the distance, their collaboration continued, especially after Penn temporarily served as a Consultant in Plastic Surgery at Addington Hospital, Durban worked with Gillman in his laboratory at the university.[41] Rabbits were used in this study and had pieces of skin and underlying tissue removed under anaesthesia with various forms of dressings applied to test the rate of healing as well as infection. The conclusion

[37] Summary of J. Penn and T. Gillman, "Plastic Surgery in the Service of the Leper with Some Comments on the Clinical and Microscopic Features of the Skin of 'Healed' Lepers", Presented at *Congresso Internazionale per la Difesa e la Rehabilitazione Sociale del "Lebbroso"*, Rome, April 1956, *Plastic and Reconstructive Surgery*, 18, 6, December 1956, pp495–496.

[38] Theodore Gillman, Jack Penn, Doris Bronks and Marie Roux, "Closure of Wounds and Incisions with Adhesive Tape", *The Lancet*, 945–946, 5 November 1955.

[39] Theodore Gillman, Jack Penn, Doris Bronks and Marie Roux, "Reactions of Healing Wounds and Granulation Tissue in Man to Auto-Thiersch, Autodermal, and Homodermal Grafts", *British Journal of Plastic Surgery*, 6, 153–223, 1953–1954.

[40] "Obituary: Theodore Gillman", pp271–272.

[41] Penn, *The Right to Look Human*, p112.

was that plastic dressings were efficacious in the immediate treatment of injury such as burns without any recourse to homografts (skin grafts provided by a donor).[42] This productive research collaboration came to an end in 1960 when Gillman left South Africa permanently, settling in Britain and serving as the head of the department of experimental pathology at the Agricultural Research Council Institute of Animal Physiology at Cambridge. Part of the motivation for his emigration was his disillusionment with the increasingly repressive climate of apartheid South Africa and his belief that "it was not possible to work in an environment in which he could no longer contribute to the alleviation of suffering".[43] The last was not mentioned by Penn in his autobiography although he emphasised the value of Gillman as a research partner, acknowledging that it was unlikely that he would again experience such a fruitful research relationship.[44]

The clinic gained a special place in the history of plastic surgery in South Africa when it became the site of the formation of the Association of Plastic Surgeons of Southern Africa in 1956, now known as the Association of Plastic, Reconstructive and Aesthetic Surgeons of Southern Africa (APRASSA).[45] Early in his career, Penn had attempted to draw attention to plastic surgery and its important role, appearing on radio to publicise the work of the Brenthurst Military Hospital during the War.[46] The Association, however, symbolised recognition for the specialisation as a distinct field. As plastic surgery was a relatively new field in the country, the initial group forming the Association consisted of Penn and five other surgeons. He served as the first president and Dennis Walker as the Honorary Secretary and Treasurer. James Cuthbert drew up the Association's constitution, having also had the experience of being present at

[42] Theodore Gillman, Michael Hathorne and Jack Penn, "Is Skin Homografting Necessary?: A Re-examination for the Rationale for Auto- or Homo-Grafting of Cutaneous Injuries and a Preliminary Report on the Action of Plastic Dressings", *Plastic and Reconstructive Surgery*, 18, 4, 260–274, October 1956.

[43] "Obituary: Theodore Gillman", pp271–272.

[44] Penn, *The Right to Look Human*, p112.

[45] Chris Snijman, "The History and Development of Our Society", http://www.drsnijman.co.za/association-plastic-reconstructive-aesthetic-surgeons-southern-africa/, accessed 20 April 2021; "History", *APRASSA*, https://aprassa.co.za/history/, accessed 20 April 2021; "Discipline of Plastic Surgery: More About Plastic Surgery", University of KwaZulu-Natal, https://plasticsurg.ukzn.ac.za/aboutus/, accessed 20 April 2021.

[46] "Broadcasting Programmes", *Rand Daily Mail*, 19 April 1943.

the formation of the British Association for Plastic Surgeons a decade earlier. The other three plastic surgeons who made up the cohort were Norman Petersen and David S. Davies from Groote Schuur Hospital in Cape Town and B.W. Franklin Bishop of Wentworth Hospital and the University of Natal.[47]

The only member unable to attend the initial meeting was Norman Petersen—about whom very little is known. Petersen, however, was one of the two plastic surgeons sent to England during the War—the other being Jack Penn. He studied at the University of London, graduating with his Bachelor's Degree, in 1920, and three years later was made a fellow of the Royal College of Surgeons in Scotland and England respectively.[48] During the Second World War he was based in Durban at the Springfield Military Hospital before moving to Groote Schuur in Cape Town—and was thus a contemporary of David Davies. The latter had spent sixteen years working as a plastic surgeon in Iran and, upon the end of the War, returned to South Africa. Cuthbert, also a graduate from the University of London, was specialising in Orthopaedics at Edinburgh University when the War broke out and subsequently found himself working under Gillies where he remained for the duration. He applied his skills for a brief period in Yugoslavia before returning to South Africa and was based in Johannesburg. His student was Dennis Walker who had only been registered as a plastic surgeon for two years before the formation of the Association.[49]

Franklin Bishop had briefly studied under one of the "Big Four", Thomas Pomfret Kilner earlier in the decade, becoming the first plastic surgeon in Natal in 1953. While he served the various hospitals in the province, he was based at Wentworth Hospital with the unit there set up for white patients. It was at Wentworth Hospital that he organised the first meeting of plastic surgeons a year after the formation of the Association in 1957. A guest of honour was Pomfret Kilner who, on behalf

[47] Snijman, "The History and Development of Our Society"; "History", *APRASSA*; "Discipline of Plastic Surgery: More About Plastic Surgery".

[48] "Petersen, Norman August Marais", *Plarr's Lives of the Fellows*, Royal College of Surgeons of England, https://livesonline.rcseng.ac.uk/client/en_GB/lives/search/detailnonmodal?qu=LIVES_OCCUPATION%3D%22Maxillofacial+surgeon%22&qf=LIVES_HONOURS%09Titles%2FQualifications%09MRCS+1920%09MRCS+1920&d=ent%3A%2F%2FSD_ASSET%2F0%2FSD_ASSET%3A378202~~0&ic=true, accessed 6 May 2021.

[49] Morris, "The Plastic Surgeons of Southern Africa", p2.

of the British Association of Plastic Surgeons, gifted the new Association with a gavel crafted in silver and ebony.[50]

The Association underwent a number of name changes that reflected the changing name of the specialisation from "Plastic Surgery" to "Plastic and Reconstructive Surgery" with the latest incarnation occurring in 2016. The "Southern Africa" in the title reflected the hopes of the members that it would serve as a parent organisation for plastic surgeons beyond the borders of South Africa. The later requirement by the Medical Association that members belong to its body as well, made this a challenge and only one "Southern African" joined the organisation. This was Bertram Owen-Smith, a member of McIndoe's Guinea Pig Club. Owen-Smith, a bomber pilot, was burned when his Whitby bomber crashed during a training exercise and caught fire. Two of the other three crew members were also burned and treated at East Grinstead.[51] Owen-Smith underwent two years of treatment and numerous operations and, a clerk before the War, was subsequently inspired to become a plastic surgeon, qualifying under McIndoe's tutelage before moving to present-day Zimbabwe.[52]

In 1962, with a membership that had grown to ten surgeons, the Association applied to the Medical Association for formal recognition which was subsequently awarded, setting the scene for the expansion of plastic surgery in the country.[53] In this way, Penn was able to initiate the formalisation of the specialisation, following in the footsteps of his British and American counterparts. Today, APRASSA still bears a reminder of its beginnings at Brenthurst. Its logo is that of the mythological phoenix rising from the flames—the symbol chosen by Penn for Brenthurst and, later, for the Association as a reminder of the origins

[50] Snijman, "The History and Development of Our Society".

[51] Chris Webber, "Son's Emotional Journey to Site Where "Hero" RAF Father Crashed in the Second World War", *The Northern Echo*, 20 July 2015, https://www.thenorthernecho.co.uk/news/13464833.sons-emotional-journey-site-hero-raf-father-crashed-second-world-war/, accessed 6 May 2021.

[52] Morris, "The Plastic Surgeons of Southern Africa", p3; Emily Mayhew, *Guinea Pig Club: Archibald McIndoe and the RAF in World War II* (Barnsley, Greenhill Books, 2018), p197.

[53] Snijman, "The History and Development of Our Society".

of plastic surgery in the flames of war.[54] An international connection was made in 1967 in Rome when Penn became part of the Executive Council of the International Confederation of Plastic and Reconstructive Surgeons, an organisation that included representatives from the United States, Europe, South America and New Zealand.[55] The Confederation was established in Sweden in 1955 to foster a sense of engagement and exchange of knowledge between plastic surgeons based all over the world and held meetings every four years. Its membership consisted of one delegate representing each member nation and the executive committee was made up of delegates of various regions, with Penn representing Africa.[56]

Other changes were on the cards for Penn. In 1956, his lease in Hillbrow was up for renewal and the new rental fee was prohibitive, so much so that Penn felt it was no longer financially viable to maintain the clinic there. By 1957, plans were drawn up for the construction of a new Brenthurst Clinic at Clarendon Place in Parktown, a suburb close to Hillbrow and just north of the city centre. While Penn was able to purchase the acre of land on which to build the clinic, his new project was more ambitious than the last and he needed financial assistance—and turned again to John Schlesinger.[57]

Schlesinger had inherited an empire from his father, Isidore William Schlesinger, at the relatively youthful age of 26. The elder Schlesinger—born in New York—arrived in South Africa at the end of the nineteenth century and took to selling life insurance, travelling through the country in a horse-drawn buggy. His success enabled him to turn his hand to real estate with a focus on cinemas and then hotels.[58] With his introduction to Johannesburg contextualised by the city's growing urbanisation and in the middle of the heyday of the goldmining industry, Isidore had a vision of the modernisation of Johannesburg that he sought to implement:

[54] "History of APRASSA", https://aprassa.co.za/history-of-the-association.php#, accessed 3 May 2021.

[55] *South African Medical Journal*, 16 December 1967, p1203.

[56] "International Confederation for Plastic, Reconstructive and Aesthetic Surgery (IPRAS)", *Yearbook of International Organizations Online*, https://uia.org/s/or/en/1100065003, accessed 24 May 2021.

[57] Penn, *The Right to Look Human*, p113.

[58] "South Africa: His Father's Son", *Time Magazine*, 2 August 1963, http://www.time.com/time/magazine/article/0,9171,870366,00.html, accessed 15 April 2021.

> Schlesinger became the engine for Americanisation and modernisation in Johannesburg—and ... in the 1920s and 1930s the two terms were largely interchangeable. He was a man, people were fond of remarking, who "made things hum". He was at his office at daybreak in order, as he said, to "make the world go round".[59]

Upon his death, Harvard-educated John Schlesinger inherited an empire worth 84 million dollars and proceeded to expand it. His attention was largely on the development of modern high-rise buildings in South Africa's urban centres. Like his father before him, Schlesinger clearly saw the importance of development and modernisation. His political philosophy, to some extent, mirrored that of Jack Penn, which focused on the importance of white agency in facilitating modernisation:

> There will have to be changes here...The government's policy of separate development is not the answer. South Africa must eventually become multiracial, but in the first instance whites will have to play the dominant role.[60]

Schlesinger's observation was little different to Albert Schweitzer's notion of the "younger brother"—as discussed later. Both relate to "trusteeship". With its origins in the colonial period and the "civilising mission", trusteeship was used "to legitimate rule of the *capable* on behalf of the *uncapable*" and was associated with a paternalism that rendered those under colonial rule infantile, requiring the guiding hand of whites to eventually ready them for "civilisation" and self-determination. Associated with liberalism, Allsobrook and Boisen argue that in the South African context, its link with eventual integration was subsequently used to reinforce segregation that would culminate in the system of Bantustans or "independent" homelands under apartheid.[61]This notion of trusteeship would be expressed in Penn's political views and work on the President's Council—addressed in the final section. In South Africa in the

[59] "Schlesinger, Izidore Williem: Business Magnate and Property Mogul", *Artefacts.co.za*, https://www.artefacts.co.za/main/Buildings/archframes.php?archid=6355, accessed 16 April 2021.

[60] Quote attributed to Schlesinger in "South Africa: His Father's Son".

[61] Christopher Allsobrook and Camilla Boisen, "Two Types of Trusteeship in South Africa: From Subjugation to Separate Development", *Politikon*, 44, 2, 265–285, 2017, pp265–267.

mid-nineteenth century, colonial administrators took as self-evident the superiority of British ideas of property, law, education and medicine. The justification for colonial rule then was not the blatant economic exploitation of indigenous peoples but the imposition of British "civilisation" with the aim of eventually incorporating these people into white society. As the mineral revolution in South Africa in the late nineteenth century promoted industrialisation, modernisation and with it, a demand for labour, there was the growing marginalisation of a black middle class that had embraced the aspirational and liberal possibilities of assimilation. Trusteeship became instead associated with segregation and separate development along culturally distinct lines. Scientific thinking was used to emphasise cultural differences. Contextualised by decolonisation, trusteeship—as articulated by Schlesinger—was the means by which the narrative of "development" was used to deny political and economic equality.[62]

After Penn had exhausted his financial resources in purchasing the land for the Clinic, he approached Schlesinger for a loan to construct the Clinic itself. He had little in the way of collateral and the Clinic was as yet an unproven entity. However, Schlesinger had little qualm in financing its construction—and as Penn observed, would eventually find that his investment reaped rewards.[63]

Penn was not a small thinker and his project was an ambitious one. The plans for the Clinic drew inspiration from Arthur Stephenson—who also provided direct input. Stephenson had qualified as an architect in London and from 1924, focused on the designing of institutions, especially hospitals. He worked in consultation with medical professionals, taking their needs into account in his construction or renovation of major hospitals in Australia. During the Second World War, he was involved in the building of military hospitals and in the post-war era, the construction of the first atomic energy reactor in Australia.[64] The contractor responsible for the erection of the Clinic was Jrachmil Miodownik who had emigrated from the Middle East two decades earlier and become a part of South Africa's post-war property development boom, taking on increasingly lucrative contracts including the building of the President Hotel which cost a hefty

62 Ibid., pp272–274, 283.

63 Penn, *The Right to Look Human*, pp113–114.

64 J.D. Fisher, "Stephenson, Sir Arthur George (1890–1967)", *Australian Dictionary of Biography*, https://adb.anu.edu.au/biography/stephenson-sir-arthur-george-8646, accessed 16 April 2021.

four million rand. Miodownik was also involved in the construction of factories and building projects in present-day Zimbabwe.[65]

While the Brenthurst Clinic may have been more modest in scope, Penn had very clear ideas of what the clinic should look like—key areas for the efficient running and administration of the hospital were on the ground floor, the nursing area was divided according to function, a centralised area was created solely for the purpose of sterilising equipment and there was provision for eight operating theatres, each with the surgical equipment required for specialised surgery. The wards were subdivided into units and each of these had a unique role such as orthopaedics, for instance, with a dedicated medical team. In this way, Penn was able to maintain his preference for the "cottage hospital" within the larger institution. The hospital was also designed to allow ease and efficiency of movement for the nursing staff. Patients were not neglected either—those waiting for surgery could look at "soothing patterns" on the ceiling to alleviate their anxiety and priority was given to "post-operative care". Always appreciative of his nursing staff, Penn purchased an apartment block nearby to serve as a residence for nurses.[66]

The Brenthurst Clinic opened its doors on 1 January 1958, the ceremony presided over by Penn's teenage son, John. At pride of place in the foyer was Penn's sculpted bust of Albert Schweitzer.[67] Six years later, further additions were made to the Clinic as well as the nurses' residence.[68]

In addition to the organisational elements, the aesthetics of the hospital were an integral part of Penn's vision—and reflected his belief in the harmony between surgery and art. He applied his mind to everything—the absence of bare metal in favour of "warm colours", and the use of the latest technological comforts and gadgets. This created an environment that unified cutting-edge technology with a more holistic approach to healing that combined medicine and art.[69] When the new wing was completed in 1964, it comprised 27 new wards and was described in

[65] "Builder Who Never Saw His 'Plum' Contracts", *Rand Daily Mail*, 20 October 1967.

[66] Penn, *The Right to Look Human*, pp114–115.

[67] Ibid., p113.

[68] Ibid., p116.

[69] Ibid.

sumptuous terms by the *Rand Daily Mail*, as the epitome of luxurious hospital living:

> Luxury, air-conditioned rooms with bathrooms en suite. Telephone and radio (L.M. and F.M). Selected and matched French walnut panelling, writing desk and full-length mirror. Rocking-chair view of rolling gardens and splashing fountains.[70]

Even more compelling was the coupling of patient comfort with the latest technology that appeared almost futuristic, emblematic of the new "space age":

> The air-conditioning unit can be controlled by the patient pressing a button...The patient presses a button to talk directly to the sister in the duty room...In each room is a padded, collapsible chair, specially designed for the hospital, which puts the patient into any relaxing pose by slight pressure of the hands.[71]

While the ultimate in high-tech luxury was not simply envisaged for an elite but was touted as the ideal form of rest and recuperation afforded to all patients,[72] the Clinic did attract an elite clientele, including its first black patient, a Swazi royal prince, Prince Pinda Dhlamini admitted in September 1971.[73] The reasons for the exception are not clear; however, the acceptance of Prince Dhlamini may be contextualised by the historical relationship between Swaziland[74] and South Africa. The small kingdom is geographically largely bounded by South Africa and has been dependent on its larger neighbour for the provision of goods, services and employment. It was historically perceived to be "compliant" with the apartheid state whose superior military forces presented a coercive element to this "compliant" relationship. By the late 1970s into the following decade, Swaziland also served as an ally for South African Defence Force (SADF) raids against the African National Congress in neighbouring African states. Neo-Marxists have also alluded to the shared economic worldview

[70] "Luxury Clinic has Executive Wing", *Rand Daily Mail*, 31 March 1964.

[71] Ibid.

[72] Ibid.

[73] "Clinic is Silent on Prince", *Rand Daily Mail*, 31 September 1971.

[74] Now known as Eswatini.

of the Swazi ruling elite and the apartheid state, making both hostile to the radical ideologies of black nationalist movements.[75] Once again, events in Penn's medical career were enmeshed in wider national and ideological concerns.

The treatment of a black patient in a "white" hospital also emphasised the contradictions between the idealised humanitarian vision of medicine and its implementation in a racially oppressive system. As Baldwin-Ragaven et al. demonstrate so persuasively and powerfully, the inadequate provision of facilities and funding in health care for black South Africans as well as the unhealthy working conditions for African mineworkers, for instance, compounded by poverty and other social ills, meant that black South Africans had a dramatically higher mortality rate than white South Africans. Segregation practised at hospitals led to overcrowding and inadequate treatment in "black" spaces. Ambulances were strictly segregated, regardless of emergency, and white hospitals could—and did—refuse treatment to seriously ill or injured black patients. Blood itself was segregated. This disjuncture between the humanising impulse of medicine and the dehumanisation of the apartheid state would be marked by both compliance and resistance.[76]

There were other prominent patients at Brenthurst. While Israeli Defence Minister Moshe Dayan's treatment by Penn was much publicised, his wife Rachel, was also a patient at the hospital in 1974, using a pseudonym, "Mrs Nayad" to confound the gossip columnists. The Clinic did not give details about her procedure but made clear that her visit did not relate to having elective cosmetic surgery[77]—indicating the stigma of frivolity and vanity associated with elective plastic surgery.

A major component of the convivial atmosphere of the hospital was its aesthetic appearance and in particular, the tapestries. In this, Penn collaborated with artist Ernest Ullmann. Ullmann was born in Munich and studied at the University of Munich and the Academy of Fine Arts. With the rise of Nazism in 1933, his Jewish origins meant that he was deemed to be "not fit to contribute further to German culture". While he

[75] Cf. Albert Domson-Lindsay, "South African-Swazi Relations: A Constructivist Reading", *South African Journal of International Affairs*, 21, 3, 391–411, 2014.

[76] Laurel Baldwin-Ragaven, Jeanelle de Gruchy and Leslie London, *An Ambulance of the Wrong Colour: Health Professionals, Human Rights and Ethics in South Africa* (Cape Town, University of Cape Town Press, 1999), pp20–42.

[77] "Mrs Dayan Has Plastic Surgery", *Rand Daily Mail*, 26 August 1974.

continued sculpting, his work had either to be left anonymous or signed by a "ghost artist". With the continuing repression of his artistic expression, Ullmann left Germany in 1935. Unable to obtain permission to work in England and faced with high quotas on Jewish immigration in the United States, Australia and South America, he turned to South Africa. While he was initially unimpressed with his first sighting of Johannesburg, he developed a fondness for the harsh landscape of the highveld and was soon capturing his interpretation of it in art.[78]

Ullmann's work brought him to the attention of the Smuts intellectual cohort—Jan Hofmeyr, Basil Schonland, E.G. Malherbe and Raymond Dart. He was offered a position on a new magazine, *Forum*, as the "director of art content". The magazine was to be a publication that would address the pressing socio-political and cultural issues of the day, drawing upon the "best brains in the country".[79] It was the brainchild of R.J. Kingston Russell, the editor of the *Natal Mercury* and upon his retirement, fell to John Patrick Cope, a former reporter with the *Rand Daily Mail*, political correspondent at the *Natal Mercury* and a founder of the Progressive Party.[80] The Progressive Party was formed in 1959, eventually coming to represent a strong liberal opposition to the National Party. It would, however, only advocate a universal franchise in 1978, believing beforehand in a qualified franchise based on property ownership and education.[81] *Forum*, however, came to an end long before that with the changing political climate after the Second World War. During the War Ullmann—unable to serve due to being medically unfit—worked in the Educational Corps and drew public attention to Nazi discrimination against the Jews in the *IC Digest* produced by Military Intelligence. In the following decade, he was the key designer for the South African exhibit at the second Atomic Energy Exhibition.[82] The "Second United Nations

[78] Derek Jooste, "The Life of Iconic Artist, Sculptor and Designer Ernest Ullmann", *The Heritage Portal*, August 2016, http://www.theheritageportal.co.za/article/life-iconic-artist-sculptor-and-designer-ernest-ullmann, accessed 19 April 2021.

[79] Ibid.

[80] "Cope, John Patrick", brief biographical history as part of archival note at *Archive Hub*, https://archiveshub.jisc.ac.uk/search/archives/f281acd6-0589-3943-ac90-67bdd9eaf4e2, accessed 19 April 2021.

[81] Saul Dubow, *Apartheid 1948–1994* (Oxford, Oxford University Press, 2014), p127.

[82] Jooste, "The Life of Iconic Artist, Sculptor and Designer Ernest Ullmann".

International Conference on the Peaceful Uses of Atomic Energy"—popularly known as "Atoms for Peace"—was held in Geneva, Switzerland in 1958 and looked both at beneficial uses of nuclear power and how to make available nuclear research in the "spirit [of international] scientific co-operation". One of the attendees was Edward Teller,[83] father of the hydrogen bomb and later acquaintance of Penn.

Ullmann also shared, in part, Penn's admiration for the work of Albert Schweitzer at Lambarene—the settlement that Penn first visited in 1956. Ullmann created drawings of Lambarene depicting both the patients treated at the hospital as well as Schweitzer's work. The drawings—described by a reviewer as a "supreme example of brain control" by the artist—were housed at the South African Institute of Race Relations and the exhibition—in the absence of the artist—was opened by Jack Penn in 1959.[84]

Ullmann was later also a patient of the Brenthurst Clinic, admitted while the new wing was still under construction, after suffering a heart attack. As he was recuperating, Penn asked him to create tapestries for the hospital which also served usefully to distract him from his illness. The tapestries were a collaboration between Ullman and his wife, Jo—Ernest conceptualised each piece and designed it while Jo transferred them to cloth. Out of this collaboration arose the defining representation of the Brenthurst Clinic—a tapestry depicting the history of plastic surgery from ancient Egypt to the modern surgical art with the Clinic's motto, "It is the divine right of man to look human".[85] Penn described the symbolism of the main tapestry in a brief article in the *British Journal of Plastic Surgery* where the centre motif of two trees—"one with a broken branch and withered leaves and the other with a grafted branch and flowering leaves" represented the restorative role of the plastic surgeon—and was flanked by three figures on each side. The figures on the left represented the early origins of plastic surgery—ancient Egypt, India and the work of

[83] Sabina Griffith, "Two Weeks in September, 1958: Atoms for Peace Conference in Geneva", *Iter Newsline*, 47, September 2008, https://www.iter.org/newsline/47/680, accessed 19 April 2021.

[84] "Amazing Drawings from Lambarene", *Rand Daily Mail*, 10 April 1959.

[85] Penn, *The Right to Look Human*, pp116–118.

Tagliacozzi in sixteenth-century Italy. The figures on the right were of a surgeon, a patient and a nurse in the modern era.[86]

With the opening of the new wing, the Clinic held a "private showing" of the tapestries. The Ullmanns' tapestries would also grace the Chamber of Mines Pavillion and they were awarded a commission to create tapestries for the South African embassy in France,[87] with their art thus gracing sites of economic, political and in the case of Brenthurst, medical significance.

Penn's financial commitment to the Clinic reflected his fervent belief in his method of practising medicine but he was nonetheless relieved when the Clinic not only achieved financial stability from the outset but acquired a reputation for both research and teaching. It attracted medical professionals from all over the world—and this was likely helped in part by Penn's own visits abroad. In addition, the medical staff reflected this cosmopolitanism with many nationalities and languages represented.[88]

Yet this idealised state-of-the-art medical facility was also subject to the vagaries of medical treatment in twentieth-century South Africa. In 1968, a trial took place of a young nurse employed by the Clinic charged with culpable homicide in the death of a three-year-old in June 1967. The nurse was alleged to have administered potassium chloride directly into the vein of the child rather than through a "vacelitre" that would have regulated the dosage. The influx of the drug into the child's system was believed to have caused death due to cardiac arrest five days later.[89] The nurse, however, was exonerated as negligence could not be proven and the magistrate pointed out that there were no warning labels or instructions on the ampoules containing the potassium chloride, describing the incident as "a chapter of accidents".[90] Little could be done to avert human error and poor judgment as a result of inexperience.

Despite Penn's desire to have the best and most qualified medical personnel available, the training of staff was one of the mandates of the Clinic which was a registered training site for nursing assistants. This also

[86] Jack Penn, "The Brenthurst Clinic Tapestry", *British Journal of Plastic Surgery*, 20, January 1967, pp104–105.

[87] H.E.W., "Why Must They Be Sent Away?", *Rand Daily Mail*, 3 April 1964.

[88] Penn, *The Right to Look Human*, p118.

[89] "Nurse Wept as She Told of Injection", *Rand Daily Mail*, 29 March 1968.

[90] "Nurse Is Cleared of Death", *Rand Daily Mail*, 8 May 1968.

led to its implication in the apartheid policies of discrimination and in particular, the differential pay scale for black and white nurses. It was only in 1976 that the state permitted the employment of black nurses in white hospitals with the proviso that:

> ...no qualified white staff were available...they were paid the same salaries as whites and the hospitals were not saving money; that the patients had no objection, and the appointment was not made merely to antagonise the Government.[91]

The history of black nursing in South Africa demonstrates the convergence of race, class and gender, as evident in the work of Shula Marks and Simmone Horwitz.[92] In the nineteenth century, medicine was part of the "civilising mission" against what was perceived to be the malign influence of "witch-doctors"; it was the triumph of science, a healthy lifestyle and Christian faith. The "Native" nurse was an exemplar of "Native womanhood" in this context, the epitome of the triumph of "civilised" values. Yet the use of African nurses in segregated spaces raised questions of propriety where they were subject to the harassment of "European males of an unsuitable type" who saw them as little other than women who could be sexually exploited in contrast to white nurses. This contributed to segregation and the limited role of black nurses in "white" hospitals.[93]

Yet nursing also became the preferred occupation for an educated African elite—it was associated with respectability and the idealised nurturing role of women. In the twentieth century, therefore, viewed as a high-status occupation, the number of African nurses increased dramatically. Yet the increase in numbers belied the unequal state of education in segregationist South Africa where schooling opportunities remained limited—especially for African women—for a great part of the twentieth century. Along with a racial belief in the inferior mental capability of African women, there were perpetual concerns regarding the affording of

[91] Penny Cummins, "Why the Gap?", *Rand Daily Mail*, 4 August 1977.

[92] Cf. Shula Marks, *Divided Sisterhood: Race, Class and Gender in the South African Nursing Profession* (Johannesburg, Witwatersrand University Press, 1994); and Simmone Horwitz, "'Black Nurses in White': Exploring Young Women's Entry into the Nursing Profession at Baragwanath Hospital, Soweto, 1948–1980", *Social History of Medicine*, 20, 1, 131–164, 2007.

[93] Marks, *Divided Sisterhood*, pp81, 85.

black nurses the same professional status as their white counterparts. By the 1950s—the period in which the Brenthurst Clinic was established—apartheid policy was increasingly evident in the field of nursing, replacing early liberalism. Ideas of white student nurses falling under black nurses and of "social fraternizing" were anathema. The Nursing Amendment Act of 1957, emphasised segregation in nursing, where nurses would be best suited to working with their "own people".[94] The history of nursing then demonstrated a shifting and contradictory vision of modernity—linked to the modernising project and "civilisation" in the nineteenth century, their role was increasingly marginalised, rendering them unequal and incompatible with the apartheid state's vision of modernisation based on racial exclusion.

For young black women, nursing was a high-status form of employment that had the benefit of earning them a salary while they trained. However, despite having to engage in the same level of training and take on the same type of work, their salary was markedly lower than their white counterparts when they were employed in state facilities. At private hospitals such as Brenthurst—which depended to a tremendous extent on its nursing staff—they were only permitted to use black nurses in particular contexts such as "the central sterile area or other parts of the hospital where they have no contact with white patients". And, while they were paid more than the rate stipulated by the Transvaal Provincial Administration, it was still less than the salary of white nurses. For white nursing assistants at Brenthurst, however, their salary upon qualification was almost twice that of those employed in government institutions.[95] During his career, Penn acknowledged the immense value of nurses in providing medical care and had little reservation in promoting black nursing as well, evident in the various sculptures created celebrating the nursing profession.

With the construction of the Brenthurst Clinic, it is possible to get a sense of the intellectual and cultural world that Penn inhabited—he had forged connections with like-minded members of Jewish society—Oppenheimer, Schlesinger, Ullmann. He was a devotee of modernisation that permeated all aspects of the Brenthurst Clinic in its various incarnations, as evident in the initial conception of the project, its structural layout

[94] Ibid., pp88, 90–93, 148, 150.

[95] Cummins, "Why the Gap?".

and the provision of the latest medical technology for the treatment of patients. And Penn and his various acquaintances inhabited an intellectual milieu that demonstrated similarities in thinking regarding socio-political and economic conditions in South Africa, the uses of atomic energy and even the idealised role of medical care and philanthropy as practised by Albert Schweitzer. However, Penn's range was wider than the southern tip of Africa.

Iran

The Brenthurst Clinic was the culmination of Penn's work as a surgeon yet it still fell short of his great vision—the establishment of a great centre of medical knowledge and treatment, the vision that he had had on the banks of the Thames. A vision of such breadth, however, required resources and a state amenable to such a large project. Penn pictured his medical centre—described as the "Disneyland of technology"—as an international centre established through contributions by various donor countries, "apolitical" and independent. A pre-requisite then was that it be situated in "neutral" territory and Penn considered Iran as a possible site. He mentioned the project to an Iranian plastic surgeon encountered at a conference in Jerusalem in 1973 which led to a subsequent invitation to meet with the monarchy in Tehran.[96]

Prior to the royal audience, Penn drew up a memorandum for the perceived project which bears detailed replication, symbolising both his idealism and vision for medical care and the transmission of knowledge.

> A garden centre to be chosen and presented by His Majesty the Shah to the world as a technological headquarters under his personal patronage.
>
> This centre to be completely apolitical and in no way connected with the United Nations Organisation.
>
> The city to consist of the following units:
>
> 1. Secretarial offices for international technological bodies, medical, engineering, architecture, strategic studies etc. Each group is to be given facilities by invitation only. The general administrative organisation is to be maintained by the controllers of the projects.

[96] Penn, *The Right to Look Human*, pp200–201.

> Secretarial work, stationery etc. to be maintained by the members' subscriptions.
> 2. International museums.
> 3. International libraries.
> 4. Rooms for symposia and conferences.
> 5. Hotels, apartments and houses for guests and permanent staff.
>
> CONTROL
>
> Their Majesties to sponsor and maintain this "garden city" which would be a vocational centre for the families attending any congresses, the practical controlling body to be chosen from international experts. No political candidate should be involved.[97]

Penn's vision was breath-taking even as it combined the idealistic with the mundane (viz. stationery) but it also demonstrated a certain naivete, a sense that the practice of medicine was ideologically neutral. During Penn's audience with Farah Pahlavi, the Queen, he explained that his choice of Iran as the ideal site was due to its rich cultural and intellectual past—this would not be a "modernistic innovation" but instead a "renaissance of technology", a revitalisation of the millennia-old Persian culture.[98]

During the reign of the Shah, however, Iran was engaged in a very complicated and fraught interaction with modernity. Described by David Edgerton as a "brutal, modernising monarchy",[99] Iran at the time of Penn's visit was hardly "neutral" territory. On the Shah's accession to power (after his father's abdication) during the Second World War, Mohammad Reza Pahlavi's rule was subject to the implementation of modern reforms made at the behest of the Allies. This included rule as a "constitutional monarch" rather than autocratic rule, the establishment of sanitation infrastructure and money spent on medical training, research and treatment. Yet power was concentrated in the hands of an

[97] Ibid., p200.

[98] Ibid., p201.

[99] David Edgerton, *The Shock of the Old: Technology and Global History Since 1900* (London, Profile Books, 2008), p153.

elite.[100] The monarchy thus remained the potent force, driving Iranian modernisation in the second half of the twentieth century.

Iran's modernisation cannot be divorced from its links with the United States. During the Cold War, the anticommunist Iranian state was a strategic ally of the United States due to its proximity to the Soviet Union and increasingly, its vast oil reserves. The Shah met with President John F. Kennedy in Washington in April 1962. At this point it was clear that the two sides had different visions of modernity with American concerns that economic development was key to maintaining a stable society—and one less inclined to be swayed by communist influence. For the Shah, on the other hand, economic development could only occur once society had already been rendered stable and his view of modernisation necessitated the prioritisation of the military to maintain order and stability. Maintaining the Shah's rule was a paramount feature of US-Iranian relations and so it would be the Shah's view of modernisation that would prevail.[101]

This became particularly evident during the Johnson administration due to the deteriorating situation in Vietnam as well as the conflict between India and Pakistan where the Americans intervened by cutting off their military supplies to Pakistan, much to the Shah's disapproval. This led to the Shah's increasing reliance on military strength and Iran's purchasing of weapons from the Soviet Union.[102] The Shah's support for the American war effort in Vietnam, American strategic need to establish "CIA listening posts" in Iran as well as growing détente between Iran and the Soviet Union, meant that the Shah became increasingly assertive in the relationship between Iran and the United States.[103] A token effort on the part of the Shah such as the sending of a surgical team—two surgeons and a handful of nurses—to Vietnam was an important tactical ploy, demonstrating the support of the developing world for a war effort increasingly mired in controversy.[104] Over the subsequent

[100] Ervand Abrahamian, *A History of Modern Iran* (New York, Cambridge University Press, 2008), pp98–98.

[101] Ben Offiler, *U.S. Foreign Policy and the Modernization of Iran: Kennedy, Johnson, Nixon and the Shah* (Basingstoke, Palgrave Macmillan, 2015), pp1–5, 9.

[102] Ibid., pp93–94.

[103] Ibid., pp96–97.

[104] Ibid., p104.

decade, as Iran began to exploit its oil reserves to a greater degree, American influence declined even further. During the Six Day War in 1967 when Arab states placed an embargo on oil exports, Iran continued to supply the West—and the United States—with oil, thereby confirming to the Shah the importance of Iran.[105] There was no longer the need for Americans to provide aid to Iran—which had created a relationship of dependency. By 1968, the United States had acceded to the Shah's view of modernisation by extending military credit to Iran for the next five years.[106] At the same time, while not prioritised to the same extent as military development, the Shah had attempted to carry out modernisation projects in Iran—"the nationalisation of Iran's water and forests", a focus on greater rights for women (if only to challenge the strong religious element within the country) and an improvement in literacy.[107] By the time of Penn's visit, the Shah's project of modernisation had led to improvements in port and rail infrastructure, the building of hydroelectric dams, two steel mills (one built with Soviet assistance), a nuclear plant and an expansion in industry.[108] A Literacy Corps had been set up and the level of literacy was increasing rapidly, now covering nearly half the country's population. On the health front, there was an increase in the number of clinics, medical personnel and success rates in ridding Iran of famine and childhood diseases. Women were enfranchised and able to hold office, given greater equality in marriage with control over their children and restrictions were placed on polygamy.[109]

Yet this was a vision of modernisation that had a different focus to that held by the West. Iran's emphasis was on military spending and the maintenance of an elite stranglehold on power with the associated systems of patronage.[110] It could perhaps account for Penn's assessment of Iran as a neutral state based on the Shah's ability to assert Iranian needs and his own vision of modernisation against the dictates of the West. For Penn, Iran was a compromise solution—he would have preferred to realise his

[105] Ibid., p119.

[106] Ibid., p116.

[107] Ibid., pp131–132.

[108] Abrahamian, *A History of Modern Iran*, p133.

[109] Ibid., p134.

[110] Ibid., pp126–127.

vision in London or in Israel but was aware of the Shah's wealth and influence as an absolute ruler and rather idealistically hoped that this would make him inclined to "donate a large area on the Caspian Sea to be an International Centre for this purpose".[111]

The surgeon's meeting with the Queen took place at her palace which he described as akin to "an episode in the *Arabian Nights*". The issue of the loss of educated Iranians was raised with Penn's solution that the means of keeping the best and brightest in the country would be the allocation of scholarships that would tie the recipient to the state for five years. His proposed centre could also be the site of learning for these students and the congregation of an Iranian intellectual elite.[112]

While the Queen lent a sympathetic ear to Penn's proposal as did the Court Minister, Penn was unable to gain a direct audience with the Shah himself. His view of the Shah as "a benevolent dictator—in the best sense of the word…[and as] fearless and a man of integrity"[113] was perhaps less a reflection of the Shah's rule than it was of Penn's own views regarding the implementation of full democracy—views that were extremely ambivalent in the context of decolonisation and apartheid.[114] Like South Africa too, modernisation in Iran had taken a different path with power held in the hands of an elite. By 1973—the year of Penn's visit—Iran had one of the highest rates of economic inequality in the world. Its improvements in education still placed it well below par with the rest of the Middle East and there were insufficient tertiary opportunities for those able to apply to universities. As a result, many of the educated elite left the country—the so-called "brain drain" which was such a source of concern to the Queen.[115] Penn's view of the "benevolent dictator" was misguided and a few years later the monarchy was overthrown in Iran, with an Islamic state taking its place.

[111] "We Can't Always Win!" in "Philosophy is Fun" (Unpublished manuscript), December 1983, File: Penn, Jack—Writings (3), AMUW.

[112] Penn, *The Right to Look Human*, p201.

[113] Ibid.

[114] This is addressed in the following section.

[115] Abrahamian, *A History of Modern Iran*, pp141–142.

Penn's vision of a medical city would not come to pass yet in the example of Iran, were the warning signs that would apply to his own country and here too, Penn would advocate a different vision of modernisation.

PART II

The Surgeon Ambassador

CHAPTER 7

The Heart of Darkness? Albert Schweitzer and Lambarene

> He is a visionary; a teacher; and a philosopher; and a deeply religious man....but unlike any ecclesiastical head I have ever heard of, his parish is not the city but the jungle; his cathedral is not a magnificent stone affair built by the exploited parishoners [sic], but a wood and iron hospital built for the parishoners [sic] by himself personally; his home is not a palace but a wood and iron room with no more comforts than anyone else; his councellors [sic] are not cardinals, bishops, rabbis, or what have you but simple decent folk who feel as he does but come to him for leadership. He is their mouthpiece.[1]

Jack Penn's description of Dr Albert Schweitzer to Caroline Oppenheimer during his initial visit to Schweitzer's hospital at Lambarene demonstrates an almost hagiographical admiration of Schweitzer with religious overtones. The reality of the encounter, however, would be more complex and at the heart of it, lay different views on the practice of medicine and the ideal role of white, medical professionals in the African context.

[1] Jack Penn, Excerpt from Letter to Lady Oppenheimer—5 April 1956, BC748 A1.10, Dr Jack Penn Collection A1.1–A1.81, Correspondence between Dr Jack Penn and Albert Schweitzer and Others, Mainly at Lambarene, 1956–1957, University of Cape Town Libraries (hereafter UCTL).

S. Chetty, *Reconstructive Surgery and Modernisation in Twentieth-Century South Africa*, Medicine and Biomedical Sciences in Modern History, https://doi.org/10.1007/978-3-031-38673-2_7

While presenting a paper in Rome on leprosy[2] in 1956, Penn was approached by Clara Urquhart, Schweitzer's administrative assistant and interpreter. Schweitzer requested Penn to visit his hospital in Lambarene, an invitation which Penn accepted enthusiastically.[3]

Yet, subsequent correspondence suggested that Schweitzer was ambivalent about his initial invitation:

> I am delighted that you have the intention to realise your plan and come to us from March 3rd—April 12th. I think you are touching [sic], that you want to sacrifice your time and help to our natives. Yet there are objections I feel obliged to tell you:
>
> 1) We live in the jungle. It is not easy to gather together the cases, interesting your art. They are disseminated in the forest. I fear that you would not find cases enough to give you satisfaction.
> 2) The sterility is not as you are accustomed to. We have no windows in the operating room, because the heat would be unbearable.
>
> I am obliged to tell you all this, I feel it my duty to speak about it. Maybe your visit here could be a desillusion [sic]. You alone know if you want to risk it. Lambarene is not a big agglomeration. You cannot find the surgery cases, interesting you, in sufficient number, in spite of all efforts to gather them.
>
> It is my duty to tell you how is the situation here. Kindly decide now what you want to do.[4]

Schwitzer's hesitation was possibly due to the ways in which his hospital differed significantly from the conventional standards of Western medicine and aroused no small amount of criticism from his contemporaries. It would also be a point of contention in Penn's own analysis of the conditions at Lambarene and provide the basis for his subsequent efforts to

[2] Leprosy is also known as Hansen's Disease, however, here and elsewhere, it is referred to by the former name by Penn.

[3] Jack Penn, *The Right to Look Human: An Autobiography* (Johannesburg, Hugh Keartland Publishers, 1976), p134.

[4] Excerpt from Letter from Albert Schweitzer to Jack Penn, 23rd January 1956, BC748 A1.4, UCTL. The Dr Jack Penn Collection contains Schweitzer's hand-written correspondence in German along with a typed English translation. This chapter makes use of the latter.

intervene. Yet Lambarene was a product of Schweitzer's ambiguous position—the convergence of the religious and the secular, the colonial and the post-colonial, individual redemption and the common good.

Born in Alsace in 1875, Albert Schweitzer had strong religious influences from a young age. Both his father and maternal grandfather were Lutheran ministers and Schweitzer studied theology at the University of Strasbourg before lecturing in the subject at the Lutheran college. Not content with the role of an academic, he decided to become a missionary, displaying a special interest in the Lambarene mission station in the French colony of Gabon which was under the aegis of the Paris Evangelical Missionary Society.[5] Schweitzer's decision to go to Gabon was based on his avowed dedication to a moral and spiritually uplifting life. He had initially hoped to put these beliefs into practice in Germany—possibilities included the rehabilitation of prisoners and the care of orphans and the indigent—yet these were already addressed by existing institutions and Schweitzer desired greater autonomy for his work. It was in 1904 that he came across an advertisement by the Paris Missionary Society requesting volunteers to carry out its missionary activities in Gabon. After some soul-searching, he raised the funds to set up his own hospital and to travel to Gabon. He was able to work out an arrangement with the Paris Evangelical Missionary Society that would allow him access to Gabon under the auspices of the Society yet still remain largely self-sufficient. His decision to work with the Society was based on what was perceived to be a joint dedication to Christian humanitarian duty.[6]

At the time of Albert and Helene Schweitzer's arrival in Africa in 1913, Gabon was a French colony and Lambarene—where Schweitzer was to build his hospital—was in the equatorial forest and geared towards the export of hardwood, a trade that had succeeded rubber and ivory. Despite the French administration's belief that the provision of medical services would make the indigenous population more amenable to colonial rule, the African population had had very little experience of European medicine and access to doctors outside the more established

[5] James Carleton Paget, "Albert Schweitzer and Africa", *Journal of Religion in Africa*, 42, 2012, pp279–280.

[6] Ibid., pp282–284. *Cf* Albert Schweitzer, *My Life and Thought: An Autobiography*, C.T. Campion (translator) (London, George Allen and Unwin Ltd, 1933, 1948), pp103–106, 137.

towns was minimal. Moreover, these medical practitioners were not always the most qualified or effective. Schweitzer's presence was to change that.[7]

His beliefs also meant that he had a profound commitment to the use of Christianity as a guide to "ethical" behaviour. It was less about converting Africans than it was about the philanthropic work to make amends for the imperial exploitation that had had such a detrimental impact on European colonies in Africa—and medicine was a key component of this. Yet, so too, was the propagation of Christianity—both in the face of the growing influence of Islam and as a means of introducing indigenous Africans to Christian morality.[8] After the end of the First World War and prior to his return to Africa, Schweitzer wrote *The Decay and the Restoration of Civilization*.[9] Contextualised by the War itself and colonialism, he drew attention to the loss of humanity, an increasing "light-mindedness about war and conquest, as if these were merely operations on a chess-board". There was also the dehumanisation of the "coloured races".[10] Modernity had permitted the submergence of the rational and ethical individual within the masses and it was this lack of individual agency and "judgment" that led to the justification of violence and exploitation.[11] For Schweitzer, "civilization" had been reduced to "mere material progress" devoid of spirituality and morality[12]—and colonialism exemplified this.

His initial cutting criticism of colonialism became more nuanced as he came to understand the distinction between the inherently exploitative nature of colonialism—the use of labour, natural resources and associated social and economic ills—and the civilising project. While not condoning colonialism and the role of the concession companies, his ability to place them within context gave him a greater sense of understanding. This also brought him to the realisation that the indigenous African was best suited to their "traditional" way of life, ensconced in their village and away from the corrupting influences of modernity. This goes some way to explaining

[7] Paget, "Albert Schweitzer and Africa", pp280, 285–286.

[8] Ibid., pp287–288.

[9] Published in German as *Verfall und Wiederraufbau der Kultur* in 1923.

[10] Albert Schweitzer, *The Philosophy of Civilization 1: The Decay and the Restoration of Civilization* (London, Adam and Charles Black, 1950), p25.

[11] Ibid., p32.

[12] Ibid., p38.

his failure to adequately engage in the training of African nurses and doctors, due to his belief that they were essentially "unreliable". Simultaneously, he considered them to be "children of nature" with an intuitive grasp of Christian morality once they had been introduced to it.[13] Initially sceptical regarding "whether [Africans] were mere prisoners of tradition or beings capable of really independent thought",[14] Schweitzer came to believe that their simplicity of understanding meant that they could surpass European corrupted notions that permitted mass warfare and violence, demonstrating a sense of spiritual ethics that was increasingly difficult to achieve in Western civilisation.[15] Yet he paid little heed to this "traditional" way of life, demonstrated no interest in African culture and religion and acquired no proficiency in the dominant indigenous languages of Lambarene.[16] He instead made use of an assistant, a former cook, Joseph Azowani, who also served as a translator. Azowani assisted in acquainting Schweitzer with the cultural expectations and beliefs of African patients in relation to medical treatment.[17] Schweitzer thus developed an understanding of the context of local beliefs and adapted his hospital in a manner best suited to African sensibilities—regardless of the way this would be perceived by more conventional Western medical practitioners.[18] His hospital contained consulting and operating rooms as well as a dispensary and the prevalent illnesses treated ranged from leprosy to pneumonia. White patients were segregated from their black counterparts, with whites housed in the mission itself and in Schweitzer's quarters, and bamboo huts built for black patients.[19] In the case of the latter, the hospital did not follow the European model and resembled a "village" where families lived with, cooked for and assisted with taking care of the patient. With this model, Schweitzer helped circumvent indigenous distrust of Western medicine and its practitioners.[20]

[13] Paget, "Albert Schweitzer and Africa", pp289–291.

[14] Schweitzer, *My Life and Thought*, p168.

[15] Ruth Harris, "The Allure of Albert Schweitzer", *History of European Ideas*, 40, 6, 804–825, 2014, pp814, 815; *Cf* Schweitzer, *My Life and Thought*, pp171–172.

[16] Paget, "Albert Schweitzer and Africa", pp292–293.

[17] Schweitzer, *My Life and Thought*, p165.

[18] Paget, "Albert Schweitzer and Africa", pp292–293.

[19] Schweitzer, *My Life and Thought*, p163–164.

[20] Harris, "The Allure of Albert Schweitzer", p813.

Yet he knew that the clock could not be turned back. Once exposed to the forces of colonialism, Africans irrevocably became part of it. This then, is where the paternalistic leadership of Europeans was needed to rule benevolently and provide the necessary moral counselling. Now, colonialism became a moral imperative as Schweitzer believed that Africans were not ready to be granted their autonomy in the foreseeable future. This view was less than welcome in the mid-twentieth century amidst the growth of anti-colonial movements and increasing agitation for African independence. For Schweitzer, however, economic independence was a necessary pre-requisite for political independence. He also believed that African "tribalism"—which would experience a resurgence in a post-colonial environment—would form a volatile mix when combined with political autonomy.[21] This would be echoed by Penn in his own thinking about apartheid and African enfranchisement. Schweitzer felt that the basis of ethics lay in the empathy that human beings have for each other. Drawing upon his experiences at Lambarene, he concluded that, for the "primitive", however, this sense of empathy and compassion extended at most to the tribe.[22] Human history was also characterised by notions of difference based on ideology, race and nationalism. The Christian prioritisation of love, however, allowed for a wider identification and one that would ultimately include all living beings.[23] Allied with love was the reason emanating from the Enlightenment which created the conditions for the improvement of society.[24] For Schweitzer, ideas of science and progress were, however, distinct from ethics—science served a pragmatic purpose, ethical action a spiritual one.[25] It is largely this philosophy as articulated in *The Teaching of Reverence for Life* that explains Schweitzer's emphasis on Christian morality at Lambarene, his disinterest in training Africans as medical practitioners and his unfashionable belief that Africa—and Africans—were not ready for political independence. And it was the last which would resonate with Jack Penn who would echo it almost two decades later.

[21] Paget, "Albert Schweitzer and Africa", pp294.

[22] Albert Schweitzer, *The Teaching of Reverence for Life* (London, Peter Owen Limited, 1965, 1966), p9.

[23] Ibid., pp11, 17.

[24] Ibid., p19.

[25] Ibid., pp24, 41.

First Impressions

Prior to his arrival in Lambarene on 2 April 1956, Penn spent the night in Brazzaville, the capital of French Equatorial Africa. His impressions of the city were mixed where "The Africans are clean and well dressed...and very surly to the point of rudeness to all white men". The efforts of French colonialism were subsequently accorded a dismissive, "So much for liberte, fraternite and egalite".[26]

Penn left for Lambarene the following day aboard a Dakota—a remodelled military transport—on an event-filled flight that demonstrated both the inaccessibility of Schweitzer's settlement as well as the constant effort of bringing some semblance of Western modernity to this part of Africa. Tiny airstrips had been carved out of the verdant jungle and the French pilots made several landings in far from ideal conditions, already creating the impression of the hardy and adventurous traveller distant from civilisation. This impression was confirmed by the contingent sent to transport Penn across the river to the Lamberene settlement. A mahogany canoe, which Penn dubbed "Schweitzer's 'Cadillac'", and which had been apparently built by Schweitzer himself, was crewed by a number of lepers who proceeded to row Penn on what was evidently a lengthy journey.[27] Penn was aware of the image presented of the white adventurer travelling down the river, flanked by jungle, describing himself as akin to "the central figure of a Somerset Maugham play".[28] He was also uneasy about the use of lepers as rowers, considering this to likely take a toll on their already vulnerable extremities. While the use of a motorboat seemed to Penn to be a far more efficient option, it clearly did not harmonise with the image that Schweitzer seemed intent on portraying. This was reinforced by the first meeting between the two men. Schweitzer appeared at the dock surrounded by his nurses, all dressed "in spotlessly white uniforms and white pith helmets".[29]

While what Penn described as Schweitzer's "stage-setting" —a portrayal of white dominance and civilisation in hostile Africa that would not have been out of place in the late nineteenth century—implied that

[26] Excerpt from Letter by Penn to Family (Di, Joan and John), 2 April 1956, BC748 A1.8 and A1.14, UCTL.

[27] Excerpt from Letter by Penn to Family, 2 April 1956.

[28] Much of Maugham's writing focused on Asia during the colonial period.

[29] Penn, *The Right to Look Human*, p136.

the missionary/doctor was hopelessly out of touch with the contemporary period, his first perception of Schweitzer belied this crude impression. While initially reticent about his impression of Schweitzer in his correspondence, other than describing him as an imposing presence despite his age, Penn was more forthcoming in his autobiography written almost two decades later. He emphasised a certain sense of melancholy and power which was nonetheless lightened by a sense of humour.[30] Penn also displayed an increasing fondness in his description of and dealings with Schweitzer yet this did not detract from his criticism of conditions at the hospital.

And Penn did not mince his words:

> The physical environment of the hospital has been described a dozen times by better pens than mine. All are agreed that it is primitive. My own first reaction was one of horror, for although I was unused to squalor, the indescribable filth associated with this temple of healing was worse than any other African hospital I have ever seen. The wards were dank, dark and overcrowded, without running water or sanitary facilities. Everywhere, inside and out, were the droppings of goats, and the families of patients, with their animals, were all over the place. Leaves and debris were everywhere.[31]

Yet, his first impressions were soon ameliorated, and he came to the realisation that context was key, "this was not a hospital in the ordinary sense, but a native village with doctors and nurses working in it".[32] In spite of the conditions that were in such contrast to Western medical and sanitary practices, Penn concluded that the hospital at Lambarene worked. Despite the high infection rates, there was little evidence of sepsis in patients recovering from surgery nor was there "cross-infection". Penn attributed this to less exposure to antibiotics and hence less resistance on the part of patients. The unhygienic conditions were due to a lack of sufficient cleaning staff and Schweitzer asserted that the fallen leaves served

[30] Excerpt from Letter by Penn to Family, 2 April 1956; Penn, *The Right to Look Human*, p137.

[31] Penn, *The Right to Look Human*, p137.

[32] Ibid.

as a means of "[binding] the soil" in the face of the erosive rain which "would wash the hospital into the river".[33]

Lambarene: A Day in the Life...

In 1956, Penn wrote an article for the journal, *Plastic and Reconstructive Surgery*, where he presented his impressions of his first visit to Lambarene. At the heart of it is, of course, the figure of Schweitzer, an almost saintly "Moses" who used the money from his Nobel Prize to build a leper village and was familiar with all the wildlife of the jungle, taking care not to harm even an ant. The clinic itself seemed to provide medical treatment for both indigenous Africans and animals alike. It is an image of childlike obedience to the dictates of Western medicine:

> At one end the patients line up to see the doctor and in the queue you may see a dog with a torn ear, or a goat with a lacerated leg waiting patiently for his turn. At the other end is another queue waiting for their medicines. Patients who can walk are summoned by a bell. They open their mouths and the necessary pill or mixture is put into it by the nurse. They must swallow it on the spot as they are not above spitting it out if they don't like the taste.[34]

Schweitzer's view of his African patients as childlike as well as being "lazy and unappreciative" was endorsed by Penn who emphasised their lack of "initiative", and their reluctance to assist either themselves or others, demonstrating a passivity and lack of empathy that necessitated them being led. It was a perception that challenged that of "the armchair philosophers who clamoured for their rapid emancipation".[35]

Meals at Lambarene were eccentric, to say the least. Presided over by the paternal figure of Schweitzer accompanied by his wife, dinner included the staff as well as Schweitzer's dog and a gorilla, the chimpanzee having temporarily been banished. The meal was largely fruit-based with meat served twice a week. Once the meal was concluded, Schweitzer would say

[33] Ibid.

[34] Jack Penn, "A Visit to Albert Schweitzer", *Plastic and Reconstructive Surgery*, 18, 3, September 1956, pp162–164.

[35] Ibid., p165.

a prayer, then there was the singing of hymns with his piano accompaniment. He then left, with his wife remaining behind to oversee the more social aspects of the gathering.[36]

Penn reserved much of his empathy for the European volunteers who worked at the hospital, amongst them Schweitzer's wife. He bemoaned her lack of recognition especially as her role had been key as Schweitzer began his mission in Africa. The impression given is that she had been increasingly marginalised as more staff were drawn to the hospital. This was compounded by Schweitzer's own controlling nature and a hierarchical system at the hospital that placed him at its apex. Subsequent ill health—rheumatism and tuberculosis, largely due to the environment—had restricted her mobility. Penn portrayed an intelligent woman, confined to an ailing body, and one who was increasingly isolated, both from other members of staff and from her distant husband who, "almost ignored her and did not speak to her with any great deference".[37] Nevertheless, Helene Schweitzer demonstrated an interest in Penn's work, making what was obviously an arduous journey to the theatre to observe him as he operated.[38] The figure of Helene Bresslau Schweitzer—who would die soon after—strikes a discordant note in Penn's description of the almost saintly figure of Albert Schweitzer and his mission that rendered her "a tragic passenger in a venture which she had started with such courage".[39]

Penn also paid attention to the female nursing staff. The conditions in tropical Africa were not ideal and Schweitzer's settlement left much to be desired, with no electricity or running water. The environment was hostile—unremitting heat and humidity and insects that carried with them dangers of malaria and "sleeping sickness":

> And yet in this environment I have worked with the kindest and sweetest people I have ever met. None of them get paid—they work like hell all

[36] Ibid., pp163, 166–167.

[37] Penn, *The Right to Look Human*, pp139–140.

[38] Jack Penn, Excerpt from Letter to Di, Joan, John, family and friends, 4 April 1956, BC748 A1.9, UCTL.

[39] Penn, *The Right to Look Human*, p140.

> day—they have to be in by 8 p.m. because of mosquitoes etc and everybody lies on their beds gasping like newly caught fish. Yet they are happy, kindly and considerate, even to the tiniest animal.[40]

Further, there was no social outlet for these women and their work was long, difficult and materially unrewarding. This only emphasised their dedication and spirit of volunteerism. The majority had left behind a comfortable life in Europe inspired by Schweitzer's vision and a desire to serve. Some had braved the adverse conditions for more than three decades. Simultaneously, Penn was not impressed with the methods employed to treat leprosy as the head nurse did not observe adequate protocol to prevent infection and used mercurochrome to treat the lesions resulting from the disease. The hardship endured by these nurses was thus undermined by his assessment of their "devoted, fruitless service".[41]

His disapproval of the treatment methods extended to those employed by Schweitzer's "chief assistant", a doctor from Holland. While acknowledging her dedication and talent, her youth and lack of formal surgical training led to her showing poor judgment in preserving the leg of a leprosy sufferer when the best form of treatment would have been amputation. Hospital resources had therefore been used in an unproductive manner—with the patient confined for eighteen months in an effort to delay the inevitable. However, it was less the poor judgment exercised by the unnamed doctor, than Schweitzer's own lack of intervention in the matter.[42] The image of Schweitzer presented by Penn is of a combination of dominance yet distance and reflects Penn's views regarding the role of the surgeon in terms of supervision as well as the use of cutting-edge therapeutics and technology.

Penn also painted a picture of an ailing African population, tormented by the diseases produced by social, economic and environmental conditions—Kwashiorkor due to malnutrition, venereal disease, elephantiasis and leprosy. Patients were portrayed as passive, in a state of torpor, waiting for the inevitable end. Briefly, this seemed to provoke a similar

[40] Excerpt from Letter to Di, Joan, John, family and friends—4 April 1956, BC748 A1.9, UCTL.

[41] Penn, *The Right to Look Human*, p138.

[42] Ibid., pp139–140.

sense of inertia in Penn, "...nothing here could be judged by normal standards".[43]

However, his apathy was fleeting. Prior to his arrival at Lambarene, Penn had outlined his motive in undertaking the visit. The treatment of a few leprosy sufferers was secondary to his ambition to provide comprehensive treatment for the many suffering from "deforming diseases", preferably with the assistance of international agencies such as WHO. Penn had a vision of groups of medical practitioners setting up mobile treatment centres that could potentially reach millions.[44] Yet his vision would be frustrated by Schweitzer's recalcitrance, with the latter focusing on his medical and humanitarian efforts as a means of achieving his own salvation. To Penn's dismay, Schweitzer demonstrated little interest in broader issues—for instance, in "medicine or science" where "nothing new has ever been contributed by Dr Schweitzer to scientific journals".[45] More significantly, "it was his intention to help the Africans, not to elevate them", a view that led to him refusing Penn's offer of a "South African Bantu doctor" that Schweitzer felt would upset the racial dynamic at the hospital.[46]

Penn's Modern Mission

Between mid-May and July 1956, upon his return, Penn wrote three successive letters to Schweitzer, outlining his plan to improve the hospital. In the first, Penn had an ambitious plan for improving the operating facilities of the hospital—even as he assured Schweitzer that this would not mean altering the "character of the hospital":

> ...I am glad to state that the representatives of the W.H.O. and the British Empire Leprocy [sic] Association were very keen on the idea of mobile units. I have had discussions with Dr Muir of the B.E.L.A. in London and am in contact with Dr Bonne of the W.H.O. in Geneva.

[43] Ibid., p138.

[44] Jack Penn, Excerpt from Letter to Albert Schweitzer, 1 February 1956, BC748 A1.6, UCTL.

[45] Penn, *The Right to Look Human*, p140.

[46] Ibid., p144.

It is my suggestion that such a team should consist not only of Surgeons but also personnel for matters of Public Health and prevention, occupational therapy and research—pathology. I feel that the team should spend a 6 months probationary period in Pretoria under me or in Vallore, India under Brand before considering sending them into the "field" for about 2 years.

As I see it, the total cost of such a project should be under £100,000 which should not be difficult to collect from any of half a dozen sources. But before suggesting ways and means to them I feel I would like to discuss the following propositions with you.

The wisdom of Christ would have been unknown if it were not for the propaganda of the disciples and your own message to the world would have been loot [sic] if it were not for your ability to write. I feel that if a truthful, dignified and modest film were made of your Hospital at Lambarene an additional service would be given not only to the cause for which you have devoted your life but also to those who do not read books but do go to the films. It would give every strata of society a true sense of values.

If your permission were given I feel sure that the expenses involved would be borne by some film company of note so that all the earnings of such a film could be donated towards a Schweitzer fund for the rehabilitation of Lepers which could finance the mobile team discussed above. I need hardly add that I would be glad to help in these arrangements if you so desire.

I am afraid that ignorant and unqualified observers may, for their own profit attempt to interpret your Lambarene set up in their own ways and so give a twisted idea of the situation. One fully sanctioned documentary film would counteract against any such interference.

Please give this idea your early consideration so that I should know how to carry out my further discussions. I may add that I have discussed this idea with **nobody** so that you need not fear that a negative reply would embarrass me at all.

You will be interested to know that the Students of the University of Jerusalem have indicated to me that they would like to assist your young Doctors in building up a modern medical library at your hospital. They will probably send down a number of books and journals shortly. If there are any specific books or journals that they may want please let me know and I shall be pleased to send their requests through.[47]

[47] Jack Penn, Excerpt from Letter to Schweitzer, 14 May 1956, BC 748 A1.17, UCTL.

In a subsequent letter, Penn mentioned a meeting with WHO in South Africa with an enthusiastic response to his suggestion of mobile units dispatched to treat leprosy, with a possible similar setup for the treatment of elephantiasis.[48] The letter addressed the reports that Penn had received from Lambarene medical staff regarding the patients he had treated while at the hospital. Penn also offered to assemble another team of experts and return to Lambarene to treat the "eye conditions" which were prevalent in the region.[49]

It was only at the end of August that Schweitzer responded to this slew of correspondence, citing "exhaustion" and "writer's cramp" for the delay. In his response, he indicated his pleasure at the prospect of various specialists going to Lambarene but preferred that they not do so *en masse*. This suggests a possible apprehension on the part of Schweitzer of having control over Lambarene medical practices wrested from him. He further refused to consent to the film Penn had envisaged that would result in publicity and possibly funds to support Lambarene, citing a dislike for the "limelight".[50] He concluded by indicating his pleasure at the possibility of books donated by medical students to the hospital and thanked Penn for his efforts. There is an element of weariness in Schweitzer's response as he discussed overseeing a building project, which is in marked contrast to Penn's enthusiasm, "…I am looking forward to the time when these materialistic matters will be behind me. I did not think that I would still have to be dealing with such matters at the age of 80".[51] Schweitzer's brief response also indicated a level of recalcitrance at the changes proposed by Penn. Faced with the lack of co-operation from the revered missionary doctor, Penn's subsequent efforts would be more modest, yet also indicate his continuing commitment to the provision of adequate medical care at the hospital.

[48] Jack Penn, Excerpt from Letter to Schweitzer, 21 June 1956, BC748 A1.21, UCTL.

[49] Jack Penn, Excerpt from Letter to Schweitzer, 16 July 1956, BC 748, A1.26, UCTL.

[50] In 1957—just a year later—a documentary was made of Albert Schweitzer's life with the first half a dramatisation of his early life and the latter half portraying him in Lambarene. Directed by Jerome Hill, *Albert Schweitzer* went on to win an Academy Award the following year, https://www.imdb.com/title/tt0050109/, accessed 25 June 2021.

[51] Albert Schweitzer, Excerpt from Letter by Schweitzer to Penn, 29 August 1956, BC748 A1.29, UCTL.

In September 1956, Penn wrote to Schweitzer requesting permission to send medical personnel on temporary sojourns to Lambarene to assist with the treatment of cases that challenged the capabilities of the permanent staff at the hospital. Penn had already approached Lady Oppenheimer who agreed to create an "Albert Schweitzer Society" to fund the scheme, provided the missionary doctor gave his consent. This would subsequently lead to the dispatch of teams of specialists from South Africa.[52]

In 1957, British anaesthesiologist Dr Bobby Roberts, who was based in Johannesburg, was asked by Harry Oppenheimer to join a South African medical team going to Lambarene to provide medical assistance. Based on Penn's description of conditions at Lambarene, the younger Oppenheimer had sent regular contingents of medical personnel to address the more challenging cases at the hospital. Roberts's experiences of the journey to Lambarene in an Air France Dakota (light-heartedly nicknamed "Air Chance") only a year after Penn's first visit, mirrored the latter's experiences. After numerous stops, they landed at the airport at Lambarene where they were met by Schweitzer and taken by boat to their destination.[53]

The living conditions for the staff were spare with no running water and limited electricity provided by a generator used only for medical procedures. During this three-week stint at Lambarene, Roberts was all too aware of the paucity of adequate medical supplies: a non-functioning and outdated X-ray machine which Schweitzer seemed to have taken little initiative in having repaired as he "did not think it was really necessary", limited blood supplies due to the indigenous population—and closest donors—having contracted various tropical diseases and the use of outmoded methods of administering anaesthetic. Roberts had taken the precaution of bringing with him supplies of anaesthesia as well as a machine to administer them, an "EMO (Epstein Macintosh Oxford) apparatus". He was, however, faced with the hurdle of a senior nurse reluctant to embrace the new technology.[54]

[52] Jack Penn, Excerpt from Letter by Penn to Schweitzer, 11 September 1956, BC 748 A1.41, UCTL.

[53] F.W. Roberts, "Working with Albert Schweitzer", http://www.nigel-roberts.info/Working-with-Schweitzer.htm, accessed 5 August 2020.

[54] Ibid.

While medical professionals found themselves exasperated by conditions at Lambarene, Schweitzer's efforts and charisma attracted numerous adherents termed "Schweitzer addicts". One of these was a young heiress who had joined the Lambarene settlement on a whim and apparently to find a sense of purpose— she was assigned the task of arranging the drugs. Roberts's experiences concurred with those of Penn—Schweitzer was clearly the central figure around which the life of Lambarene revolved. It was his attitude towards a medical practice that influenced the treatment at the hospital and his sense of increasingly outdated paternalism that shaped the interactions with the indigenous people who congregated around Lambarene, "The black man is my brother, therefore I must love him as a brother, but he is my younger brother and he must do as I tell him!".[55]

The Cult of Personality

Schweitzer's obvious reluctance to improve the conditions at Lambarene was attributed by Penn to a "subconscious" desire to emphasise the role of the individual and his sense of mission.[56] Schweitzer was clearly a man of contradiction—self-effacing yet creating a hospital that retained him as its focus and following a personal philosophy from which he refused to deviate. While Penn recognised this ambiguity, he was nevertheless swayed by the image of Schweitzer, using powerful religious imagery in his description of the man, "He has no favourites, but is gentle with everything created by God. Savages and animals of the jungle come to him with trust. He has an appearance worthy of a Michelangelo; a vision worthy of a Moses; and a soul worthy of Christ".[57] While the religious imagery is more overt in his correspondence with Lady Oppenheimer, it is as apparent in his biography. Penn presented an image of a saviour and healer of "savage" and beast alike, who inspired the trust of those he treated and led them into the light of modernity. This would form the backdrop for Penn's sculpture of Schweitzer.

[55] Ibid.

[56] Penn, *The Right to Look Human*, p144.

[57] Jack Penn, Excerpt from Letter to Lady Oppenheimer – 5th April 1956, BC748 A1.10, UCTL.

Inspired by the visage of Schweitzer which Penn described as that "of a handsome and rugged individualist", he was able to persuade Schweitzer to sit so that he could make sketches of him that would be used to create a bronze bust.[58] The bust depicts a face that is lined and care-worn, symbolic of the suffering martyr. While Schweitzer did not see the finished product, Penn sent him a photograph of it and he subsequently wrote to Penn to express his pleasure at the artist's ability to give him "a spiritual view of myself".[59] With Schweitzer's approval, the bust was presented to Schweitzer's alma mater, the University of Strasbourg, at a formal ceremony where tribute was paid to the humanitarian—who did not attend.[60]

The casting of Schweitzer's features in bronze also reflected Penn's own ambivalence towards him and their disagreement over the ideological role of the medical professional in Africa: "He has the gentlest and the saddest eyes I have ever looked into and yet certain parts of his make-up are as hard as granite".[61]

Schweitzer was a representative of the medical missionary as epitomised by David Livingstone in the nineteenth century. Missionaries were an integral part of the "civilising mission" and the mission station became the means by which Western culture, education and medicine were disseminated to the indigenous peoples of Asia and Africa. Through Western medicine, the medical missionary was able to demonstrate the superiority of Western science over indigenous knowledge systems. The healing arts were also associated with Christianity, thereby also serving to propagate religious beliefs.[62] But Schweitzer also departed significantly from this image. Penn was at pains to point out that little time was given to proselytisation and the hospital at Lambarene—rather than being a beacon of Western medicine in the heart of West Africa—aroused instead the criticism of Western-trained medical professionals, Penn included. Schweitzer was also reluctant to promote the creation of a "Schweitzer Institute" to

[58] Penn, *The Right to Look Human*, p140.

[59] Ibid., p143.

[60] Ibid.

[61] Penn, Excerpt from Letter to Di, Joan, John, family and friends, 4 April 1956, BC748 A1.9, UCTL.

[62] Pratik Chakrabarti, *Medicine and Empire, 1600–1960* (Basingstoke, Palgrave Macmillan, 2014), pp129–130.

train doctors to treat specifically African tropical diseases, "He would not consider the suggestion. Anything done after his death would throw out of focus his personal effort".[63] Schweitzer's role in Gabon centred on individual salvation—his own. It was instead the more secular Penn who promoted Western medicine and modernity, even as Schweitzer refused to yield.

Gabon: Post-Schweitzer

Just a few weeks before his death in September 1965, Schweitzer wrote to Penn requesting him to pay another visit to Lambarene, now part of independent Gabon. Penn only received the letter after Schweitzer's death and was unable to comply but was subsequently able to return to Gabon along with prominent South African heart surgeon Christiaan Barnard in 1969.[64] Penn would go on to remark on the resemblance between Barnard and Schweitzer, not just in terms of their physical attributes but due to their background and their characteristics, "...superior intelligence, egocentric and self-assured, with a sense of mission, courageous and honest, and too proud to dissemble".[65]

Less than two years earlier, Barnard had become the face of South African medical achievement by carrying out the first successful heart transplant. In an interesting convergence, it was the Second World War and plastic surgery that provided some of the important research on rejection that is an integral part of the transplant process. This was evident in the work of Medawar and Gibson.[66] The case that marked a seminal moment in the understanding of rejection was of a young woman who had been severely burned after a bomb attack. Taken to Glasgow Royal Infirmary, the men responsible for her treatment at the Glasgow Burns Unit were surgeon Thomas Gibson and a 24-year-old zoologist and graduate of Oxford University, Peter Medawar. Both were attempting to resolve the issue of rejection of skin grafts and the efficacy

[63] Penn, *The Right to Look Human*, p144.

[64] Ibid., p145. Penn would also return to Lambarene after his initial trip in 1956.

[65] Ibid., p148.

[66] James-Brent Styan, *Heartbreaker: Christiaan Barnard and the First Heart Transplant* (Johannesburg and Cape Town, Jonathan Ball Publishers, 2018), p71.

of skin allografts—or skin grafts taken from another individual—particularly important for the treatment of pilots during the Battle of Britain. Conventional belief was that the rejection of skin grafts was due to infection. Their young patient was treated with skin grafts donated by her brother. She subsequently rejected these. Another set of grafts was put in place and the rejection occurred even more quickly. Gibson and Medawar came to an important realisation—rather than infection, rejection was due to the response of her immune system. This was a breakthrough in the understanding of rejection and would not only make an impact on plastic surgery but would underpin organ transplant.[67]

Barnard's biography, portrayed in some media reports as the rags-to-riches story of an impoverished, rural Afrikaner boy achieving the heights of success, seemed to personify the triumphalist spirit of Afrikaner nationalism.[68] Dr Laurie (Lapa) Munnik, a leading figure in the Cape provincial health services who would later serve as Minister for Health, described the heart transplant in December 1967 as a "surgical Sputnik", placing Barnard's success firmly within the context of Cold War rivalry.[69] This made Barnard the ideal ambassador for the scientific prowess of the apartheid state as well as its proposed beneficence for Africa, countering the communist influence on the continent.

Yet the narrative of Barnard's success had papered over the complexities that underlay the operation. Barnard's celebrity status—also noticed by Penn who observed the press attention lavished on the heart surgeon—obscured the contributions made by other members of the research and medical team, including those classified as "Coloured" and "Bantu" in apartheid nomenclature. These figures were prominent in the laboratory experiments conducted on animals, preparatory to the first human procedure. They were not medical doctors, however, and would not have been

[67] James F. George and Laura J. Pinderski, "Peter Medawar and the Science of Transplantation: A Parable", *Journal of Heart Lung Transplant*, International Society for Heart and Lung Transplantation 20, 2001, p927; Thomas E. Starzl, "Peter Brian Medawar: Father of Transplantation", *Journal of the American College of Surgeons*, 180, 3, March 1995, pp332–336; H. Conway, W.H. Reid, J.J. Beaton and D.A. McGrouther, "Thomas Gibson, Plastic Surgeon (1915–93): Allograft Rejection by the Immune System and Prediction of Free Tissue Transplantation", *Journal of Plastic, Reconstructive and Aesthetic Surgery*, 65, 2012, pp1447–1450.

[68] Saul Dubow, *A Commonwealth of Knowledge: Science, Sensibility, and White South Africa, 1820–2000* (Oxford, Oxford University Press, 2006), p263.

[69] Styan, *Heartbreaker*, p115.

permitted to treat white patients.[70] The members of the transplant team itself were ethnically diverse, including the senior anaesthetist, Joseph Ozinsky who from 1967 to 1992, would be involved in approximately a thousand open-heart procedures.[71]

The first heart transplant had necessitated the use of a white donor and recipient to avoid any possible backlash from international circles regarding the use of black donors. To apartheid critics cognisant of the restrictions on political rights and liberties of black South Africans, this would suggest "experimentation on black patients".[72] The third heart transplant, carried out in early January 1968, however, brought the issue of race to the fore. A white dentist, Philip Blaiberg, received the heart of Clive Haupt, a 24-year-old coloured man who had succumbed to a brain haemorrhage. In a country where inter-racial blood transfusions were not permitted, the operation led to a storm of controversy with opinions veering between two extremes: the incongruity of the life of a white man dependent on that of the historically subjugated and whether Blaiberg "would still be classified white".[73]

Nor was Barnard simply a pliant tool of the state. The visit of Penn and Barnard to Gabon had coincided with industrial upheaval in Durban and the resignation of numerous black doctors in protest against their lower salary which was 68% of their white counterparts. While in Gabon, Barnard spoke out against the unjust pay scale whilst urging black doctors to remain at their posts as the government sought to redress the imbalance.[74] As Vanessa Noble has shown, there was an increasing radicalisation amongst black medical students at the Natal Medical School in Durban with members of the SRC in 1966 including Steve Biko. The Black Consciousness Movement had its origins here and the radicalisation was based on the common experience of discrimination and a segregated education system by black students drawn together from all over

[70] Ibid., pp52–54.

[71] Ibid., p84.

[72] Ibid., p89.

[73] Ibid., pp132–137.

[74] "Wrong to Pay by Colour—Barnard", *Rand Daily Mail*, 22 April 1969.

the country.[75] More than an instrument of apartheid propaganda then, Christiaan Barnard's work had highlighted the ambiguities and tensions that marked apartheid South Africa in the 1960s. The propaganda or public relations element was nonetheless a prominent feature of his trip to Gabon.

For his visit to Gabon, Penn had three aims: the first of which was to investigate the camps set up for Biafran refugees. In early 1966, the Nigerian government was subject to a coup that brought to power a largely Igbo-led government. This ethnic group originated in the south of the country and key members of the ousted government hailed from the north. The coup was thus perceived as ethnic conflict, leading to a "counter-coup", attacks on civilian Igbo and the outbreak of outright war in 1967, termed the Nigeria-Biafra war, which lasted until January 1970.[76] Acts of violence carried out against Igbo civilians were considered genocide, resulting in many fleeing both to Gabon and the Ivory Coast, both states having allied themselves to the Biafran attempt to break away from Nigeria and create an independent state.[77] As Kevin O'Sullivan argues, Western aid to the Biafran refugee camp and the role of NGOs such as Oxfam, Christian Aid as well as various missionary organisations in both alleviating and drawing attention to the humanitarian crisis, were symbolic of global action to address suffering. This was reinforced by the increasing media attention focused on the camp. However, the intervention of these organisations also created a new dichotomy in the relationship between the West and Africa in the wake of independence, one that involved both "paternalism" and "dependence".[78] For Penn, the treatment of the Igbo was an indictment of African independence.

[75] Vanessa Noble, *A School of Struggle: Durban's Medical School and the Education of Black Doctors in South Africa* (Scottsville, University of KwaZulu-Natal Press, 2013), pp210–213.

[76] Douglas Anthony, "'Ours Is a War of Survival': Biafra, Nigeria and Arguments About Genocide, 1966–70", *Journal of Genocide Research*, 16, 2–3, 205–225, August 2014, pp205–206.

[77] Thomas J. Hamilton, "5 000 Children Evacuated from Biafra in Civil War will be Repatriated from Gabon and Ivory Coast", *New York Times*, 11 October 1970, https://www.nytimes.com/1970/10/11/archives/5000-children-evacuated-from-biafra-in-civil-war-will-be.html, accessed 6 August 2020.

[78] *Cf* Kevin O'Sullivan, "Humanitarian Encounters: Biafras, NGOs and Imaginings of the Third World in Britain and Ireland, 1967–70", *Journal of Genocide Research*, 16, 2–3, 2014, pp299–315.

When visiting the Igbo refugee camp, Penn gave a heartrending description of the refugee children suffering from malnutrition. Their plight was, however, attributed to the actions of the United Nations (UN) as well as major powers who encouraged the Nigerian "genocide" against the Igbo[79] population. For Penn, these actions were viewed as even more reprehensible due to what he considered the racial superiority of the Igbo, "The Igbos have often been called the Jews of Africa, for they are intelligent and crave for education. If left alone, they could create the only self-viable State in the Continent…"[80] Barnard was described by Penn as being particularly "shocked and horrified" by his visit to the camp, with a desire to return to assist.[81]

The experience of the Igbo related to Penn's second reason for his visit—assessing the independent government of Gabon. Penn's observations were also an indictment of newly independent African states that were in danger of succumbing to communist influence, served as a site of struggle over natural resources and were disinclined towards multiparty democracy. The dominance of the single political party was evident in Gabon with Penn's description of its charismatic president who was inclined to opulence and authoritarianism. Penn's audience with the president was not, however, a simple assessment of the government. He was clearly interested in using science and medicine as a means of fostering ties between the South African government and that of Gabon in line with improving South African "[relations] to Black Africa". President Omar Bongo indicated his willingness to establish ties with South Africa based on "medicine and commerce" and three Gabonese doctors subsequently paid a visit to South Africa—a visit that Penn described as a "social success".[82] Penn's use of science as a means of establishing relations between South Africa and the rest of the African continent has to be contextualised by the priorities of the apartheid state in the 1960s. After the events of Sharpeville and the banning of national liberation movements, the South African state was faced with international condemnation. South Africa left the Commonwealth and declared a republic in

[79] Whereas Penn refers to this group as the "Ibo", they are termed the "Igbo" in current academic literature and it is the latter terminology employed here.

[80] Penn, *The Right to Look Human*, p146.

[81] "Gabon is ready to co-operate with S.A.", *Rand Daily Mail*, 26 April 1969.

[82] Penn, *The Right to Look Human*, pp146–147.

1961. Increasingly internationally isolated, the decade was nevertheless the period at which apartheid reached its zenith, bringing with it unparalleled prosperity for the minority white population. Simultaneously, the growth of independent states in Africa presented the possibility and threat of South Africa being surrounded by potentially hostile neighbours. As a result, there was a desire to reach out to these states to establish friendly relations and establish South African leadership in Africa—and Penn was evidently part of this.

Philippe Doumenc had arranged the visit in response to an invitation by the Corps Medical Gabonaise. He reported that the motive for Penn and Barnard's visit to Gabon was "to establish links between South Africa and a black African country which was sympathetic to the Republic".[83] According to Doumenc, the visitors were greeted by a cheering throng at Libreville Airport and at a later event, African doctors drank a toast to the Republic and its leader, Prime Minister John Vorster. The success of Penn and Barnard's medical ambassadorial roles was evident by Bongo's willingness to work with South Africa "in the economic and medical fields" and the assurance that Gabon would "never oppose South Africa in any international assembly".[84] South African attempts to build relations with other African states—as evident in the trip to Gabon—can also be contextualised within an increasingly public division between the *verkrampte* (or conservative) and *verligte* (literally meaning "enlightened") elements within the National Party in South Africa. This split was evident with Vorster's leadership espousing unity between English and Afrikaans-speaking white South Africans and a willingness to consider diplomatic ties with African states that was in contrast to the challenges posed by conservative elements such as Andries Treunicht.[85] According to an editorial appearing in the *Rand Daily Mail*, the *verkramptes* were a minority and the visit to Gabon—and perhaps later overtures to other African states as well as prospective economic ties with Latin America and Mauritius—indicated an end to South African "isolationism" driven in part by the country's scientific and technological development.[86]

[83] "Gabon is ready to co-operate with S.A.".

[84] Ibid.

[85] James Barber and John Barrett, *South Africa's Foreign Policy: The Search for Status and Security, 1945–1988* (Cambridge University Press, 1990), pp109–110.

[86] "Towards a Climax", *Rand Daily Mail*, 28 April 1969.

For Penn, the culmination of his trip to Gabon was his return to Lambarene where he found the situation much altered. There no longer seemed to be any place for the philosophy of Albert Schweitzer in post-independent Gabon. Prior to his journey, Penn was exposed to the thinking of the Gabonese political leaders who relegated Schweitzer's efforts to a colonial past defined by inequality, "They went so far as to state that Schweitzer kept the hospital in a primitive state in order to indicate his superiority over the Gabonese—certainly a complex and twisted interpretation".[87] Penn's assessment of the ingratitude of Africans can be traced to what he believed to be the cause of Schweitzer's own disillusionment, "I have the impression that he is deeply disappointed with his impact on the African and that his message has not reached them for in spite of giving his life to their welfare they are lazy and unappreciative".[88]

Penn's second trip to Lambarene was made in vastly different circumstances with a motorboat taking him to his destination. While the original structures were still in evidence, they were being replaced by contemporary buildings which to Penn, only highlighted the unsuitability of Schweitzer's old hospital. Albert Schweitzer's work was being slowly expunged and Penn was clearly ambivalent about it—on the one hand, the modern version was preferable to what had existed in the past and Penn had himself attempted in vain to effect the transition earlier. Yet there was a sense of erasure and of loss as Lambarene engaged in "eliminating the spirit of Schweitzer from its core".[89]

While acknowledging that Schweitzer's role would be marginalised in an independent Gabon eager to break from its colonial past, Penn would subsequently make overtures to prominent figures in Paris to initiate an Albert Schweitzer Prize.[90]

Jack Penn's interaction with and perception of Albert Schweitzer reveals as much about Penn as it does about Schweitzer. The latter represented a sense of paternalism and a vision of white leadership in Africa, as he introduced the benefits of Western medicine to a population in dire need of it. Yet the combination of the environment and its people as well

[87] Penn, *The Right to Look Human*, p147.

[88] Jack Penn, Excerpt from Letter to Di, Joan, John, family and friends, 4 April 1956, BC748 A1.9, UCTL.

[89] Penn, *The Right to Look Human*, p147.

[90] Ibid., p148.

as Schweitzer's idiosyncrasies meant that Lambarene fell short of the standards of modern medicine espoused by Penn. Despite Penn's attempts to broaden Schweitzer's project and thus make a significant claim for the dominance of white medical expertise and guidance in Africa, he was thwarted by Schweitzer himself. It is ironic that the modernisation of Lambarene would only occur after independence. Penn's ultimate assessment of Schweitzer therefore reflected an admiration that bordered on the hagiographic but one that was nevertheless tinged with a hint of frustration, "Dr Schweitzer framed his existence in Africa within definite boundaries and kept to those boundaries stubbornly, courageously and even ruthlessly, but always honestly".[91]

[91] Ibid., p144.

CHAPTER 8

Fallen Blossoms: Hiroshima, Nagasaki, Nagashima and an Engagement with Modernity

Physician Michihiko Hachiya was at home on the morning of 6 August 1945 when he was surprised by a bright light. His subsequent experiences were of disorientation—staggering outside, bleeding, his clothes gone, his home almost destroyed.[1] When he reached the hospital, he was struck by the silence of people making their way there, a sign of their utter shock and incomprehension:

> There were the shadowy forms of people, some of whom looked like walking ghosts. Others moved as though in pain, like scarecrows, their arms held out from their bodies with forearms and hands dangling. These

[1] Michihiko Hachiya, *Hiroshima Diary: The Journal of a Japanese Physician, August 6–September 30, 1945*, Warner Well (translator and editor) (Chapel Hill and London, The University of North Carolina Press, 1955, 1995) pp1–2.

The title is paraphrased from a poem penned by "Hiroshima Maiden", Michiko Sako in Henry Kamm, "A 'Hiroshima Maiden' Conquers Bitterness", *New York Times*, 22 May 1977, The *New York Times* Archives, https://www.nytimes.com/1977/05/22/archives/a-hiroshima-maiden-conquers-bitterness-a-hiroshima-maiden-overcomes.html?searchResultPosition=1, accessed 10 August 2020.

S. Chetty, *Reconstructive Surgery and Modernisation in Twentieth-Century South Africa*, Medicine and Biomedical Sciences in Modern History, https://doi.org/10.1007/978-3-031-38673-2_8

> people puzzled me until I suddenly realized that they had been burned and were holding their arms out to prevent the painful friction of raw surfaces rubbing together.[2]

Michiko Sako was thirteen years old in August 1945 and living in Hiroshima. Along with other children in her class, she was about one and a half kilometres from the epicentre of the atomic bomb explosion. Without shelter, she experienced severe facial burns from the blast, lacking the ability to smile and unable to close her eyes. So disfigured, her grandmother removed all the mirrors so that she could not see her own reflection, Michiko was a recluse for the next decade, writing poetry to articulate her psychological pain.[3]

In 1955 she was one of the "Hiroshima Maidens", a contingent of 25 Japanese women injured in the attack and sent to the United States for treatment and reconstructive surgery to address the burns and the resultant scar tissue. These women were housed with American families for the duration of their treatment.[4]

Their arrival in the United States aroused mixed feelings, both in the United States as well as Japan. As Penn commented, the Japanese were aggrieved at their removal to the United States for treatment as well as the selection of only women.[5] As Michiko pointed out however, facial disfigurement had severe repercussions for women in a society that valued physical beauty, subjecting them to discrimination that did not apply to the men who were similarly afflicted.[6]

The "Hiroshima Maidens" project was the brainchild of Norman Cousins who would also be instrumental in sending a group of Polish concentration camp survivors to the United States for treatment.[7] Cousins had begun as a reporter with the *New York Evening Post* in

[2] Ibid., p4.

[3] Kamm, "A 'Hiroshima Maiden'".

[4] Ibid.

[5] Jack Penn, *The Right to Look Human: An Autobiography* (Johannesburg, Hugh Keartland Publishers, 1976), p149.

[6] Kamm, "A 'Hiroshima Maiden'".

[7] William H. Honan, "B. E. Simon, 'Hiroshima Maidens' Surgeon, 87", *New York Times*, 5 August 1991, The *New York Times* Archives, https://www.nytimes.com/1999/08/05/nyregion/b-e-simon-hiroshima-maidens-surgeon-87.html?searchResultPosition=2, accessed 10 August 2020.

1934 and became editor of the *Saturday Review of Literature* in 1940. As editor-in-chief of the publication in 1942, he ushered in sweeping changes, focusing on contemporary issues—which was reflected in his own writing. Shortly after the atomic bombing of Nagasaki in 1945, he wrote an editorial appearing in the *Saturday Review* which was later expanded into a full-length book, *Modern Man is Obsolete*.[8] In the piece, Cousins reflected on the destructive capability of science with the attacks on Hiroshima and Nagasaki representing a sombre indictment of war which was viewed as a product of humankind's inherently "competitive nature". This competitive streak that could be traced throughout history, rendered "man obsolete" in the modern era unless there was an acknowledgement of the potential abuse of science as well as a corresponding will to change.[9] With an inherently optimistic view of human nature in terms of its ability to reflect and its capacity for moral improvement, Cousins personified change through his attempts to address the harsh effects of war. It was this thinking that underpinned the treatment of the Polish women—known as the Ravensbruck Lapins—as well as the Hiroshima Maidens. Cousins and his wife, Ellen, would eventually adopt one of the latter, Shigeko Sasamori.[10]

The "Hiroshima Maidens" were treated at Mount Sinai Hospital in New York by plastic surgeons who volunteered their services. In total 140 surgical procedures were performed, many focused on facial reconstruction, and patients underwent multiple operations. Shigeko Sasamori remembered, "One third of my body was burned, especially my neck and hands...Dr [Bernard Everett] Simon and his colleagues operated on me more than a dozen times. I was then able to marry and give birth to a son".[11] This was a theme that would echo in Penn's work—the importance of reconstructive surgery in allowing patients to lead "normal" lives which, in the case of the "Hiroshima Maidens", took on a gendered dimension as well.

Just as the use of atomic weapons against Japan had led to Cousins reflecting on the nature of humankind, the same was true of Jack Penn.

[8] https://biography.yourdictionary.com/norman-cousins, accessed 14 August 2020.

[9] Norman Cousins, "Modern Man is Obsolete", Editorial obtained from https://rachelcarsoncouncil.org/wp-content/uploads/2018/01/RCC.Cousins.-SatRev.ModernMan.pdf, accessed 14 August 2020.

[10] https://biography.yourdictionary.com/norman-cousins.

[11] Honan, "B. E. Simon, 'Hiroshima Maidens' Surgeon, 87".

He remembered the historical moment on 6 August 1945 when he had heard the news—as he was operating on a pilot who had severe burns. The moment caused Penn to reflect on humanity's ambivalent relationship with science where technological progress had exceeded "wisdom".[12]

Cousins approached Penn to travel to Hiroshima in 1957. Penn's response to the request was a qualified one and reflected his desire for control over treatment, a desire that had been as evident in his clashes with the military bureaucracy and hierarchy years earlier. Penn demanded and was granted the freedom to choose a team that he would lead. Subsequent investigation of American candidates suggested to Penn that there were no anaesthetists familiar with his preferred low-pressure anaesthesia.[13]

Low-pressure or hypotensive anaesthesia was the innovation of George Edward Hale Enderby. During the Second World War, Hale Enderby had worked at Basingstoke under Gillies and in 1951, at East Grinstead with McIndoe. The development of new drugs in the late forties, especially related to muscle relaxation, underpinned hypotensive anaesthesia. While the drop in blood pressure was considered undesirable, Hale Enderby believed in its efficacy in reducing blood flow and hence bleeding during surgical procedures. The anaesthetist was also responsible for the "head up tilt of the operating table" that also reduced blood flow and was particularly apposite for plastic surgeons due to the focus on operations on the neck and head. First publishing his use of hypotensive anaesthesia in 1950, he went on to tour the world, giving lectures on the efficacy of the revolutionary—and controversial—method.[14]

Hale Enderby visited South Africa and Penn was quick to adopt the method in his private practice, demonstrating over the course of more than twenty thousand procedures, that low-pressure anaesthesia had little adverse effect, such as the brain damage that deterred more cautious anaesthetists from adopting it.[15] Bental and Penn co-authored an article on hypotensive anaesthesia based on their extensive use of the method. It

[12] Penn, *The Right to Look Human*, p29.

[13] Ibid., p149.

[14] "George Edward Hale Enderby: Pioneer and Architect of Modern Anaesthesia", *The BMJ*, https://www.bmj.com/content/suppl/2004/05/20/328.7450.1263.DC1, accessed 4 February 2020.

[15] Penn, *The Right to Look Human*, pp128–129.

presented challenges where it was difficult to reduce the blood pressure of younger, more able-bodied patients and they were certainly aware of the complications that could result from its use. Its benefits however, such as a reduced operating time, increased surgical precision and lessening of bruising compensated for the potential complications which could be addressed through a judicial selection of patients, careful monitoring of blood pressure throughout the operation and good post-operative care. It required "team work".[16] And Penn had an established team so he therefore requested the use of his own anaesthetist, Speedy Bental, as well as theatre nurse, Marie Roux, as the salary of prospective nurses exceeded the budget available. His South African team would provide their services on a purely voluntary basis.[17]

While Penn travelled to Japan at the behest of Cousins, he was also doing so as a South African who would eventually use medical knowledge to promote South African scientific expertise. There were strong trading links between the two countries that dated to the First World War. By 1913 however, a trade imbalance which favoured Japan coincided with anti-Asian sentiment in South Africa and the Immigration Act of 1913 was used to restrict Japanese economic influence. Almost two decades later however, as the Great Depression hit and South African wool exports were taking strain, Japan was willing to absorb wool exports. The trade-off was the recognition of Japanese citizens as having equal status to that of white South Africans as well as the removal of the restrictions that applied to the Japanese under the Immigration Act.[18] After the Second World War, a devastated Japan embarked on a formidable process of economic recovery by taking advantage of the importation of resources from Africa as well as trading opportunities with South Africa.[19] Four years after Penn's visit, South Africa faced international condemnation after the Sharpeville Massacre, making it even more amenable to strengthening economic ties with Japan. With the formation of the Republic of South Africa in 1961, the Japanese were designated "honorary whites"

[16] Jack Penn and H. Bental, "Hypotensive Anaesthesia in Plastic Surgery: A Report on 500 Cases", *South African Medical Journal*, 9 May 1953, pp405–406.

[17] Penn, *The Right to Look Human*, p149.

[18] Richard T. Payne, "Japan's South Africa Policy: Political Rhetoric and Economic Realities", *African Affairs*, 86, 343, 167–178, April 1987.

[19] Chris Alden, "The Chrysanthemum and the Protea: Reinventing Japanese-South African Relations after Apartheid", *African Affairs*, 101, 365–386, 2002, pp366–367.

and thus not subject to the legal and economic discrimination experienced by other "non-white" groups.[20] Over the ensuing decades, Japan would maintain its ties with the apartheid state, importing the minerals with which the sub-Saharan country was amply endowed and which were necessary to drive Japan's economic development. In return Japan exported to South Africa the technological consumer end-products such as cars and appliances.[21]

On agreeing to lead his contingent to Japan, Penn found himself unwillingly part of a wave of media attention centred on the controversy about the American use of atomic weapons against Japan. Yet to prepare for his visit, Penn had read extensively on the circumstances that contextualised the decision. He was moreover acquainted with the personal experiences of the victims of the atomic blasts, having read Hachiya's *Hiroshima Diary*. Although not overtly stated in his biography, there is an indication that the use of atomic weapons could be economically and militarily justified—the money spent on the development of atomic weaponry could only be defensible to the American taxpayer if these weapons were deployed. The military rationale was even more compelling—the fears of a possible Japanese-Russian alliance in the latter days of the war necessitated the United States acting pre-emptively to remove the Japanese threat and force a surrender.[22] Further, the use of the atomic bombs precluded the invasion of Japan which would likely have incurred a far higher death toll on both sides.[23] However, Penn refused to be publicly drawn into the debate, fearing his views would be a "condemnation of the very people who sent me".[24] Yet it is also important to note that Penn's theoretical understanding of the use of atomic weapons as a strategic military tool sat uneasily with his indictment of atomic warfare, especially when confronted with its very real repercussions.

He exhibited an empathetic understanding of these repercussions from early on. Upon his arrival in Hiroshima, an early stop for Penn

[20] Payne, "Japan's South Africa Policy", pp168–169.

[21] Ibid., pp169–170.

[22] Penn's reasoning here should also be contexualised by the period during which he wrote his biography decades later and his pressing concerns with communist expansion during the Cold War.

[23] Penn, *The Right to Look Human*, p150.

[24] Ibid., pp149–150.

was Hiroshima Peace Memorial Park. The focal point of the park is the Hiroshima Peace Memorial (Genbaku Dome). It is the remains of the Hiroshima Prefectural Industrial Promotional Hall which was the only building left standing near the epicentre of the blast and serves as mute testimony to the destruction wrought by the atomic bomb—"Genbaku" being the Japanese word for the atomic bomb.[25] Part of the park is the cenotaph which was the work of architect, Kenzō Tange.[26] It is to the latter that Penn paid particular attention, "The main memorial was a simple arch, the ultimate in good taste, and characteristic of Japanese simplicity in such things".[27] He would be less complimentary about the Nagasaki memorial which was dismissively described as "rather heavy and hideous" and not in keeping with Japanese "taste".[28]

The Hiroshima arch, however, was more than a reflection of "simplicity" in Japanese culture and instead suggestive of a complex engagement with modernity—that had marked Japan since Commodore Perry's arrival in the mid-nineteenth century. The architect, Tange, was part of the modernist school yet also incorporated "traditional" elements in his work, "Creative work is expressed in our time as a union of technology and humanity".[29] While the arch therefore indicates minimalism, it was also designed in homage to the clay saddles that were found in Japanese tombs.[30]

Penn was moved by the cenotaph yet also considered how it departed from his own vision for a memorial to the Hiroshima dead. He would realise his mental image when he returned to South Africa, casting in bronze a sculpture of a mother and child that he named "Hiroshima". The sculpture depicted a woman cradling her infant—which symbolised "the future generations". The woman is wearing clothing that is torn and possibly burned, indicative of Penn's experience with Hiroshima victims

[25] "Hiroshima Peace Memorial (Genbaku Dome)", https://whc.unesco.org/en/list/775/, accessed 13 August 2020.

[26] https://www.britannica.com/place/Hiroshima-Japan#ref289199, accessed 13 August 2020.

[27] Penn, *The Right to Look Human*, p153.

[28] Ibid., p157.

[29] AD Editorial Team, "Spotlight: Kenzō Tange", 4 September 2019, https://www.archdaily.com/270043/happy-birthday-kenzo-tange, accessed 13 August 2020.

[30] https://www.britannica.com/place/Hiroshima-Japan#ref289199.

where injury was largely caused by clothing catching fire.[31] The sculpture follows Western conventions in the depiction of mother and child, even as the woman looks to the left and upward—from whence death came. It therefore was not as far removed from Tange's depiction with its amalgamation of "tradition"—albeit a European artistic tradition that can be traced as far back as the religious iconography of the Renaissance and even earlier—and the modern epitomised by the atomic bomb. As with the "Hiroshima Maidens", Penn emphasised the civilian casualties of Hiroshima and women in particular, with the defining aspects of their femininity—their beauty, their role as mothers—negatively affected. It was the role of reconstructive surgery to restore this.

The effects of the atomic bombs on the civilian population were of great interest and Hiroshima and Nagasaki presented a unique opportunity for scientific and medical study. A month after the blasts and mere weeks after the Japanese surrender, the Americans had already assembled three medical teams, drawn from the Army, Navy and Army Corps of Engineers, to study the effects on the civilian population. This initial core would be expanded and incorporate Japanese scientists, eventually becoming the Atomic Bomb Casualty Commission.[32] Collaboration between American and Japanese scientists was undermined by language and cultural differences, a sense of mistrust as well as the tensions implicit in the relationship between the victor and the defeated. These factors were exacerbated as scientists engaged with the civilian population.[33] Most controversial however, was the "No-Treatment policy". The Atomic Bomb Casualty Commission was a purely research-orientated body which meant that the medical personnel employed by the Commission were not permitted to provide medical assistance to the victims. The Commission was subjected to criticism for reducing patients to objects of scientific study. For many Japanese it was a sign of dehumanisation. Moreover, by focusing on pure science rather than healing, the impression was that the Americans were distancing themselves from any acts suggestive of expiation. From the American perspective however, the "No-Treatment

[31] Penn, *The Right to Look Human*, pp153–154.

[32] Gerald F. O'Malley, "The Grave is Wide: The Hibakusha of Hiroshima and Nagasaki and the Legacy of the Atomic Bomb Casualty Commission and the Radiation Effects Research Foundation", *Clinical Toxicology*, 54, 6, 526–530, 2016, pp526–527.

[33] Ibid., pp527–528.

policy" was a means of ensuring the objectivity of the data.[34] Scientific disinterest, however, did little to alleviate the human suffering and Penn's work in Japan was a means of remedying this.

In consultation with the various hospitals as well as the administrators of the city, a decision was taken to have Penn work on a rotational schedule between five hospitals. Prospective patients were then requested to travel to these hospitals and make an appointment. To Penn's surprise, he was not as inundated as expected with only eighty-four patients in total. He attributed the low number to the lower survival rate, painting a horrific picture of people dying from falling debris, third-degree burns, radiation sickness and drowning as they attempted to escape. His patients then, were those fortunate enough to live some distance from the epicentre as well as escape the secondary effects of the blast.[35]

While treating his patients, Penn exhibited a scientific interest in the specific injuries incurred by the atomic bombs such as radiation poisoning and related to his area of expertise, burns. The latter were largely of a superficial nature however, if dark clothing was worn, this absorbed the heat, caught fire and led to more serious burns. Those wearing white clothing were more fortunate as their clothing reflected the heat. Moreover, burns tended to be focused on the back as they turned away from the blast in an attempt to shield themselves. In this way, Penn was able to determine some of the injurious effects of the atomic bomb. Serious burns were also caused by the fires that had broken out in the city.[36] Penn also determined that the burns were confined to the skin with little penetration to the muscle and bone and that there was a period between the explosion and its effects when "patients were able to protect themselves to a certain extent by curling up in a sort of foetal position". There also appeared to be little difference between atomic burns and regular burns.[37]

Penn and his staff had two aims in Hiroshima—the first was the treatment of survivors and the second was the provision of reconstructive surgery skills to Japanese medical staff. In the case of the former,

[34] Ibid., p528.

[35] Penn, *The Right to Look Human*, p154.

[36] Ibid., p153.

[37] Jack Penn, "Hiroshima and After", *Transactions of the Association of Plastic Surgeons of Southern Africa*, 3, 21, 500–509, 12 October 1957, pp503–505, 508, AMUW.

his methods were relatively simple and dealt largely with the scar tissue formed on the burns. In most cases, the scar was surgically removed, and a skin graft was placed over the affected area. A key concern for burn victims was the formation of keloids. These form over a wound either soon after injury or later and may exceed the area of the wound itself. These growths can cause some discomfort and as with the Hiroshima survivors, they appeared to be particularly prevalent on the upper body. Moreover, while the cause of their formation is still not clearly understood, they tend to be less likely to form in populations termed Caucasian.[38] Penn challenged the orthodoxy that the scars that had formed on the Hiroshima survivors were keloid in nature, considering them to be largely hypertrophic and a result of either infection of the wound or the inadequacy of the skin graft application.[39] A hypertrophic scar is scar tissue formed directly over the site of injury with varying thickness that over time, becomes less prominent.[40] The latter, due to being less hardened than keloids, proved less of a challenge for Penn who applied skin grafts to the affected areas. Ironically, it was the delay of medical treatment that made Penn's work easier. The intervening twelve years had "softened" the scars thus requiring less drastic surgery—the use of "local flap adjustments" rather than the "massive flap surgery" that would have been necessary if they had undergone plastic surgery a decade earlier. Moreover, there was very little need for pedicle grafts.[41] His reconstructive work took approximately six weeks and he then moved on to assisting with the treatment of leprosy sufferers before travelling to Nagasaki.[42]

Penn's experience of working in Hiroshima was positive. Interpreters served as go-betweens between doctor and patient, but Penn also acquired rudimentary Japanese to facilitate communication. For him, the barriers of race, class and culture were ephemeral when compared to the common aim of easing suffering. Patients were co-operative and Japanese doctors proved keen to adopt Penn's techniques.[43] On his arrival in

[38] Amanda Oakley, "Keloid and Hypertrophic Scar", *Dermnet NZ*, https://dermnetnz.org/topics/keloids-and-hypertrophic-scar/, accessed 24 August 2020.

[39] Penn, *The Right to Look Human*, p155.

[40] Oakley, "Keloid and Hypertrophic Scar".

[41] Penn, "Hiroshima and After", pp507–508.

[42] Penn, *The Right to Look Human*, p155.

[43] Ibid., p156.

Hiroshima, he realised that training was paramount—in the intervening twelve years since the atomic bomb explosion, there had been no attempt at plastic surgery as there were no trained plastic surgeons available. During his time in Japan, he would train some one hundred Japanese doctors in the basic skills necessary to carry out plastic and reconstructive surgery.[44]

Penn also made the acquaintance of *Hiroshima Diary* author, Michihiko Hachiya, who came to exemplify for the South African the spirit of service that he held dear, with the proceeds from the sale of the book going towards the education of children orphaned by the bomb, "The actions of such gentle, quiet men give life on this planet a meaning".[45] After two months in Hiroshima, Penn described the moving scenes at the railway station where both medical staff and patients assembled, bowing in unison to bid him farewell.[46]

In Nagasaki, Penn found a similar pattern of injury to that of Hiroshima—although at twelve, the numbers were even less, due largely to the lower death toll. Despite the last however, Penn would offer a greater indictment of the bombing of Nagasaki. Part of this may have stemmed from his interaction with the Japanese Professor of Surgery with whom he worked and who had had both his young sons killed, leaving behind little trace other than a belt buckle. Penn emphasised that the Americans had missed the military installations with the bomb falling instead on the valley that housed the universities and schools, thus taking a disproportionately high toll on the youth.[47]

In addition to the effects of the bombing, Penn also paid attention to Nagasaki's cultural and historical past. Christianity had made greater inroads into Nagasaki than elsewhere in the country due to a more extended period of contact with the West.[48] Under the rule of the formidable Tokugawa from the early seventeenth century, Japan had been able to control and dictate the terms of European interaction with the

[44] Val Carter-Johnson, "SA Plastic Surgeon Relives A-bomb Horrors", *Sunday Times*, 10 August 1980, File: Biography—Jack Penn, AMUW.

[45] Penn, *The Right to Look Human*, p32.

[46] Ibid., p156.

[47] Ibid., p157.

[48] Ibid., p156.

country. Concerned about the influence of Christian missionaries, particularly the Spanish and Portuguese, the Japanese constructed the island of Deshima to house the Portuguese. This lasted for three years until the Portuguese were driven out. The Dutch then occupied Deshima in 1640.[49] The Europeans at Deshima were themselves objects of curiosity with Japanese illustrations of them at work and play and European physicians also provided the Japanese with early and rudimentary knowledge of Western medicine.[50] A German surgeon, Casper Schamberger, began treating and training the Japanese in Western medicine with a particularly adept Japanese surgeon, Kawaguchi Ryon, spreading these techniques much further afield over the ensuing decades. Four decades later, surgeon Engelbert Kaempfer's medical skills (along with his ready access to European liquor) allowed him rare access to the Japanese landscape and his writings became the authoritative texts for Europeans, providing a "window" into Japanese geography, flora and medicines.[51] While curiosity would eventually outweigh caution, not all Japanese were enamoured by Western ideas with some warning against the adoption of Christianity as well as European "novel gadgets and rare medicines". These were seen as potentially subversive and serving as a prelude to conquest. An opposing view was that it was only through the adoption of Western technology that Japan could hope to retain its independence and effectively defend against Western incursion, a lesson that the Chinese had failed to learn.[52]

By the mid-nineteenth century however, Japan was forced increasingly to accept Western trading concessions, particularly on the part of the Americans—but later, by the European powers as well. These changes were accompanied by the fall of the Tokugawa shogunate, the ending of feudalism in Japan and the elements of government put in place to underpin the creation of a nation state. This modernisation also occurred

[49] Jayant S. Joshi and Rajesh Kumar, "The Dutch Physicians at Dejima or Deshima and the Rise of Western Medicine in Japan", *Proceedings of the Indian History Congress*, 63, 1062–1072, 2002, p1063.

[50] William G. Beasley, *The Rise of Modern Japan: Political, Economic and Social Change Since 1850* (New York, St Martin's Press, 1990), p22.

[51] Joshi and Kumar, "The Dutch Physicians at Dejima", pp1063–1064.

[52] Beasley, *The Rise of Modern Japan*, pp24–25.

in the areas of the military, education and science and technology with Japan embracing the developments of the Industrial Revolution.[53]

The practice of medicine underwent extensive modernisation as well. By 1870, Germany was at the forefront of scientific medicine—with an emphasis on empiricism, proof and the collection of data that would influence the Americans. The Germans were the first to both accept and implement Lister's views on sterilisation in operating theatres.[54] It was also in 1870, during its process of modernisation, that Japan sent thirteen medical students to Germany and seven years later, established its own medical school, initially using German professors until the Japanese had acquired sufficient expertise to fulfil the teaching requirements—which they subsequently did by the turn of the century. The Japanese focus on sanitation in military medicine meant that for the first time, more soldiers died from actual war wounds than from infection—in contrast to the mortality ratios incurred by most armies throughout history. Japan's success at adopting modern medical practice gave it a singular advantage over Russia, contributing to its victory.[55]

The Japanese process of modernisation set it on a very different path from other territories in Asia and Africa that had been confronted by European imperialism. Japan itself became an imperial power, defeating the Chinese in the late nineteenth century and defeating Russia in 1905, the first non-Western country to triumph in modern warfare. Modernisation and militarisation would also set the Japanese on the path to the Second World War—culminating in the bombing of Hiroshima and Nagasaki. Penn also incorporated in his assessment a cultural tendency of subservience to strong leadership.[56] While modernisation did not preclude authoritarianism as was evident in the case of Nazi Germany or the Stalinist Soviet Union, it was less a cultural bent towards strong leadership that shaped the path of modernisation of Japan.

It was instead a fervent avowal of modernisation—that became almost ideological in nature—that defined Japan in the pre-war period. With the convergence of Confucianist thinking and Japanese Protestantism, an

[53] R. Taggart Murphy, *Japan and the Shackles of the Past* (Oxford, Oxford University Press, 2014), pp57–64.

[54] Richard A. Gabriel, *Between Flesh and Steel: A History of Military Medicine from the Middle Ages to the War in Afghanistan* (Lincoln, Potomac Books, 2016), p180.

[55] Ibid., pp203–204.

[56] Penn, *The Right to Look Human*, p33.

emphasis was placed on a Spartan lifestyle devoted to the rewards of hard labour. Not only was this portrayed as part of a cultural mindset but also key to modernisation. And culture was secondary to the all-consuming modernisation with the abolition of "the evil customs of the past" that had hindered Japan from becoming a modern power.[57] Modernisation was harnessed to nationalism.

Science and medicine remained a significant part of the modernisation programme with religious sects that had arisen in the twentieth century repressed for being "superstitious" and engaging in "spiritual healing" that contradicted modern medical practice. They were a particular target of the League for Women's Suffrage who wanted instead the widespread implementation of "scientific" medical practices.[58] Spearheaded by a new middle-class elite—who had replaced the feudal samurai—widespread reforms were initiated to introduce Western-style modernity in terms of diet, dress, work and even encourage the adoption of American appliances. In the 1920s and 1930s efforts were made by women's organisations, religious reformers, intellectuals and bureaucrats to encourage both urban and rural Japanese to adopt "rationality" and as was the case in the West, women were encouraged to become "scientific mothers", adopting rationality in the home and in child-rearing.[59]

On a darker note, the forces of science and technology were harnessed to war. As Japan went about a process of imperialist expansion, occupying Manchuria which was renamed Manchukuo, experiments related to germ and chemical warfare were conducted on the resident Chinese population.[60] With the Japanese defeat and American occupation in 1945, the process of modernisation continued but with the American-influenced move towards liberalism.[61] Scientific and technological development was geared towards the economy and society and away from the military.

[57] Sheldon Garon, "Rethinking Modernization and Modernity in Japanese History: A Focus on State-Society Relations", *The Journal of Asian Studies*, 53, 2, 346–366, May 1994, pp349, 354.

[58] Ibid., p353.

[59] Ibid., pp356, 360.

[60] Bill Sewell, "Reconsidering the Modern in Japanese History: Modernity in the Service of the Prewar Japanese Empire", p285, https://www.researchgate.net/publication/254167793, accessed 25 August 2020.

[61] Michael Auslin, "Japan's Endless Search for Modernity: What the anniversary of the Meiji Restoration Tells us About the Country's Uncertain Future", *The Atlantic*, 3

Modernisation was therefore as significant to Japan's post-war recovery as it had been in the interwar period and the overwhelmingly positive reception to Penn's efforts by the Japanese was a significant part of this.

With the completion of his work on Hiroshima survivors, Penn turned his attention to leprosy—a condition with which he already had some familiarity after his sojourn in Lambarene in West Africa. He was permitted to visit the island of Nagashima, site of the National Leprosarium Nagashima Aiseien. In 1930 the Japanese Public Health Bureau made provision for the fifteen thousand Japanese diagnosed with leprosy. The National Leprosarium was founded in the same year on Nagashima Island and additional leprosaria were created during the 1940s. From its inception, the National Leprosarium attracted visitors including the District Secretary of the American Leprosy Mission as well as an Indian doctor, Isaac Santra in 1934. These visitors gave favourable reports of the leprosarium which was under the control of Dr Kensuke Mitsuda. Strict control was maintained on the island with the belongings of prospective patients sterilised, autopsies performed on the deceased and voluntary vasectomies performed on married men.[62]

Later accounts by the inhabitants of Nagashima were however, imbued with a sense of isolation and the discrimination experienced by those afflicted with leprosy which belied the idealised image of the leprosarium. In 1948, fourteen-year-old Shinji Nakao who had been diagnosed with leprosy was taken to the island. Designated Patient 4973 on his arrival—a designation that was used throughout his internment—Nakao, along other patients, endured a process of dehumanisation where they:

> ...were taken into quarantine, stripped of their clothes and valuables and photographed, before being made to lower themselves into a bath of hot water and cresol disinfectant. They spent a week to 10 days being observed in hospital wards, segregated by sex, age and the severity of their symptoms.[63]

January 2018, https://www.theatlantic.com/international/archive/2018/01/japan-abe-meiji-restoration-china/549536/, accessed 25 August 2020.

62 "Nagashima (Japan)", https://leprosyhistory.org/geographical_region/site/nagashima, accessed 24 August 2020.

63 Justin McCurry, "'Like Entering a Prison': Japan's Leprosy Sufferers Reflect on Decades of Pain", *The Guardian*, 13 April 2016, https://www.theguardian.com/world/2016/apr/14/like-entering-a-prison-japans-leprosy-sufferers-sue-government-for-decades-of-pain, accessed 24 August 2020.

Nakao was placed in a dormitory of seventy children and likened his experiences there to a "prison". Further, under legislation implemented in 1953, leprosy sufferers were forcibly held in isolation and quarantine facilities. This was built on existing policy that had been in place before the Second World War and would continue for decades until the law was repealed in 1996—yet drugs had existed for the successful treatment of leprosy sufferers from the mid-twentieth century. The accounts of patients being compelled to endure sterilisations and abortions, the exploitation of their labour and their confinement for infractions painted a very different picture to that witnessed by Penn—and other international visitors.[64]

Penn encountered a number of patients while on Nagashima Island, with a particular incident making enough of an impression on him to be recorded in his memoirs. He examined a slightly built man who, through the ravages of leprosy, had lost an eye, both feet and had the use of only one hand. His constant companion was another sufferer—a larger man, completely blind who had lost both his hands but with his lower limbs intact. In what Penn describes as an act of "symbiosis", the larger man carried on his back the smaller, providing mobility to both while his companion provided limited sight. An extremely touching story, it was used by Penn to indict self-serving individuals who lacked an ethos of service. The notion of service underpinned Penn's assessment of the leprosarium with his description of the director who was described as having devoted sixty years of his career to the settlement. The image portrayed was of a harmonious environment with a "remarkable atmosphere of *esprit de corps* as both patients and staff carried out their duties in relaxed and contented fashion".[65]

Penn was also aware of the stigma that had historically been attached to sufferers of leprosy for much of Japan's history—a stigma from which medical professionals were not immune. The doctor who had organised Penn's visit to Nagashima was part of a family tradition that had produced doctors for more than six hundred years. However, the unnamed doctor was reluctant to involve himself in the treatment of leprosy, having never been to the island himself. Penn described his attitude as a "strange fear of the disease", one that clearly had no basis in medical science. It was Penn's example that convinced the doctor to change his mind set, leading

[64] Ibid.

[65] Penn, *The Right to Look Human*, pp26, 28.

to his subsequent involvement in the treatment of leprosy sufferers. Here, Penn symbolised rational medical knowledge challenging and successfully overcoming the irrationality of stigmatisation.[66]

Penn's affording of his expertise to the Japanese continued in more academic vein. He delivered lectures at universities based in Hiroshima and the Japanese capital. And in Tokyo he was invited to "launch the Japanese Society of Plastic Surgery", contributing further to the recognition and professionalisation of reconstructive surgery in the country.[67] The early basis of the Japan Society of Plastic and Reconstructive Surgery lay in its interaction with Western medicine—the importation of medical equipment and the provision of skills provided by Western-trained medical experts such as Penn (who also remarked on the enthusiasm and willingness to learn on the part of Japanese doctors). Later, Japanese doctors would go to the United States to develop their skills in reconstructive surgery. Penn had earlier and unsuccessfully attempted to foster this medical relationship between Japan and the United States. Before his departure, he contacted the Committee of the Hiroshima Peace Centre Associates with a proposal to have fifty Japanese plastic surgeons trained in the United States as this "would develop Japanese plastic surgery on good clean lines".[68] For Penn, not only was the impartation of Western medical skills in this field a necessary one—and in line with efforts he made in Africa and elsewhere for the training of indigenous doctors—it was what he felt was a necessary part of the process of American atonement for the destruction caused.[69]

Penn's initial visit to Japan in 1957 and his follow-up visit in 1963 can be contextualised by a historically strong economic relationship between South Africa and Japan that would continue over the ensuing decades. When Penn returned to Tokyo—accompanied by his wife—to participate in a conference, he was pleased at the legacy of his original visit. Japanese reconstructive surgery skills had improved markedly, his previous patients were doing well and he was received with acclaim in Hiroshima. Penn noted that young surgeons cited him as their inspiration in specialising in

[66] Ibid., p155.

[67] Ibid., p157.

[68] Ibid., p155; "Japanese Society of Plastic and Reconstructive Surgery", https://jsprs.or.jp/english/background/, accessed 25 August 2020.

[69] Penn, *The Right to Look Human*, pp157–158.

reconstructive surgery and moves were afoot to ensure that each district or "prefectural hospital" would have its own contingent of reconstructive surgeons.[70] Penn's work in Hiroshima was therefore evidence of a further exchange between the two countries—this time in the form of medical expertise—with his belief that the training of Japanese doctors in the art of reconstructive surgery was the end-product of a "chain reaction" that he had set in motion in 1957.[71]

Three features therefore underlay Penn's experiences in Japan—US-Japanese relations and with them, the Japanese experience of modernisation as well as the historical ties between Japan and South Africa that continued—and were strengthened—under the apartheid state. In the case of the former, and as mentioned earlier in this chapter, it had been the Americans who "opened up" Japan and it would be the Americans who "conquered" it in 1945, serving as an occupying force. Penn's assessment of the medical treatment provided to the Japanese—both by the Americans and by himself—can also be attributed to a moral imperative and an ethos of service. At the same time, the unique features of Japanese culture gave it an ideological bent. He pointed out that the Japanese were themselves not motivated by ideology—be it religious or political. This explained the lack of success in the propagation of Christianity by missionaries even as the Japanese adopted various elements of modernisation.[72] And while the Japanese had a martial tradition that had only been enhanced by the adoption of modern military techniques and weaponry, their rationale for war was not based on "abstract causes" but arose from a sense of national identity related to cultural distinctiveness as well as a subservience to authority. For Penn, this was the reason that the Japanese had accepted their conquest by the Americans with little dissent.[73] While Penn viewed Japanese compliance in a simplistic light, it was what he perceived to be the lack of ideological inclination in Japanese culture that

[70] Ibid., p158.

[71] Ibid.

[72] Ibid., p156.

[73] Ibid., p33.

was the weak point that could allow for communist infiltration. The provision of modern surgical techniques and the training of Japanese doctors could thus serve to minimise communist influence as, "It needs no great stretch of imagination to realise that a shift from one side of the Iron Curtain to the other would just as easily be tolerated".[74]

[74] Ibid.

CHAPTER 9

"The Brotherhood of Pain": Israel

In Benedict Anderson's seminal work on nationalism, *Imagined Communities*, his view of a nation is one that is not necessarily confined to a specific territory. It does, however, promote a sense of identity and of belonging amongst people united by the elements that they hold in common such as culture and history. This gives the members of a nation a particular sense of "community", even as the bonds that hold them together is an "imagined" one.[1] The notion of an imagined homeland exerted a particular power on the diasporic Jewish community. This was related in part to the centuries of persecution in Europe, turning many into refugees in countries that implemented anti-Semitic policies. Often singled out for historical enmity for being culturally and religiously distinct, the Holocaust had shown that even acculturation was of little benefit, rendering Jews the ultimate outsider in the land of their birth.[2]

[1] Benedict Anderson, *Imagined Communities: Reflections on the Origin and Spread of Nationalism* (London and New York, Verso, 2006), pp6–7.

[2] Ibid., p149.

"The Brotherhood of Pain": Quote taken from Jack Penn, *The Right to Look Human: An Autobiography* (Johannesburg, Hugh Keartland Publishers, 1976), p29.

S. Chetty, *Reconstructive Surgery and Modernisation in Twentieth-Century South Africa*, Medicine and Biomedical Sciences in Modern History, https://doi.org/10.1007/978-3-031-38673-2_9

The fate of Jews in Eastern Europe was of great concern to South African Jews with older generations particularly distraught by the rising levels of anti-Semitism in Europe in the interwar period, culminating in the slaughter of millions. The Holocaust was therefore a significant feature in the consciousness of the minds of the South African Jewish population in the early post-war years who set up organisations to provide aid to their European counterparts.[3]

In mid-twentieth century South Africa, a number of factors contributed to Jewish nationalism or Zionism: the anti-Semitism as a result of increasing Jewish immigration from the late nineteenth century, the rising tide of nationalism after the Second World War, the attempted genocide perpetuated by Nazi Germany and finally, the concretisation of the imagined homeland with the founding of the state of Israel, the ultimate aim of Zionists.[4]

In November 1947, the UN sanctioned the partition of Palestine into a Jewish and Arab state. Six months later, the independent state of Israel was created, and David Ben-Gurion recorded the following in his diary: "The State of Israel was founded at four o'clock in the afternoon. Its fate lies in the hands of the army".[5] The conflict that had preceded the declaration of the independent state of Israel in May 1948 did not end with independence. Almost immediately the fledgling state was plunged into a series of wars with its hostile Arab neighbours that would play out for much of the twentieth century. Jack Penn would travel to the war-torn country many times over the next thirty years—and was present during the conflicts in 1948, 1956, 1967 and 1973—to provide surgical assistance to the war wounded.[6] Penn was only one of a number of South African personnel who travelled to the Middle East to provide medical assistance to the Israelis. Another was his former classmate, Lionel Melzer. In Melzer's contingent was orthopaedic surgeon Arthur Helfet who made

[3] Milton Shain, "Jewish Cultures, Identities and Contingencies: Reflections from the South African Experience", *European Review of History*, 18, 1, 89–100, February 2011, p92.

[4] Ibid., p92.

[5] Michael Brenner, *In Search of Israel: The History of an Idea* (Princeton and Oxford, Princeton University Press, 2018), pp138–140.

[6] Jack Penn, "A Surgeon's Story: It Is the Divine Right of Man to Look Human" (Unpublished Manuscript), p3, Brn No 12057, 617.95 PEN, BL.

the dangerous journey with an ample supply of very necessary medical instruments.

Just two years older than Penn, Helfet had also been born in the Cape Province. He studied at the University of Cape Town and received his medical degree from Liverpool University, specialising in orthopaedics. His war service was distinguished—serving in the RAMC in Sierra Leone and as the orthopaedic consulting surgeon for the entire Allied contingent based in Africa. During the War, he had acquired familiarity with the tropical bacterial disease, yaws, that was prevalent in West Africa and affected bone. In April 1948, he left for Israel to bring his vast experience to bear during the conflict, as he had already spent a year in the Middle East during the War. While he would later describe his time in Israel as "the most romantic moment of my medical career", he was not unaware of the inherent dangers associated with it—and neither was Penn who wished him farewell. Both knew of a recent incident where a convoy of doctors travelling to Hadassah Hospital and the Hebrew University had been ambushed, with a number of doctors killed, including an acquaintance of Helfet, Dr Haim Yassky, director of the Hadassah Medical Organisation. It had been Yassky who had made the request to Helfet to come to Israel and assist in organising the treatment for the large number of casualties predicted.[7]

Lionel Melzer was key in getting together the necessary medical personnel to serve as volunteers in Israel and was also made second in command of the Israel Medical Corps under Chaim Sheba.[8] Melzer, an anaesthetist, had been part of Penn's graduating class from Wits in 1932. As a student, he was also a talented athlete and captain of the athletics team, with Penn as the vice-captain.[9] During the War, Melzer commanded the 11th and later, the 20th Field Ambulance, serving in East

[7] Henry Katzew, *South Africa's 800: The Story of South Africa's Volunteers in Israel's War of Birth*, Joe Woolf (ed) (South African Zionist Federation, 2003), p74; "Helfet, Arthur Jacob (1907–1989)", *Plarr's Lives of the Fellows*, Royal College of Surgeons of England, https://livesonline.rcseng.ac.uk/client/en_GB/lives/search/detail nonmodal/ent:$002f$002fSD_ASSET$002f0$002fSD_ASSET:379507/one, accessed 20 March 2021; Judy Siegel-Itzkovich, "Victims of Hassadah Massacre to be Memorialized", *The Jerusalem Post*, 7 April 2008, https://www.jpost.com/Jewish-World/Jewish-News/Victims-of-Hadassah-massacre-to-be-memorialized, accessed 20 March 2021.

[8] Philip Gillon, *Seventy Years of Southern African Aliyah: A Story of Achievement* (Israel, Adar Productions, 1992), pp100–101.

[9] Penn, *The Right to Look Human*, p46.

Africa, North Africa and Italy. It was during his service in North Africa that he had the opportunity to see Palestine.[10] It was also while stationed in North Africa that he was awarded the Military Cross in 1942 and two years later, while in Italy, received the Order of the British Empire.[11] With his wartime experience, Melzer was the driving force behind the first South African medical contingent in Israel.

In 1948, cloak-and-dagger methods were employed to get South Africans into Israel and not all were successful, with one group arrested and detained in Egypt until two of the detainees claimed to be Dutch Reformed ministers on their way to France.[12] Melzer also discovered that the South African state was aware of their activities when he was called to a meeting with a high-ranking member of the Medical Corps, Brigadier Du Plessis, who requested reports on the state of the Israeli medical services as well as the experiences of serving South Africans in the hopes that this could be of relevance to South Africa.[13] As Penn would later do, Melzer travelled throughout Israel, often in the wake of conflict and under dangerous combat conditions, both to inspect and to improve the treatment of injured troops. Based on his own experience in the 11th and 20th Field Ambulance, he is accredited with introducing the field ambulance to Israel—a system of mobile units that provide early treatment to the injured in combat zones.[14]

Prior to the War of 1948, Penn had already operated on Israeli patients sent to South Africa for plastic surgery. Their injuries were a product of the violence that preceded the declaration of independence.[15] His first trip to Israel was made at the request of a man referred to as "Palgi" who highlighted the need for Penn's services in aiding the increasing numbers of wounded at a time when Israel had no plastic surgeons of its own and none appeared to be forthcoming from Britain or the United States.

[10] "Dr Lionel Melzer", http://www.machal.org.il/index.php?option=com_content&view=article&id=533&Itemid=879&lang=en, accessed 29 August 2020.

[11] WO 373/18—21 October 1941–24 February 1942 (DCM) and WO 373/72—Italy: 21 December 1944—19 April 1945, War Office and Ministry of Defence, National Archives, https://discovery.nationalarchives.gov.uk/results/r?_q=lionel+melzer, accessed 28 April 2021.

[12] Gillon, *Seventy Years of Southern African Aliyah*, p20.

[13] "Dr Lionel Melzer".

[14] Ibid.

[15] Gillon, *Seventy Years of Southern African Aliyah*, p99.

The decision to go to Israel was not a simple one for Penn and necessitated him weighing his own responsibilities at Wits (where he was still employed) and ensuring the financial stability of his young family with his "conscience".[16] As Penn recorded in his "Palestinian Diary" while still in Johannesburg, he was not motivated by any religious impulse as he was instead a believer in philosophical principles and "Hebraism holds no bond for me in its outmoded methods of approach". A motivating factor was instead the humanitarian impulse to assist people in need and significantly, an early desire to understand "world politics" and "whether there is definite progress towards a real civilised state".[17]

With the approval of his wife, Diana, "conscience" won the day and Penn travelled to Israel, arriving in Tel Aviv.[18] While in both his autobiography and diary, Penn does not claim any ideological sympathies, his sister, Milly, along with her husband, Abraham Levy, had been living in Israel for more than a decade. Abraham was based at the Migdal Insurance Company and Milly was described as a "passionate Zionist".[19]

Penn's arrival was not as uncomplicated as his itinerary would suggest. While on the flight to Tunis, he was propositioned by an apparently famous actress described as "blonde, burnished and buxom" and landed in Tunisia a few hours later where he was confronted with the sight of an Arab population with the visible indicators of disease that had long since been eradicated in the West.[20] The theme of modern medicine and old diseases would resurface later during his time in Israel. The outbreak of war also meant that upon landing in Rome, Penn discovered that flights to Israel had been cancelled. Stranded, he ran into a South African identified only as Griffiths whose first child had been delivered by Penn in Benoni—it was a small world. Griffiths, a pilot, was scheduled to fly

[16] Penn, *The Right to Look Human*, pp165–166.

[17] Jack Penn, "Palestinian Diary", 2 July 1948, Johannesburg, File: Penn, Jack—Writings (4), AMUW.

[18] Penn, *The Right to Look Human*, pp165–166.

[19] David Susman, *An African Shopkeeper: Memoirs of David Susman*, Leni Martin (ed) (Fernwood Press, 2004). Excerpt taken from http://www.machal.org.il/index.php?option=com_content&view=article&id=287%3Adavid-susman&catid=45%3APersonal+Stories+&Itemid=392&lang=en, accessed 29 August 2020.

[20] Penn, "Palestinian Diary", 8 July 1948, Tunis.

to "Oklahoma"—as Israel was termed in a manner straight out of spy novels—and included Penn as a passenger.[21]

Upon arriving in Tel Aviv, Penn made the acquaintance of Chaim Sheba. Sheba had been appointed the Director General of Medical Services of the Israeli armed forces after independence. Born in the Austro-Hungarian empire, he qualified as a doctor in Vienna before emigrating to Palestine in 1933.[22] During the Second World War, he served as a major in the British army and upon its end, was a member of Haganah. A committed Zionist, he was the ideal choice to lead and reform the Israeli army's medical corps.[23] Sheba would later become the Director General of the Ministry of Health.[24]

Before 1948, there were three main trends in the Israeli health care system—the British health care services that included the building and running of hospitals during the Mandate, independent Jewish health services such as the Hadassah Medical Organisation and the input provided by skilled Jewish doctors fleeing Nazi persecution. The latter comprised a professional class who also contributed to other fields such as education, law and commerce. With independence, the state of Israel assumed control of the earlier British hospitals and medical care in general was under the Ministry of Health.[25]

With Sheba serving as a guide, Penn visited medical units across the country where he also treated patients, often in very rudimentary conditions that necessitated him operating at times on the floor. At the ancient city of Tiberias alongside the Sea of Galilee where the Israelis were battling the Syrians, Penn encountered another South African surgeon, Jack Wilton. Wilton had been part of the first contingent of South African medical personnel under Melzer and was similarly a veteran of the Second

[21] Katzew, *South Africa's 800*, p90.

[22] "Israelis You Should Know: Dr Chaim Sheba", *International Fellowship of Christians and Jews*, https://www.ifcj.org/news/fellowship-blog/israelis-you-should-know-chaim-sheba-2/, accessed 25 May 2021.

[23] Penn, *The Right to Look Human*, p167.

[24] "Israelis You Should Know: Dr Chaim Sheba".

[25] A. Mark Clarfield, Orly Manor, Gabi Bin Nun, Shifra Shvarts, Zaher S. Azzam, Arnon Afek, Fuad Basis and Avi Israeli, "Health and Health Care in Israel: An Introduction", *Lancet*, 389, 2503–2513, 24 June 2017.

World War.[26] Wilton had learned to make do with the basics and adapt what was available for medical purposes. Penn related his use of a desk and its drawers to serve as an orthopaedic table, setting and immobilising the fractured limb until a plaster cast was applied, all done without the aid of morphine.[27] Due to the shortage of doctors, Wilton worked in rotation with other doctors at facilities in Tel Aviv, Jerusalem and a convalescent facility at Nahariya.[28] His role in the war was to establish and organise the casualty clearing stations and hospitals close to the frontlines of conflict. As Penn observed, South African medical personnel were key in the evacuation and treatment of the wounded, "A great percentage of the cases pass therefore from the firing lines, through to the Regimental aid-posts to forward hospitals and back to us – through the hands of South African doctors all the way".[29]

After his tour of the various medical facilities throughout Israel, Penn had a better understanding of the state of medical care in the country, finding that many were ill-equipped to meet the demands of war. The facilities were largely left-over structures from the British occupation and were haphazard such as Tel Hashomer—now named after Chaim Sheba. While today considered an internationally recognised medical facility, it was a very different prospect in 1948. It reflected the area's history—first a set of barracks erected by the Americans in 1941 which was then used as a British military hospital. In 1948, "Army Hospital No 5", as it was called, was used to treat wounded civilians and military personnel. Its evolution was symbolic of Israel's modernisation and transformation in health care during war—in 1948, almost half the wounded soldiers succumbed to their injuries; sixty years later, this had dropped to 15%.[30] However, this lay far into the future and Penn's description of the hospital as "not yet…fully functioning" meant that it could not serve as his base. Tel Hashomer however, assumed significance for Penn

[26] Penn, *The Right to Look Human*, pp167–168; Gillon, *Seventy Years of Southern African Aliyah*, p100.

[27] Penn, *The Right to Look Human*, p168.

[28] Katzew, *South Africa's 800*, p317.

[29] Penn, "Palestinian Diary", 15 July 1948, Tel Aviv.

[30] Maayan Hoffman, "Growing with Israel: 70 Years of Sheba Success", *The Jerusalem Post*, 17 April 2018, https://www.jpost.com/israels-70th-anniversary/growing-with-israel-70-years-of-sheba-success-550038, accessed 21 March 2021.

as it was where he first encountered Moshe Dayan, the formidable military commander: "His personality was electric and it was not long before I realised that I was talking to a born leader, intelligent, forthright and unwavering".[31] Dayan was also Penn's patient and would "require extensive plastic surgery to a face that once was very handsome". Two years previously, he had been denied an entry visa to Britain to be treated by Archie McIndoe—an incident that raised Penn's ire.[32] Dayan would later become a patient at the Brenthurst Clinic in Johannesburg.

When in Israel, Penn requested the assistance of a South African nurse, Ray Brunton, based at Djani Medical Hospital. The hospital was the site of a previous nursing home in Jaffa. When Brunton arrived, she discovered that while the building was a solid one, the Arabs had buried the instruments and the operating table and she, along with another nursing sister, had a formidable task ahead to prepare the hospital to receive patients. Beds were obtained from nearby residences; medical supplies were sourced from where available and Brunton even made use of crochet cotton to substitute for gut in suturing wounds. Added to these challenges was the "inexperience" of Israeli medical personnel who tended to resort to drastic methods such as amputation with an ease she found disconcerting and in stark contradiction to her medical training in South Africa. She was even more appalled to find a nurse delivering penicillin injections to patients—not only reusing the syringe but not sterilising it before each use. As Katzew described it, "She found herself profoundly involved in Israel's trials, tragedies, mistakes and rawness".[33] Impressed by her capability in extremely adverse conditions, Penn requested her assistance. On the day of her transfer however, the doctors at Djani threatened to go on strike unless she remained. When she finally did leave for the Kfar Giladi hospital, Djani had three operating theatres and a cohort of well-trained nurses.[34]

Denied Brunton, Penn sent for two of his nurses from South Africa—Audrey Benedict and Marie Roux. Their trip was a protracted one—a

[31] Penn, *The Right to Look Human*, p171.

[32] Penn, "Palestinian Diary", 21 July 1948. Dayan was subsequently treated in Paris in 1947, "Letters Describing Dayan Losing His Eye to be Auctioned", *The Times of Israel*, 27 July 2015, https://www.timesofisrael.com/letters-describing-dayan-losing-eye-to-be-auctioned/, accessed 25 June 2021.

[33] Katzew, *South Africa's 800*, pp126–127, 142.

[34] Ibid., p144.

flight to Rome, another to Greece and then a landing at Tel Aviv that proved eventful when Benedict was initially refused entry and both women were detained until the following day when Lionel Meltzer intervened. Neither woman was Jewish, but Roux would accompany Penn on his various travels, providing medical assistance, and Benedict professed Zionist sympathies, "I was not a Jew, but I am a Zionist…"[35] Both women were stationed at the Bat Galim Hospital in Haifa overlooking the Mediterranean.[36]

The hospital—today known as the Rambam Medical Centre—was built in 1938 while Palestine was still under British mandate. Its role was a strategic one—due to its rail links to Egypt and Syria, it was the ideal location for the treatment of sailors in the British Navy stationed in the Mediterranean. The construction of the hospital—that the British high commissioner for Palestine, Sir Harold Macmichael described as "the finest medical institution in the Middle East"—was therefore part of British preparations for the likely outbreak of war with Nazi Germany. Taking three years to construct, the hospital was designed by German-trained architect Erich Mendelsohn and comprised space for the residence of medical personnel as well as operating theatres and a laboratory. The extensive use of glass meant a breath-taking view, but the architecture also reflected the contemporary segregationist attitudes as separate residence facilities had been built for the British wounded.[37] It was here then, that Roux and Benedict joined Penn. With independence, the hospital had become a civilian one but with an increasing number of war injuries. Its medical staff were volunteers from all over the world with English as an important mode of communication—although the nurses began learning Hebrew, the better to communicate with patients. The wartime emergency conditions also meant that medical supplies were at a premium and dressings, for instance—usually discarded after a single use—had to be sterilised and reused.[38]

[35] Ibid., pp92–93.

[36] Ibid., p182.

[37] Judy Siegel-Itzkovich, "Rambam: From Hospital for British Wounded in WWII to Most Developed Medical Center in North", *The Jerusalem Post*, 22 December 2013, https://www.jpost.com/Health-and-Science/Rambam-From-hospital-for-British-wounded-in-WWII-to-most-developed-medical-center-in-North-335762, accessed 11 March 2021.

[38] Katzew, *South Africa's 800*, p182.

The arrival of Roux and Benedict, however, was not without tension. When Penn decided to establish his plastic surgery unit at the hospital—despite an initial impression of lack of adequate hygiene as well as medical equipment—his request for his own nursing team was seen as an indictment on the capabilities of the existing nursing staff who were initially hostile to the South Africans. However plastic surgery cases grew exponentially, forcing Penn, Roux and Benedict to work unremitting hours in challenging conditions, eventually winning them the respect of the Israeli medical staff.[39]

The two women also found themselves exposed to the tumultuous complexities that accompanied the birth of Israel in a very real way when they witnessed the autopsies of Bernadotte and Colonel Serot of the French Air Force at the Italian Hospital in September 1948.[40] Count Folke Bernadotte was the head of the Swedish Red Cross and the mediator for Palestine on behalf of the UN, tasked with finding a compromise between Arab and Israeli interests in Palestine, that lay at the heart of the conflict in 1948. The "Bernadotte Plan" suggested that control over Arab-occupied areas of Palestine be ceded to Jordan as no provision had been made for an independent Arab state in Palestine. In addition, Bernadotte recommended the return of Arab refugees, displaced by the conflict, to their homes in Palestine. While he desired the UN control of Jerusalem, other members of his team favoured the cessation of Jerusalem to Jordan. For extremists, Bernadotte's compromise was seen as antithetical to Israeli interests. His convoy was ambushed and Bernadotte was shot, along with Serot who sat alongside him. The assassination was carried out by Lehi, a right-wing group also known as the Stern Gang, which advocated an expanding Jewish state and one from which all "non-Jewish populations" were excluded.[41] Penn had already decided to return to South Africa at the time of the assassination and the nurses, electing to remain, had been moved to the Italian hospital—a military hospital—a few weeks earlier, giving Benedict the sense that she was participating in a key moment in history.[42] Benedict would return to

[39] Ibid., p224.

[40] Ibid., p235.

[41] Carey David Stanger, "A Haunting Legacy: The Assassination of Count Bernadotte", *The Middle East Journal*, 42, 2, 260–272, 1988, pp260–264.

[42] Katzew, *South Africa's 800*, p242.

South Africa. Marie Roux returned to Israel in 1956 during the Sinai War and remained working there for another three years, eventually emigrating to the United States. In the conflict in 1967, she retained her ties with Israel by obtaining medical supplies in New York to be shipped to the Middle East.[43]

The South African community in Israel was a close one and in addition to the medical volunteers, there were the combatants who were at the other end of the scalpel. David Susman passed away in May 2010 at the age of 84. During his long career, he was renowned for his role in remodelling the Woolworths chain in the 1950s, based on a model derived from his three-year stint at Marks and Spencer in Britain.[44] In his autobiography—rather self-deprecatingly titled *An African Shopkeeper*—Susman describes another seminal moment of his life: his service as a volunteer soldier in Israel in 1948.

Susman had already served during the Second World War but the outbreak of war in Israel in 1948 took on a different personal and ideological meaning for him as it was linked both to the events of the preceding global conflict and to his own identity as a Jewish South African. As he explained to his disapproving father:

> How could a Jew stand by when the very existence of the remnants of our people was threatened after the nightmare of the Holocaust? If the Arabs succeeded in destroying the new State of Israel, no young Jew could live with the memory that he, personally, might have helped save the situation. It was, I regretted, a duty that I could not shirk.[45]

His father attempted to have his son-in-law, surgeon Jack Wilton persuade his son to the contrary but was flummoxed when Wilton also decided to join the war effort as a member of Melzer's medical team. The recruitment of South Africans to serve as combatants in Israel was done in secret as the UN had issued an embargo on young men of combat age from travelling to the country. Like Penn, Susman first flew to Rome as a "tourist" before joining with volunteers drawn from all over the

[43] Ibid., p296.

[44] "Susman's Woolworths a Legacy to be Proud of", *Newswires*, 14 May 2010, https://insurancenewsnet.com/oarticle/Susmans-Woolworths-a-Legacy-to-Be-Proud-of-a-190373, accessed 16 March 2021.

[45] Susman, *An African Shopkeeper*.

world who were then flown by chartered plane to Haifa. The men assembled at a former British Army camp, Tel Litwinsky, where they were assigned to various units in the Israeli defence force. The process was haphazard due to the shortage of manpower in the newly formed Israeli military. The enthusiastic young volunteers were described as "Machal" (external volunteers) and would comprise more than ten per cent of the 40 000-strong Israel Defence Forces. South Africa alone contributed eight hundred volunteers.[46]

Susman's motivation was a strong one, especially once he learned of the dire military situation on the ground with Israel facing the prospect of advancing troops from hostile Arab neighbours—Syria, Lebanon, Egypt and Transjordan. Added to the mix was the Arab Liberation Army of Palestine targeting Haifa. Described by Susman as "mercenaries", they were seen as motivated by pecuniary concerns with their compensation coming "from the supposedly rich loot of destroyed Jewish settlements". Susman joined the 72nd Battalion under an American, Colonel Wilson and training took place at a camp outside Haifa. He was given command of a platoon of thirty men. Forging the men into an effective fighting unit proved a challenge, not least because of the diverse linguistic backgrounds. This was compounded by lack of ammunition and combat experience of the volunteers as well as their varying degrees of fitness, "many were physically unfit—years in the Nazi concentration camps, followed by a numbing spell in D.P. [Displaced Persons] camps in Europe and Cyprus, left them undernourished and weedy".[47]

The relocation of the 72nd to another camp close to the town of Nahariya brought Susman into contact with another group of immigrants—German Jews—who Susman described as unyielding but making significant impact in areas of science and medicine. He ascribed their "inflexible" nature to their resistance to the medical techniques imported with the newly arrived medical volunteers. Susman nevertheless accredited this group with the indelible influence of Western culture on Israel.[48]

Prior to his first combat assignment, Susman spent time in Haifa with Jack Wilton (who was soon joined by his wife, Susman's sister, Osna). The area had a significant contingent of South African volunteers, including

[46] Ibid.

[47] Ibid.

[48] Ibid.

Penn's sister, Milly, and her husband, who had been in Israel for more than a decade.[49] Susman soon met Penn, relating an incident involving Penn's encounter with the German Jewish doctors, whom he described as "reactionaries". Penn demonstrated to them a new and successful surgery technique which they attributed simply to his superior equipment. The plastic surgeon's retort was that it could be performed with "a kitchen knife" and never wasting an opportunity to make a dramatic point, performed a subsequent operation with a kitchen knife, much to the consternation of his observers.[50]

Penn was also scathing in his assessment of these doctors with his description of one such figure who was in charge of a hospital in Tel Aviv:

> He calls himself Professor – to which he has no title whatsoever…His wards stink of sepsis. He handles his patients with a particular sadism…When I saw his attempt at "Plastic Surgery" I realised his qualification – head artist in Tussaud's Chamber of Horrors. This man is a hangover of the 1930s emigration from Germany, which scattered through the world a few good men and a lot of rubbish.[51]

He was just as critical—albeit with less vitriol—after inspecting a hospital run by Orthodox Jews where the staff ranged in age from 50 to 82 and "the world stands still". It brought to mind the state of the Edinburgh Infirmary a century previously before the advent of the modern antiseptic methods developed by Joseph Lister.[52] Penn represented the face of modern medicine confronted with the recalcitrant past.

Susman would eventually have first-hand experience of Penn's surgical skill. With training completed and following the end of a ceasefire, the 72nd was sent into action against the Arab Liberation Army in Galilee.[53] Susman was wounded by a "dum dum" during the encounter. A bullet that expands on impact with a surface and designed to cause serious injury, it hit below his left shoulder blade and exited from his neck. He was treated by Wilton, spending three weeks in hospital and a further six

[49] Ibid.

[50] Ibid.

[51] Penn, "Palestinian Diary", 27 July 1948.

[52] Ibid., 23 July 1948.

[53] Susman, *An African Shopkeeper.*

weeks recuperating. One of his visitors was Jack Penn who volunteered to perform the reconstructive surgery that the wound would eventually require. Susman returned to active duty in October 1948 however on his return to Johannesburg on leave, Penn made good on his word. With the assistance of his theatre nurse, Benedict, he removed the keloid that had resulted from the healed injury, leaving behind a small scar as per Susman's request as a memento of the event. The operation was a success—although the lost muscle could not be replaced and Susman's injured left shoulder hung slightly below its right counterpart.[54]

In Penn's later analysis of his experience in Israel, he drew attention to the different types of injuries incurred during the conflict in 1948—injuries that were very different from those encountered during the Second World War and bore greater resemblance to the South African War at the turn of the century. Here, the main injuries were due to small arms fire damaging the face and jaw. Moreover, unlike Penn's experience at the Brenthurst Military Hospital where there were both "battle" and "bottle" injuries, the latter—caused by fights breaking out between inebriated soldiers—was conspicuously absent in Israel. The Israeli Medical Corps was also commended for its efforts in reducing the rates of infection. At the same time, he mentioned the high rate of amputation in 1948, a feature also noted by the South African nurses and indicative of less advanced surgical skill. For more complicated cases, usually involving reconstruction of the skull and the use of plates, the patients were sent to South Africa as Penn was leery of performing these advanced procedures in Israel. His final recommendation was that Israel needed to promote the development of military plastic surgery, drawing upon various specialisations to effectively address the injuries that affected both the military and civilian population.[55]

The historic role of science and medicine in Israel was, however, more complex than simply Penn representing the modern in the face of the recalcitrant, as painted by Susman. From the outset, medicine was linked to Zionism and the creation of a modern state. In the first decades of the twentieth century, Zionism benefitted from the modernity wrought by high imperialism—transport and communications infrastructure, the

[54] Ibid.

[55] Jack Penn, "Impressions of Plastic and Maxillo-Facial Surgery in the Palestine War", *Plastic and Reconstructive Surgery*, 6, 4, October 1950, pp327–333.

modernisation of agriculture and the role of medicine in the promotion of public health. The "civilising mission" of imperialism was adapted to the Zionist aim of taming and rendering fit for human habitation the hostile Palestinian desert environment and it was the adoption of the elements of modernity—technology, science and medicine and linked to this, improvements in public health—that were the pre-requisite for the creation of a modern Zionist state able to address the needs of its citizens.[56]

Prior to the British mandate in Palestine, Dr Leo Böhm established the Pasteur Institute for Health, Medicine and Biology in 1916. Although eventually marginalised by later medical institutions, it represented both an outgrowth of the modernising elements of French colonialism as well as an assertion of a Zionist belief in the creation of an independent state underpinned by modernity.[57] While Böhm's institute drew its inspiration from the French, the role of the German Jewry in the provision of medical services in Palestine was a significant one. Based in Berlin, the Association of Jewish Physicians and Natural Scientists for the Sanitary Interests in Palestine was established in 1913. It was not a Zionist institution and included within its ambit non-Jewish organisations, as well as both scientific and religious figures. Its overall aim was the improvement of public health for the residents of Palestine—the promotion of sanitation and the alleviation of tropical diseases such as malaria. The Association joined with others to create the International Office for the Health of Jerusalem, which marked a collaboration between both German scientists as well as Jewish nationalists in the promotion of public health and eradication of disease. The International Office was a site for the dissemination of medical and scientific knowledge. It was also a symbol of Germany's rivalry with France and its imperial aspirations in Palestine through the medium of science and medicine. Yet, extensive German involvement was also criticised as undermining Zionist belief in autonomy and self-reliance.[58]

With the British mandate in 1920, German influence gave way to that of the British and the Americans. Of primary concern to the former

[56] Nadav Davidovitch and Rakefet Zalashik, "Pasteur in Palestine: The Politics of the Laboratory", *Science in Context*, 23, 4, 401–425, 2010, p404.

[57] Ibid., pp401–402.

[58] Ibid., pp407–410.

was public health with the aim of containing infectious disease and the provision of infrastructure to promote sanitation and hygiene. The arrival of the American Zionist Medical Unit in 1918—along with its medical experts and state-of-the-art equipment—was hailed as a means of addressing the medical needs of Palestine and of collaborating with Jewish medical professionals. The free exchange of knowledge and expertise was hoped to further modernise and professionalise medicine in Palestine. However, American confidence meant a dismissal of the existing medical knowledge in the region as "outdated", thereby precluding professional co-operation based on a sense of equality. Over the next decade, it was the American model—combining research with practice—that grew to dominate the practice of medicine in Palestine.[59] The relatively small number of Jewish settlers, with a corresponding dearth of skills, necessitated an influx of experts drawn from all over the world to promote scientific progress and modern medicine. The crises faced by the newly independent Israeli state from 1948 only exacerbated this demand. Jack Penn's work in Israel can therefore be seen as part of the ongoing narrative of the history of the region in terms of its engagement with modern medicine from colonialism to independence.

In addition to providing medical treatment, Penn initiated training sessions, giving lectures to the doctors at the Hadassah Hospital, academic staff at the Hebrew University and demonstrating plastic surgical techniques to the surgeons in Jerusalem. He saw great potential in his audience, considering them to be both "highly intelligent" and "eager to learn". It presented the possibility of laying the foundation for a modern medical system and even to create his idealised "Mecca of Medicine". His own work in South Africa however, the demands of his private practice and the financial welfare of his young family meant that he would unfortunately not be able to lead the modernisation of Israeli medicine.[60] He instead provided a directive for the treatment of maxillo-facial injuries in the field as well as burns and hand injuries and "recommended a first-aid dressing design which could be used effectively...by any dumb cluck". Only one page in length, it reduced plastic surgery to a basic yet necessary minimum. In the spirit of Gillies and McIndoe, he also urged the

[59] Ibid., pp413–414, 417.

[60] Penn, "Palestinian Diary", 23 July 1948.

close collaboration between plastic surgeons and dentists in the treatment of maxillo-facial injuries.[61]

Penn spent five months in Israel in 1948—the work was unremitting, the conditions arduous. He eventually developed a duodenal ulcer. Exhausted, he made plans to return home with his wife (who had joined him during the year). The journey back was just as unconventional as the flight to Israel—the assassination of Bernadotte led to a moratorium placed on departures from Israel, so Penn and Diana flew on a cargo plan to Athens and then landed in Geneva. From there, they returned to South Africa so that Penn could focus on his private practice.[62]

A year later, the war was over, Penn returned to Israel with a surgical team. His aim was two-fold—follow-up procedures as required on his wartime patients and the "rehabilitation" of the large influx of Jewish immigrants arriving from Yemen.[63] Between 1948 and 1950, almost fifty thousand Jews arrived from Yemen and Aden. The romantically titled immigration, "Operation Magic Carpet", was due to the collaboration between Israeli authorities, the American Jewish Joint Distribution Committee and the Jewish Agency. It was portrayed by the Israeli state as a flight from the "persecution" in Arab states that rendered the immigrants little more than second class citizens. The immigration, however, brought with it incredible challenges, with many unable to access adequate food supplies and health care. Large numbers died *en route* or while in refugee camps and those who arrived in Israel were in very poor health.[64] Penn had encountered the Yemenite refugees during his first trip to Israel in 1948 and had visited a "children's colony" for Yemenite Jewish children:

> The children are not backward mentally, but so many have come in from the Yemen and Arabic countries in a state of starvation and behave like animals, which is normal Arabic behaviour as children, that they have to

[61] Ibid., 6 August 1948 and December 1948, Johannesburg.

[62] Penn, *The Right to Look Human*, pp174, 176.

[63] Ibid., p176.

[64] Esther Meir-Glitzenstein, "Operation Magic Carpet: Constructing the Myth of the Magical Immigration of Yemenite Jews to Israel", *Israel Studies*, 16, 3, 149–173, 2011, pp149–150.

> unlearn these bad habits and have to learn to eat, speak and behave like normal Westernised human beings.[65]

The Yemenite refugees were an important component in Israeli nation-building ideology—the return of Jews from exile but also, significantly, Israel as a symbol of modernity in contrast to its more "primitive" Arab neighbours. Yaakov Weinstein, a medical doctor in the Jewish Agency Immigration Department, portrayed the immigrants as simplistically pious, overwhelmed with gratitude at their return to the "promised land". At the same time, he judged their ignorance harshly as well as their reluctance towards adopting modern medical practice.[66] Penn demonstrated a similar ambivalence while treating the immigrants. They were anachronistic, remnants of a distant and biblical past unchanged by time:

> These people had been locked away in the desert for 2 000 years, and one got the impression of going back to the time of Christ or the Jewish prophets. They were deeply religious and intelligent, but in other ways, primitive in the extreme. A knife or fork, a tooth brush or even a chair were foreign to them, and as they were polygamous, most of them had many wives.[67]

And these differences were more than just quaint, presenting challenges to modern medicine and public health, "They brought with them many diseases, some of them unseen in modern civilised communities. Some of them looked like pictures out of an ancient textbook of surgery".[68] One of these diseases was trachoma—a bacterial infection of the eyes that was endemic to the more poverty-stricken or underdeveloped parts of the world.[69] Israel had already eradicated it but was once again forced to contend with it due to its prevalence in the immigrants.[70] In this way, Penn—in conjunction with the Israeli state—used medicine as a means of asserting modernisation.

[65] Penn, "Palestinian Diary", 27 July 1948.

[66] Meir-Glitzenstein, "Operation Magic Carpet", p158.

[67] Penn, *The Right to Look Human*, p176.

[68] Ibid., p176.

[69] "Trachoma", https://www.mayoclinic.org/diseases-conditions/trachoma/symptoms-causes/syc-20378505, accessed 21 March 2021.

[70] Penn, *The Right to Look Human*, p176.

Penn's association with the state went further. Along with Dayan, he made the acquaintance of David Ben-Gurion. Much has been written about the founding father of Israel and Penn was no exception, devoting at least ten pages of his autobiography to the Israeli leader, along with an assessment of the man, as well as photographs and a sketch that was preparatory to Penn's creation of a bust of Ben-Gurion. Penn's description of Ben-Gurion borders on the hagiographic and he was unable to restrain himself from drawing parallels with that other saint-like figure he had encountered—Albert Schweitzer. Yet he considered Ben-Gurion superior to Schweitzer who frustrated Penn with his disinterest in continuing his legacy after his death. In contrast, the first Prime Minister of Israel felt a compulsion to "salvage what he can from the past, and pass it on to the generations of the future".[71] This is borne out in a recent biography where Ben-Gurion is portrayed as a man supremely conscious of the judgement of history.[72]

Born David Yosef Gruen in Poland in the late nineteenth century, Ben-Gurion articulated the sense of an imagined homeland of the Jewish diaspora, informing a journalist that as young as the age of three, he had the sense that he did not truly belong in the country of his birth, "And that is how all the Jews were. We knew that our land would not be the place we were living, but in the Land of Israel".[73] And Ben-Gurion was able to play a significant role in making the imagined real.

Although access to education was a significant deterrent for the young Ben-Gurion, compounded by a lack of application as well as finances, his hope was to emigrate to Palestine as an engineer, to foster the development of Palestine along the modern lines that Theodor Herzl's Zionism propagated.[74] While Penn may have demonstrated some ambivalence towards the harnessing of the atom—especially after his experiences in Nagasaki—Ben-Gurion was convinced that nuclear power was essential to the development of Israel and in 1948, was already speaking to nuclear scientists. For him, the possibilities of science were limitless and were symbolic of a Zionist view of taming the land and rendering it habitable.

[71] Ibid., pp179–180.

[72] Tom Segev, *A State at Any Cost: The Life of David Ben-Gurion*, Haim Watzman (translator) (London, Head of Zeus Ltd, 2019), Introduction.

[73] Ibid., Part I: The Road to Power.

[74] Ibid., Chapter 2: Scroll of Fire.

Ben-Gurion's Zionism was based on "a faith in a measurable, quantifiable world that could be described with facts and numbers".[75] Science and technology were also harnessed to the military machine and just prior to Israel's declaration of independence in 1948, he founded a Science Corps, using science and technology to both improve efficacy in war as well as its "opposite", "This means scientists in the fields of physics, chemistry, and technology who can expand the capacity for killing large numbers of people, or the opposite, for curing people…Both are important". Ben-Gurion's almost matter-of-fact acceptance of the double-edged sword of science and technology symbolised his faith in science, "as the highest expression of the human spirit" and more pragmatically, the means by which the new nation state would not only hold its own, but thrive.[76]

During Penn's initial trip in 1948, he was taken to the Weizmann Institute of Science in Rehovot, close to Tel Aviv. Here, in contrast to his critical assessment of the state of Israeli medicine, Penn was awestruck by this symbol of progress and collaborative scientific effort:

> This is an enormous group of buildings so well camouflaged that you don't know you're there until you are in it. Chemical, electrical and nuclear research is going on here and people from every nation in the world have their representatives on the staff…This thing, so absolutely modern and alive was such a contrast to other aspects of Palestine so primitive and dead that it is difficult to correlate them in the same country.[77]

With the freneticism of 1948 in the past, Penn's subsequent visits to Israel focused on assisting the country's doctors to develop its coterie of plastic surgeons who were to form units in the major hospitals around the country.[78] These visits strengthened his ties with and influence on Israeli plastic surgeons. In 1948, he was aided by one of the country's first plastic surgeons, Leo Bornstein who along with others, held regular meetings that eventually culminated in the Israel Society for Plastic Surgeons in 1973. Penn was accredited with fostering the development of surgery in the country. The logo of the Association also reflected the symbolism of the "divine"—a flowering tree stump surrounded by a serpent with the

[75] Ibid., Chapter 22: Yes to the Old Man.

[76] Ibid., Chapter 22.

[77] Penn, "Palestinian Diary", 19 July 1948.

[78] Penn, *The Right to Look Human*, p183.

motto drawn from the Bible, "Every mountain shall be made low, the crooked shall be made straight, and the rough places plain".[79]

In the project to develop and professionalise Israel's medical services however, Penn was not alone. Underlying South African efforts in Israel was the work of the South African Zionist Federation. Founded in 1898 as an umbrella organisation for Jewish organisations and events in South Africa, it became the most significant organisation representing South African Jews. While the ideal of Zionism was settlement in Israel, Zionism in South Africa also acknowledged a South African identity. Israel remained however, an idealised homeland and the funds contributed to the Zionist Federation by the South African Jewry were unparalleled.[80] Part of this funding went towards the construction of the Ashkelon Hospital.

As Penn described it, he first broached the idea of a "government border hospital at Ashkelon" with the then Prime Minister of Israel, Ben-Gurion's successor, Moshe Sharett. He also approached Ben-Gurion who gave the project his approval and the plans for the hospital were subsequently drawn up. Cognisance was taken of its strategic position and the hospital had to be rendered impervious to explosives and shrapnel. Despite this, Penn described it as "one of the most aesthetically attractive buildings [he] had ever seen".[81] The town of Ashkelon itself had another South African connection—architect Roy Kantorowich, a graduate of Wits.

Kantorowich had first been responsible for designing the model town of Vanderbijlpark in South Africa in 1941. Vanderbijlpark was built to house the workers of ISCOR (the Iron and Steel Corporation), a symbol of South African industrial prowess in the pre-War era. It was planned as a "symmetrical" and modern town with "parks, playing grounds, health clinics, hospitals and schools"—the idealised suburban paradise that gave little indication of its connection to industry. Kantorowich's vision was also a reaction to the uncontrollable urbanisation that had characterised South Africa over the preceding decades and had increased during the

[79] Ami Barak and Yaron Har-Shai, "The Israel Society for Plastic Surgeons: A Brief Introduction", *Aesthetic Surgery Journal*, September/October 2004, pp448–449.

[80] Gideon Shimoni, *Community and Conscience: The Jews in Apartheid South Africa* (Glosderry, David Philip Publishers, 2003), pp4–5.

[81] Penn, *The Right to Look Human*, pp185–186.

War, bringing slums, poverty, malnutrition, disease and a threat to segregation. Harmonious architectural planning was a means of returning order to physical space. It was also criticised as "a marriage of modernity and racism".[82] Yet Kantorowich's work in South Africa can also be seen as an attempt to initiate "social reform" through the regulation of space—a vision of planned black townships with all the amenities of the suburbs was the means of alleviating the poor conditions associated with informal housing as well as obviating black protest.[83] Space was not neutral territory, neither was modernity.

And the same applied to Ashkelon. The site for the model town was adjacent to Migdal-Gad, a border region that had initially contained a mixed settlement of both Israelis and Palestinians. The latter were removed, and the planned town was a reflection of Israeli policy to focus on rural origins as sites of settlement. As well as its strategic location, the town—close to the Mediterranean—would be poised to develop a tourist industry as well as secondary industry.[84] The initial plan developed by the South African architectural team was a vision of an English landscape that had to be adapted to the conditions of the Middle East. The final plan was of "five…neighbourhood units, each housing 2 500 people, with centrally located shopping centres and schools, and major transportation routes and greenbelts separating the units", that would mark the heart of Ashkelon.[85] The plan for what became known as Afridar bore great resemblance to the vision of Vanderbijlpark. There were similar ideological imperatives—middle-class, planned Jewish suburbs on the periphery of Palestinian towns that would eventually become the dominant spaces. In the South African context, although poorly implemented, model urban spaces were a means of compensating for black dispossession and creating a controlled environment that would serve the needs of development and

[82] Bill Freund, *Twentieth-Century South Africa: A Developmental History* (Cambridge, Cambridge University Press, 2019), pp144–147. Freund Attributes the Criticism to A. Mabin, "Varied Legacies of Modernism in Urban Planning" in G. Bridge and S. Watson (eds), *A Companion to the City* (Oxford and Malden, Blackwell, 2000), pp555–566.

[83] Ayala Levin, "South African 'Know-how' and Israeli 'Facts of Life': The Planning of Afridar, Ashkelon, 1949–1956", *Planning Perspectives*, 34, 2, 285–309, 2019, p297.

[84] Ibid., pp290–291.

[85] Ibid., pp293–294.

ideology.[86] To make the comparisons even more explicit, the centre of Afridar is marked by a plaque in Afrikaans, English and Hebrew detailing the origins of the model suburb as a result of funding by South African Jewish Appeal.[87]

In addition to town planning, surgery and the provision of a hospital, another South African experiment that was applied to Israel was that of social medicine—and its founding father would eventually part ways with the apartheid state to permanently settle in Israel. Sidney Kark was born in Johannesburg in 1911, the son of emigrants from Lithuania. Like Penn, he attended the medical school at Wits. But that is where the similarities ended. Kark demonstrated an early interest in political activism, joining the National Union of South African Students (NUSAS) as well as the Labour Party. Kark was particularly interested in social medicine—the ways in which socio-economic conditions affect health that in South Africa, was often based on historical inequality.[88] In the decade preceding 1948, community health care was of primary importance in social medicine and Kark was part of the vanguard focusing on a holistic view of medical care that incorporated patient, community, medical personnel and educators. This was based on his research in rural African communities that demonstrated the adverse effects of migrant labour on domestic agriculture (leading to malnutrition), the spread of disease and the breakdown of the family unit. Sidney and Emily Kark were key figures in the Pholela Health Centre in rural Zululand that attempted to not only treat the existing medical conditions of the area's residents, but engaged in preventative measures through the advocacy of effective agricultural techniques, the availability of fresh produce, feeding schemes in schools and so forth. Kark also headed the Department of Social, Preventative and Family Medicine at the University of Natal Medical School. In the pre-apartheid era, social medicine was significant for its multiracial approach with work done in diverse

[86] Ibid., pp296–297.

[87] Ibid., p286.

[88] Theodore M. Brown and Elizabeth Fee, "Sidney Kark and John Cassel: Social Medicine Pioneers and South African Emigres", *American Journal of Public Health*, 92, 11, November 2002, pp1744–1745.

racial communities. However, this collaborative effort would come under increasing pressure from 1948.[89]

Medical doctor and political activist Mervyn Susser was unstinting in his praise of Kark's influence on social medicine—the role of Pholela in serving as a model for similar health centres established across the country, the use of health care workers drawn from the community who were part of medical teams working on comprehensive solutions to prevalent health issues and preventative measures and the formalisation of social medicine. After serving during the Second World War, Susser—motivated by a vision of a better world—was profoundly influenced by Kark's work, becoming a devoted practitioner of social medicine. The exposure to the poor health conditions of Africans resulting from discriminatory racial policies exacerbated Susser's activist tendencies.[90] While based in the sprawling township of Alexandra in Johannesburg, Susser and his wife, Dr Zeina Stein, developed an understanding of the disjuncture between their medical training and the lived experience of black South Africans:

> Our medical curriculum addressed the conditions apparent in the segregated white fraction of the population...What happened in the black majority population was foreign land. We learned about that independently out of hours in outpatient clinics and wards of black hospitals.[91]

Their subsequent criticism of apartheid policy eventually resulted in them leaving the country in 1956.[92]

Kark was not spared the enmity of the apartheid state. Under the new dispensation, he served for a time as a buffer between the state and social medical practitioners, attempting to preserve the Institute of Community and Family Health. Eventually, he too was investigated by the Department of Health for possible communist ties. Within a climate of

[89] J.D. Kark and J.H. Abramson, "Sidney Kark's Contributions to Epidemiology and Community Medicine", *International Journal of Epidemiology*, 32, 5, 882–884, October 2003, p882.

[90] Mervyn Susser, "A South African Odyssey in Community Health: A Memoir of the Impact of the Teachings of Sidney Kark", *American Journal of Public Health*, 83, 7, 1039–1042, July 1993, p1040.

[91] William Yardley, "Mervyn Susser, 92, Dies; Studied Illness and Society", *The New York Times*, 26 August 2014, https://www.nytimes.com/2014/08/27/us/mervyn-susser-92-dies-studied-illness-and-society.html, accessed 22 March 2021.

[92] Ibid.

increasing repression, Sidney and Emily Kark eventually left the country. With the assistance of WHO, he brought his talents to bear in Israel, establishing the Department of Social Medicine of the Hebrew University and Hadassah Medical School. He used his South African experience and the principles formulated there in addressing the medical needs of the influx of Jewish immigrants to the country.[93] While Penn wholeheartedly endorsed Kark's work in Israel in his autobiography, he neatly glossed over the circumstances that compelled the Karks to relocate from South Africa, attributing their permanent residence in Jerusalem to the success of their medical health programmes. Moreover, in a manner that simplifies the collaborative and interactive vision of social medicine as envisaged by Kark, for Penn medical treatment and preventative measures were a means of introducing "western methods of hygiene and practice" to populations who had had little experience of them.[94]

By 1967, an interesting turnaround had occurred in expertise in military medicine. Whereas, with the conflict of 1948, South African sympathisers were drawn in to provide their medical expertise in wartime conditions, the numerous conflicts in which the Middle Eastern country had been embroiled since its inception had hastened Israeli medical expertise and organisation on the battlefield. Penn reported on what became known as the "Six Day War", along "with recommendations for our own Army".[95] Surrounded by hostile neighbouring Arab states, the War was precipitated by Israel launching a pre-emptive strike in the face of increasing Egyptian aggression. Over the next six days, the War drew in other Arab states as well and Israel would eventually make significant territorial gains while achieving astounding military success.[96]

Penn's analysis of the conflict was not simply confined to medical treatment and organisation but also focused on successful military strategy. It addressed Soviet support of the Arab forces, both in terms of the provision of weaponry as well as reconnaissance, placing the conflict within the context of the Cold War. Israel was portrayed as engaged in a titanic battle against a numerically superior enemy and its formidable ally. Penn wrote glowingly of Israeli superiority in the air, on the ground and at

[93] Susser, "A South African Odyssey in Community Health", p1042.

[94] Penn, *The Right to Look Human*, p184.

[95] Ibid., p188.

[96] Brenner, *In Search of Israel*, p188.

sea. The pilots in the Israeli Air Force flew at low altitudes to evade the radar of the Egyptians and were thus able to carry out precision strikes against strategic targets while keeping their own casualties to a minimum. If shot down, the pilots could eject safely from the plane but if caught in hostile territory, were "brutally lynched" in retaliation. The more fortunate airmen, however, were equipped with a beacon allowing rescue helicopters to locate them. As Penn observed, in contrast to the Second World War, the ability of pilots to easily eject meant that they were not trapped in the burning wreckage, necessitating little need for plastic and reconstructive surgeons.[97]

In terms of tank warfare, Penn described Israeli forces as "inferior in numbers but vastly superior in intelligence, courage, drive and training". The same could not be said for the Egyptians, hampered by inferior Russian equipment and strategies. Finding the Egyptian battle plans "rigid" and "predictable", Israeli forces were easily able to break through Egyptian lines. Also significant was the accuracy of the tank gunners as well as the undoubted bravery of tank commanders who, disdaining the use of the periscope, stood in the opened hatch of the tank to get a more accurate picture of the battlefield and advise their forces accordingly. Their actions made them vulnerable targets and often resulted in a high mortality rate amongst officers. Penn recommended the use of some form of "shield" to protect these men. Unlike in the Air Force, burns were more common in tank warfare with the greatest destruction wrought by napalm. The open hatch left officers vulnerable but also provided troops with a quick escape from a burning tank, thus minimising burn injuries.[98]

Penn accredited the success of the infantry to their training where, in contrast to 1948, the limitations of language differences were overcome over a strenuous two-and-a-half-year period of training accorded to all Israeli men leading to the instillation of strict military discipline.[99] Emphasis was also "placed on the rescue of the wounded" that minimised casualties and also likely enforced the *esprit de corps*. As in most wars, the infantry bore the brunt of the casualties, but these were largely of the orthopaedic variety due to the use of mines and the effects of shrapnel.

[97] Penn, *The Right to Look Human*, p189.

[98] Ibid., pp190–191.

[99] The use of conscript soldiers in South Africa would be an issue on which Penn had sometimes controversial opinions and is addressed in the final section.

Again, the role of the plastic surgeon was minimal, with very few facial and jaw injuries and those largely as a result of gunshot wounds.[100]

Penn was particularly taken with the medical interventions put in place to minimise casualties. All military medical doctors were given intense training in battlefield medicine and were expected to serve on the front-lines. While this subjected them to enemy fire, leading to injury and death, it permitted the early treatment of the wounded who were efficiently transported to hospitals via ambulance or helicopter. The timeous evacuation of the wounded served as a psychological boost for fighting men. For South Africa, the key lessons learned were the importance of having doctors trained in traumatology, the quick evacuation of the wounded accompanied by the application of emergency treatment on the frontlines and the use of preventative measures to minimise injury.[101]

The Israeli military ethos with its emphasis on the rescue of the wounded soldier highlighted the importance of every life and the sacrificing nature of the tank officer underscored the role of leadership from the front. Penn contrasted this to the Egyptians, with Anwar Sadat willing to sacrifice large numbers of his soldiers while remaining out of the fray. For Penn, the role of Sadat and the motivation of the Arab states opposing Israel was negligible. This was "a Russian war" and isolated and outnumbered, Israel was the lone bulwark against communism and Russian strategic interest in the Suez Canal. Penn highlighted this sense of isolation in the wake of 1973.[102]

The Yom Kippur War was a result of an attack on Israel by Egypt and Syria. Caught off-guard, the early days of the conflict were marked by major Israeli losses until the country was, once again, able to triumph militarily. The context of the War was significant—Israel's policies were coming under increasing criticism by the international community, culminating in the UN's view of Zionism as "racism" two years later.[103] In addition, the War began in early October and while it was still ongoing, six Arab oil-producing countries—who were members of the Organisation of Petroleum Exporting Countries (OPEC)—announced a reduction in their export of oil. The reduction was initially five per cent

[100] Penn, *The Right to Look Human*, p192.

[101] Ibid., pp192–193.

[102] Ibid., pp195–196.

[103] Brenner, *In Search of Israel*, p205.

but would continue in reaction to the Palestinian conflict, with each reduction increasing the price of oil.[104] The action served to hamper the intervention of Western countries in Palestine and their support of Israel.[105]

Almost a year later, Israeli Defence Minister, Moshe Dayan, paid one of numerous visits to South Africa and in an interview, regretted Israel's handling of the War, while re-iterating the lack of viability of a separate Palestinian state. His opinion—which he accredited to a broader Israeli view—was that Arabs in Palestine should instead be sent to the neighbouring Arab states, "The Arabs must look after their own".[106] During Dayan's visit, he also exhorted young Jewish South Africans to settle in Israel, manning the "strategic settlements", including that at Ma'alot, the site of a Palestinian attack four months earlier.[107]

Dayan's visit was suggestive of the increasing links between South Africa and Israel. In an article appearing in the *Rand Daily Mail* upon his return from Israel in 1967, Penn emphasised what he considered to be the similarities in the "geographical and political picture" between South Africa and Israel.[108] Like Israel, South Africa was besieged by potentially hostile neighbours tacitly supported by the communists. But the similarities ran even deeper.

South Africa and Israel

At the end of August 1957, the *Rand Daily Mail* in its list of events carried a small advertisement placed by the South African Zionist Federation for the opportunity for the citizens of Johannesburg to "Pay Tribute to General Moshe Dayan: Chief of Staff, General Army of Israel, the Hero of the Sinai Campaign". The event was to take place at 3 p.m. on 2 September at the Wembley Stadium in Johannesburg.[109]

[104] Timothy Mitchell, "The Resources of Economics: Making the 1973 Oil Crisis", *Journal of Cultural Economy*, 3, 2, 189–204, 2010, p190.

[105] Brenner, *In Search of Israel*, p205.

[106] Bob Hitchcock, "Dayan's Big Regret", *Rand Daily Mail*, 3 September 1974.

[107] "Live in Israel—Dayan", *Rand Daily Mail*, 3 September 1974.

[108] "Mid-East War 'Has Lessons for S. Africa'", *Rand Daily Mail*, 3 July 1967.

[109] Advertisement, *Rand Daily Mail*, 31 August 1957.

Dayan had arrived in the country just two days prior on a three-week visit that would take him to the major cities of the country and include a visit to Rhodesia (Zimbabwe). His arrival was at the invitation of the SA Zionist Federation and he was given an ecstatic welcome by more than three hundred people who composed part of the Jewish segment of the population in Johannesburg. Dayan however, while the key Israeli military leader, made clear to reporters that he would not be meeting with his counterparts in the South African military.[110]

The same edition of the newspaper also ran a brief biographical sketch of Dayan, portraying him in the vein of an almost Old Testament warrior, "one hand on the sword, the other on the plough", who had begun life as a farmer before being called upon to defend "his country and people" at the young age of fourteen. Dayan's parents were early "pioneers" working to make the harsh land suitable for cultivation, laying the foundations for the state that would come into being. From the age of 12, Dayan was armed and tasked with sentry duty in the event of Arab raiders. Two years later, he joined Haganah, an armed organisation to counter Arab raids. During the Second World War, members of Haganah fought alongside the British and it was in conflict against the Syrians, that Dayan received his trademark eye injury, leading to the wearing of a distinctive black eyepatch.[111]

A significant reason for Dayan's visit to South Africa in 1957 was to have reconstructive surgery at the Brenthurst Clinic. In the war of 1956, after his driver was shot by snipers, Dayan—often at the forefront of the action—believed that his eyepatch singled him out as a target.[112] The patch was however necessary due to the potential discomfort caused by sand on his exposed eye socket. Penn's solution was the removal of the "conjunctiva" and the use of a skin graft over the exposed area, making the eye socket impervious to irritating debris.[113] A year later,

[110] "General Dayan Given Great Welcome at Jan Smuts Airport", *Rand Daily Mail*, 30 August 1957.

[111] Harry O'Connor, "A Pen Picture of Dayan, Israel's Army Chief: Boy Farmer Who Became a Soldier", *Rand Daily Mail*, 30 August 1957.

[112] Dayan also acknowledged that the wearing of an eyepatch also drew unwanted "attention" when he was out in public, serving as a source of some anxiety, "Letters describing Dayan losing his eye to be auctioned".

[113] Penn, *The Right to Look Human*, p187.

Penn returned to Israel for the follow-up stage of the procedure.[114] The South African would later observe a decade later that Dayan continued his fight in close proximity to enemy lines during the Six Day War wearing dark glasses.[115]

In September 1974, Dayan returned to South Africa on a two-week visit at the behest of the South Africa Federation. In addition to the usual round of talks and meetings, he had a special purpose in his visit—the recruitment of young South African Jewish men and women to immigrate to Israel and populate its "strategic settlements".[116] Much on Dayan's mind, however, was the war the previous year and the criticism he incurred for failing to act swiftly enough to launch a pre-emptive strike against Egypt, despite observing the increased armaments and troop movements of the latter. The eventual conflict almost spelled the end of what the article described as "the plucky little state of Israel".[117] In Penn's own assessment of the Yom Kippur War, he described the conflict as a result of the belligerent actions of Anwar Sadat, the Egyptian leader willing to sacrifice the lives of his people, in contrast to the reluctant Israelis who although eventually triumphant, could ill afford to lose its people.[118] It was perhaps this loss of life and the importance of maintaining control of the land that motivated Dayan's recruitment.

Penn also highlighted Israel's increasing sense of isolation with very few countries—such as South Africa—willing to serve as an ally. The Arab states, on the other hand, enjoyed the support of Britain and France as well as the "Black African States [who] forget their indebtedness to Israel for helping their development and broke off relations to please Arabs – who had never helped them".[119] The period also marked the point of the international oil crisis and the reliance on Arab oil exports, a period when Penn—as evident in his writings—reserved his harshest criticism for the failure of the UN to take an adequate stand against Arab "irregulars" or "terrorists", accrediting this to the insidious influence of communism.[120]

[114] "Dayan Meets Eye Surgeon", *Rand Daily Mail*, 19 April 1958.

[115] Penn, *The Right to Look Human*, p187.

[116] "Live in Israel—Dayan".

[117] Hitchcock, "Dayan's Big Regret".

[118] Penn, *The Right to Look Human*, pp195–196.

[119] Ibid., p196.

[120] Ibid.

Another country that bore the effects of this isolation was South Africa—an ally of Israel. Although written almost forty years ago, Leonard Thompson's treatise on Afrikaner nationalism demonstrates many parallels with Zionism. Afrikaner nationalism had its origins in a hostile land, often in terms of environment but also due to the great majority of indigenous peoples who needed to be subjugated to allow for settler expansion. The strife and struggle that accompanied settler expansion into the interior of the country was given a religious overtone which resonated powerfully with a people who were rural, largely uneducated and Calvinist, perceiving the Bible to be the ultimate authority. The view of Afrikaners as a "chosen" people with a destiny preordained by God was thus a powerful one.[121] Afrikaner nationalism grew in strength from the nineteenth century and in the wake of the South African War, with an emphasis on a new language (Afrikaans), the notion of martyrdom and victimisation by British imperialists and the reworking of history to emphasise the struggle against indigenous peoples and the ultimate domination of South Africa in line with divine destiny. Even with the growth of urbanisation and secularisation, the mythology retained a strong hold.[122]

A diasporic group scattered across Europe for two thousand years, Jewish identity was defined by a sense of "otherness", both in how they were perceived by those around them and in how they viewed themselves. The former often manifested in anti-Semitism and the latter in a sense of identity that transcended national boundaries. And like Afrikaner nationalists, embedded in Judaism was the notion of Jews as a "chosen people" with a unique destiny that emphasised their otherness. It was thus only through the creation of an independent nation state that drew together the diaspora that a sense of belonging could be achieved.[123] There was also a distinct vision of the role of the Jewish nation state, one that was first described by one of the leading figures in Zionism—who would influence Ben-Gurion—Theodor Herzl. In Herzl's utopian vision, the "Jewish State" would not simply be a Jewish homeland but would serve as a "model state" that would be a shining beacon of civilisation

[121] Leonard Thompson, *The Political Mythology of Apartheid* (New Haven and London, Yale University Press, 1985), pp26–32.

[122] Ibid., pp29–31.

[123] Brenner, *In Search of Israel*, pp2–4.

that would have as its goal the "improvement" of all—not just its Jewish citizens.[124]

By 1975 however, Israel was the focus of international condemnation with the UN passing a resolution that described Zionism as "a form of racism and racist discrimination".[125] Like the apartheid state, Israel was caught between the old and the new, the past and modernity and just as Israel positioned itself as an exemplar of progress and improvement in the Middle East so, too, did South Africa in Africa—and both would face increasing isolation and international hostility.

The anti-Semitism of Afrikaner nationalism in the pre-Second World War era changed dramatically after the nationalists came to power in 1948. D.F. Malan's government continued to send supplies to the Zionist Federation—as had been initiated by the preceding administration—and he visited the country in 1948 with the South African state officially recognising Israel as an independent country a year later.[126] In 1948, eight hundred South African Jewish volunteers fought in Israel. Largely war veterans, many underwent additional training in camps set up near Johannesburg and at Witbank and organised by the South African Zionist Federation. While the state was aware of these activities, it did nothing to dissuade the volunteers who went on to play active roles in Israel's war as both combatants and in offering medical assistance—as discussed here.[127]

Penn helped to foster the intellectual co-operation between the two countries through the "exchange of brains". He exhorted his friends for individual contributions of £50 to finance an exchange programme—Israeli scientists were invited to South Africa to give talks and interact with South African scientists and students and their South African counterparts did the same in Israel. According to Penn, this intellectual "exchange" would eventually be adopted by the CSIR (Council of Scientific and Industrial Research) in South Africa, the Weizmann Institute in Israel and

[124] Ibid., pp51–53.

[125] Ibid., p186.

[126] Shula Marks, "Apartheid and the Jewish Question", *Journal of Southern African Studies*, 30, 4, 889–900, December 2004, p891.

[127] Gillon, *Seventy Years of Southern African Aliyah*, pp19–20.

various tertiary institutions.[128] The initially tentative but growing relationship between the two countries also manifested itself in the sharing of nuclear technology.

After the Second World War and in line with the rest of the world, South Africa developed a keen interest in the potential of nuclear power. Further, the country had a significant advantage—while South Africa does not contain natural uranium deposits, uranium is produced as a result of the gold-mining process and South Africa began exporting the product to Britain and the United States to fuel their own nuclear programmes. Jan Smuts initiated the Atomic Energy Board and the project continued under the nationalists in 1948. While South Africa's main role was as an exporter of uranium, South African scientists were sent to the United States to understand uranium enrichment and by the 1950s, South Africa had built its own nuclear reactor.[129]

In 1955, Ben-Gurion delivered an election speech in Jerusalem where he informed the crowd that the United States would be providing Israel with a nuclear reactor. However, even without American assistance, Israel still had the uranium to begin exploiting nuclear energy. It was France, that provided Israel with a research reactor, setting in motion an alliance between the two countries.[130] Ben-Gurion had developed an early understanding of the potential uses of nuclear power and was captivated by the notion of technology as a means to both "kill" and "cure", setting up the Science Corps prior to independence to develop the means of doing both. With the vision of the new state of Israel as the exemplification of progress, he met with atomic scientists in 1949 and by 1961, was convinced of the importance of nuclear power both for its potential in developing Israel but also for its military uses.[131]

This use of nuclear power to either "kill" or "cure" was familiar to the South African state which was interested in the possibilities of using nuclear weapons against their own enemies or maintaining the weapons as a deterrent. South Africa had already begun selling uranium to Israel when in 1975, a meeting was held between the South African

[128] "We Can't Always Win!" in "Philosophy Is Fun" (Unpublished Manuscript), December 1983, File: Penn, Jack—Writings (3), AMUW.

[129] Freund, *Twentieth-Century South Africa*, p172.

[130] Segev, *A State at Any Cost*, Chapter 22: Yes to the Old Man.

[131] Ibid.

defence minister, P.W. Botha and his Israeli counterpart, Shimon Peres with the former requesting nuclear warheads and the latter offering to sell the South Africans Jericho missiles that could be adapted as nuclear weapons.[132] While the sale did not go ahead, a year later South African Prime Minister John Vorster concluded a military alliance with Israel setting the scene for greater nuclear co-operation between the two countries. By 1980, South Africa had developed its own nuclear bomb and engaged in a nuclear test of its own.[133] When the country decided to disarm its nuclear weapons in 1990, South Africa had already produced at least six fully capable nuclear weapons.[134]

It was however, the importance of nuclear power as a means of furthering development that was of interest to Penn, as evident in his own writings and his engagement with Edward Teller—which is addressed in the final section. This was largely precipitated by the energy crisis of the turbulent 1970s. At the same time, Penn was on the periphery—even if not aware—of significant military alliances as well as the development of weapons technology. During the Six Day War, for instance, where Penn served in a largely consultative capacity,[135] giving him the freedom to travel across the country, he noted Egyptian manufacture of poison gas and, particularly astounding is the following claim, "I was also able to bring back to South Africa samples of poison gases with full descriptions of their use in Russian and French!".[136]

As with the development of South Africa's nuclear weapons programme, there remains a great deal of secrecy around events and much of the documentation was deliberately destroyed however South Africa evidently began its own chemical and biological weapons project to quell violent resistance to the apartheid state. Testifying before the

[132] Chris McGeal, "Revealed: How Israel Offered to Sell South Africa Nuclear Weapons", A Supplement to the Washington Report on Middle East Affairs, August 2010, Reprinted in https://www.theguardian.com/world/2010/may/23/israel-south-africa-nuclear-weapons, accessed 28 April 2021. Israel subsequently denied that the offer related to nuclear weapons.

[133] Freund, *Twentieth-Century South Africa*, pp174–175.

[134] Verne Harris, Sello Hatang and Peter Liberman, "Unveiling South Africa's Nuclear Past", *Journal of Southern African Studies*, 30, 3, 457–475, 2004, p457.

[135] A decade earlier, Penn was the visiting Professor for Plastic Surgery at the Hebrew University in Jerusalem, "Hebrew University Anniversary Banquet", *Rand Daily Mail*, 9 June 1955.

[136] Penn, *The Right to Look Human*, p188.

Truth and Reconciliation Commission the former head of forensics in the South African Police, Lieutenant-General Lothar Neethling pinpointed 1976 as the start of the chemical weapons project in the wake of the violence of the Soweto uprising. South African representatives were sent to Europe, the United States and Israel to conduct research. The rationale for the initiation of the chemical and biological weapons project—code-named Project Coast—was that the international community had done little to assist South Africa against the apparent Cuban use of chemical weapons in Angola, forcing the country to develop its own methods of defence.[137]

The various means of employing chemical and biological weapons under Project Coast included the application of toxins that could be absorbed through the skin, the growth of disease-causing bacteria such as *Bacillus anthracis* (responsible for anthrax), *E. coli*, *Yersina enterocolitica* (similar to plague-causing bacteria) and *Vibrio cholerae* (which causes cholera). There was also a "fertility project" due to concerns regarding population growth and the desire to clandestinely curb the reproduction of black women. Very early on then, the focus shifted from developing protection against chemical and biological weapons that could theoretically be used on South African troops, to developing weapons to be used against the enemies of the state.[138]

It is ironic that at the same time as Penn would be involved in attempts to implement reforms to apartheid, Project Coast was well underway, undertaking research and engaging in experiments that defied medical ethics. Penn's obtaining of a sample of poison gas from the Middle East—and his public acknowledgement of such in his autobiography—is a good indication that his belief was that the sample could be used to develop a means of protection and was likely an object of scientific interest. It also indicates his complete ignorance of the means by which those in power were willing to go in order to maintain dominance.

While Penn appeared to be largely on the periphery, his various trips to the Middle East were indicative of the growing relationship between South Africa and Israel. From the provision of medical assistance on the part of volunteers who were not sanctioned by the state—although there

[137] Marléne Burger and Chandré Gould, *Secrets and Lies: Wouter Basson and South Africa's Chemical and Biological Warfare Programme* (Cape Town, Zebra Press, 2002), pp14–15.

[138] Ibid., pp30–31.

was evidently tacit state approval—the relationship between the two countries became increasingly formalised due to their unique global positions, culminating in the sharing of military technology. As Edgerton points out, technology—the face of modernisation—is imbued with nationalism a response "to a modern, industrial and globalising world".[139] This was as true for Israel as it was for South Africa but with the transition to modernity and the concerns about maintaining security and order, science and technology were also the means by which inequality was reinforced where "Old power relations are transmitted through new technology".[140] This emphasis on security mirrored Penn's role in Israel which had begun with medical assistance offered in 1948 and who eventually exceeded this role when he drew up reports on military capability and strategy. His access to key Israeli figures such as Dayan and Ben-Gurion also suggests the conjunction of medicine and diplomacy. Simultaneously, while many Jewish South African doctors were drawn to Israel and eventually settled permanently in the country, not all shared the same ideological views held by Penn with Sidney Kark being a prominent example. Penn served instead as a medical ambassador, a representative of South African medical and scientific prowess. In the latter part of his career, the convergence of medicine and ideology would become even more explicit.

[139] David Edgerton, *The Shock of the Old: Technology and Global History Since 1900* (London, Profile Books Ltd, 2008), p106.

[140] Ibid., p159.

PART III

Utopia?

CHAPTER 10

"A Multitude of Differing Genes": Intellect, Education and Equality

In the wake of the 1913 Natives Land Act that infamously restricted Africans to seven per cent of the land, Sol Plaatje's *Native Life in South Africa* begins with the hauntingly poignant, "Awakening on Friday morning, June 20, 1913, the South African native found himself, not actually a slave but a pariah in the land of his birth".[1] More than sixty years later, Jack Penn would also articulate a sense of alienation—albeit on a far lesser scale—based on what he perceived to be the marginalisation of the English language, "I feel that I belong to my country South Africa, but my country does not belong to me".[2] It indicated an uneasy sense of belonging and identity in apartheid South Africa. Unease notwithstanding, Penn's views on apartheid racial and ethnic policies were contextualised by a belief in white dominance and superiority. First published in 1974, Penn's autobiography *The Right to Look Human* concludes with a chapter entitled "African Dilemma", an articulation of

[1] Sol Plaatje, *Native Life in South Africa* (Northlands, Picador Africa, 2007), p21.

[2] Jack Penn, *The Right to Look Human: An Autobiography* (Johannesburg, Hugh Keartland Publishers, 1976), p234.

"A Multitude of Differing Genes": Quote taken from Jack Penn, *Reflections on Life* (Johannesburg, Ernest Stanton Publishers, 1980), p35.

S. Chetty, *Reconstructive Surgery and Modernisation in Twentieth-Century South Africa*, Medicine and Biomedical Sciences in Modern History, https://doi.org/10.1007/978-3-031-38673-2_10

Penn's reflections on race relations in South Africa. At times anachronistic, it is riddled with contradiction and at the heart of it, is underpinned by Penn's beliefs regarding intellectual ability and race.

In Penn's discussion of apartheid policy, he highlighted the distinction between "grand" and "petty" apartheid, emphasising the former's continuation of the segregationist thinking that was a product of the pre-apartheid era. In what was a common refrain, the Bantustans or independent homelands served as the sites for the development of different cultures according to their "traditional lines" with the South African state providing the financial means to sustain this separate development. In this, Penn believed the state was motivated by two aims—its genuine concern for the welfare of the "Black tribes" with the state assuming the mantle of benevolent guardianship. The second overriding aim was the maintenance of "European" supremacy and culture in South Africa:

> Personally, I have no doubt of the sincerity of the National Party that in their determination to carry out this policy they have the future of the various Black tribes at heart, even though it is obvious that their main drive is to prevent European culture and the European way of life from being swamped by overwhelming African numbers should integration and too idealistic, democratic principles prevail. They consider that South Africa is in fact a piece of Europe in Africa and are determined to keep it that way.[3]

Yet Penn was aware of the contradictions of separate development, especially in "white" South Africa where Africans were employed in various capacities such as raising "vulnerable white babies" and the Prime Minister of the country, B.J. Vorster, admitted to being able to speak *isiXhosa* before he learned Afrikaans.[4] For Penn, apartheid was not based on "prejudice" but was instead a way of maintaining a cultural identity that was in danger of being "annihilated". Should the threat of being culturally and politically "swamped" by blacks be alleviated so too would the desire for segregation.[5]

[3] Ibid., pp234–235.

[4] Ibid., p236.

[5] Ibid., pp235–236.

Penn was less sanguine about "petty" apartheid which, lacking the veneer of paternalism and self-preservation, was blatant racial discrimination. Described as "humiliating and insufferable" as well as an "embarrassment" to the country, "petty" apartheid referred to apartheid legislation applied to urban areas. This was to limit the interaction between white and black in public spaces, evident in the allocation of separate amenities.[6] Penn's views went to the heart of the tensions within the notion of "trusteeship"—the inequality associated with paternalism and the racial discrimination resulting from the implementation of "petty" apartheid. As Allsobrook and Boisen have argued, the liberal yet paternalistic discourse of trusteeship during the colonial era metamorphosised into an ideology of segregation and apartheid based on separate development.[7] Trusteeship was contextualised by ideology and by economic circumstance. A further change would occur with the reform initiatives undertaken by the apartheid state, beginning in the mid-1970s and evident in Penn's work on the President's Council. As such, Penn's views do not reflect the liberalism of his contemporaries in the Progressive Party for instance who—as will be discussed—were critical of the state's attempt at limited reform, but instead the changing position of the apartheid government as it sought to address the economic and political turmoil of the 1970s, the period in which Penn's autobiography was written.

While Penn criticised "petty" apartheid, he pointed to the hypocrisy of other states that engaged in oppressive measures of their own which were not necessarily legislated. This included persecution in the Soviet Union, the affirmative action in the United States that made special provision for black students at the expense of their white counterparts and the informal segregation evident in New Zealand, the United States and Brazil. The origins of segregation lay not with the Afrikaner Nationalists but with the British who put in place the legislation that would underpin "petty" apartheid even before South Africa came into existence as a national entity. Moreover, he pointedly referred to the ethnic violence taking place in Africa in the wake of independence, suggesting that this

[6] Ibid., p236.

[7] *Cf.* Christopher Allsobrook and Camilla Boisen, "Two Types of Trusteeship in South Africa: From Subjugation to Separate Development", *Politikon*, 44, 2, 265–285, 2017.

was more prevalent than the discrimination of white against black.[8] Examples of African discrimination cited include that of Idi Amin, described as a "psychopathic personality" who was nevertheless a figure in the UN. For Penn, the most glaring example was that of the Igbo in Nigeria who had proved their ability to assimilate to Western values and were described as "highly intelligent and Christian by religion", "the elite of Africa" and on par with the "white race" in terms of their technological ability. This made their slaughter by the "less-developed Hausa tribe, Moslem by religion" a calamity of epic proportions.[9]

In contrast to the rest of Africa, which was portrayed in apocalyptic and nihilistic terms, Penn believed that the apartheid state was not all that repressive in comparison, allowing a "free press" and censure of state policies. The holding of possible insurgents without trial was attributed to the country being in a state of war against the forces of communism.[10] Penn was also able to contextualise the events of the Sharpeville "Massacre"—the use of quotation marks already hinting at his perception of the event. An anti-pass march by the Pan African Congress (PAC) in March 1960 culminated in the police firing on the crowd outside the Sharpeville Police Station. This resulted in the death of sixty-nine people and aroused international condemnation. In reaction, the apartheid state took the offensive, banning the PAC, African National Congress (ANC) and the Communist Party of South Africa, ushering in a decade of state domination and repression. Penn was sympathetic to the "bewildered police force", highlighting the hostility presented by black protestors as evident in an earlier "mob" attack in Cato Manor which resulted in "a number of policemen being hacked to pieces". He moreover referred to the "stone-throwing agitators" who placed women and children at the forefront of the Sharpeville protestors, resulting in their deaths once the police opened fire. He alluded to similar incidents that occurred in the rest of the world, even if Sharpeville was the one given prominence. The events at Sharpeville were seen as a precursor to communist "tactics", conflating black nationalist protest with communist sedition:

[8] Penn, *The Right to Look Human*, pp236–237.

[9] Ibid., p244.

[10] Ibid., pp240–241.

> The Communists will repeat these tactics. The wretched Africans will be utilised as cannon fodder; the Communists will be labelled "liberators" and the forces of law and order will be labelled "murderers", even when fighting for their lives against foreign invaders.[11]

But while Penn had strong, complex and often contradictory views of apartheid, he sought to distance himself from the policy. "Grand" apartheid was acceptable and necessary, "petty" apartheid was an exercise in humiliation; the state—and Afrikaners in particular—were engaged in a fight for racial and ideological survival which underpinned apartheid policy but, "to those of us **who are not personally involved**, the system of personal restriction is intolerable".[12]

Penn's vacillation appears to be based on a notion of racial hierarchy that was already outdated at the time of his writing. At the core of his understanding of racial difference lay intellectual ability.

For Penn, Afrikaners had attained equality in finance, industry and science first reached by South Africans of British descent—the epitome of intellectual enterprise—and had done so in a relatively short time span. His concerns regarding apartheid segregationist policy were that, while it kept Africans separate and they would also not be averse to this separation due to whites and blacks having inherently distinct and incompatible cultures, it made little allowance for the coloureds and Indians who at least had the intellectual ability of the "average European". Moreover, the need for "technologies which the Black races find difficult" meant that there would be potential difficulties in making the independent homelands self-sufficient due to the lack of skills and the inability of the "Black races" to acquire these skills.[13] On the one hand then, segregation was necessarily based on the maintenance of white dominance as well as the cultural incompatibility of white and black. Simultaneously, what he perceived to be the intellectual inferiority of Africans meant that segregation would be difficult to implement fully without the need for white assistance, thus keeping intact a paternalistic relationship between the apartheid state and the homelands.

This dilemma led to Penn contradicting himself regarding intellectual ability and race. He emphasised that those who formed the professional

[11] Ibid., p242.

[12] Ibid., p236. Emphasis added.

[13] Ibid., pp234–235.

classes in South Africa were drawn from three racial categories—whites, Indians and coloureds. Policies of job reservation however, and lack of education opportunities, had relegated Africans to the lowest rung of the workforce. This needed to be rectified for them to acquire the necessary skills required for self-government.[14] Yet while Penn considered the means by which Africans could achieve some form of self-government, he also believed that independence and democracy were incompatible with African culture and ability. Drawing upon the newly independent African states, Penn emphasised the "artificiality" of their boundaries which did not necessarily coincide with ethnic groups, leaving the way open for internal conflict. These "Stone Age", largely "illiterate" and insular cultures were therefore ill-equipped for self-government. Independence had only given them the "[freedom] to kill one another off", to revert to internecine tribalism, atrocities and genocide against which colonialism had been a bulwark.[15] The grim picture painted of sub-Saharan Africa was in contrast to the maintenance of white civilisation and "white rule" in South Africa where "Africans are better housed, better educated, are healthier and live longer than in any other part of Africa".[16]

Whether Africans would ever be ready for independence is a key consideration and despite his belief in the acquisition of the relevant intellectual and technical skills necessary for self-government, Penn's view of intellectual ability, race and genetics would not be out of place a century earlier. In 1775, Johann Blumenbach, building on the earlier work of Carl Linnaeus, set out a racial classification system based on physical characteristics. Yet the system went beyond mere classification—associated with race were physical, mental and social attributes, amongst them intelligence and "civilisation". Inherent in the system of classification was one of hierarchy. Also relevant to this—perhaps even more so for a plastic surgeon—was the notion of physical "beauty" where that which was most aesthetically pleasing was found in the "white races".[17]

Theorists of race fell into two categories—the monogenists who believed that all races had a common origin and that differences were

[14] Ibid., p238.

[15] Ibid., pp243–244.

[16] Ibid., pp245–246.

[17] Charles King, *The Reinvention of Humanity: A Story of Race, Sex, Gender and the Discovery of Culture* (London, The Bodley Head, 2019), pp79–81.

simply a matter of variation, largely a product of environment. Polygenists argued for the insurmountable differences between races brought about by their separate origins. By the mid-nineteenth century, the position of the monogenists was the accepted one with Charles Darwin pointing out in the *Descent of Man* variations within species that made it all but impossible to delineate clear racial categories.[18] Polygenesis, however, continued to exert a strong hold, particularly in the United States where anthropometric measurements were used to highlight physical difference. This underpinned eugenics which reached its zenith in the racial sterilisation policies of Nazi Germany.[19] Yet in the first decade of the twentieth century, a key figure in American anthropology, Franz Boas, through a study of the diverse immigrant populations in New York, showed the inherent shakiness of race as an absolute category. By extension, so-called associated racial attributes—such as intelligence—lacked any scientific validity.[20] However, just as racial thinking in the United States was contextualised by concerns over the rising numbers of immigrants and concomitant fears of white degeneration, in South Africa violent encounters between settler and indigenous populations, dispossession and the subsequent formation of the Union of South Africa that entrenched white minority rule, provided the backdrop for theorising about race.

In the late nineteenth and early twentieth centuries, historian George Theal wrote several works on the history of South Africa that were designed to bolster settler claims to the region at a time when clashes between expanding settlers and indigenous groups were still ongoing and in the wake of precious mineral discoveries in Kimberley and on the Witwatersrand. Theal had clear racial categories of the indigenous inhabitants of southern Africa with a set hierarchy—the "Bushmen", the "Hottentots" and the "Bantu". In this categorisation, there was little allowance for an "advanced" civilisation that challenged European dominance and, even where some challenge could be made to this racial hierarchy using the evidence of Great Zimbabwe for instance, this was accredited to outside influence rather than African agency. Theal's hierarchy was bolstered by his use of craniometrics where average cranium

[18] Ibid., pp82–84.

[19] Ibid., pp88–89.

[20] Ibid., p98.

size was related to brain size and intellectual capacity. His work did not occur in a vacuum but was used to support Social Darwinist views of the "survival of the fittest" that justified the conquest and domination by white settlers and subsequent dispossession of indigenous inhabitants and would influence subsequent thinkers on race and segregation.[21]

In 1908, in a speech delivered to the Transvaal Native Affairs Society, F.W. Bell made an early claim for segregation. Drawing upon what was believed to be African racial inferiority, he proposed the exclusion of Africans from the franchise and their separate development according to their biological/racial abilities. In a manner that Penn would echo, Bell drew upon the work of American Robert Bean who pointed out that "negroes" had made no significant contribution to the arts and sciences which demonstrated their "fundamental" incapacity in sharp contradiction to the claims of "ignorant philanthropists".[22] While Cape liberals such as Theophilus Schreiner disagreed with Bell over the exclusion of Africans from the franchise, Schreiner did not challenge the premise of racial hierarchy and difference on which these arguments were made.[23]

Prior to the formation of the Union, racial eugenics underlay South African understandings of racial difference. In the wake of the South African War and under Alfred Milner's administration as High Commissioner, the emphasis was on Anglicisation—a policy that would only serve to enhance Afrikaner hostility and contribute in no small measure to the growth of Afrikaner nationalism. But the trend was a move towards the alliance of the "white races"—English and Afrikaners—in the forging of a new country, one that would exclude the "black races". The future of the last would be contextualised within developments of anthropology which sought to essentialise cultures and by so doing, exclude groups from the modern state. Through their shared European racial heritage, collaboration between white South Africans was desirable and even necessary. Simultaneously, the importance of controlled black labour to the economic well-being of the prospective state and the preservation of white

[21] Saul Dubow, *Scientific Racism in Modern South Africa* (Cambridge, Cambridge University Press, 1995), pp68–72.

[22] Ibid., pp89–90.

[23] Ibid., p91.

minority political dominance necessitated the use of eugenics to underpin the segregation of black and white.[24]

In the interwar period, eugenics thinking was concretised in the formation of the Race Welfare Society (RWS) in 1930. With a largely intellectual membership, its emphasis was on the promotion of a healthy white population and to prevent miscegenation and degeneration. Contextualised by the Great Depression the "poor white" problem, increasing African urbanisation, poverty, poor health, high mortality and the growth of slums, as well as fears of working-class alliances across colour lines, the RWS emphasised "negative" eugenics or the eradication of attributes that were deemed inferior. Birth control clinics were established for African, Indian, coloured as well as working-class white women to prevent the reproduction of those deemed biologically inferior. Yet both eugenics and Social Darwinism would increasingly fall into disrepute, their death knell due to the racial sterilisation policies of Nazi Germany. Within South Africa, the emphasis of liberals shifted to welfare policies focusing on the well-being of these vulnerable groups.[25] The apartheid state also did not base its policies of separation on Social Darwinism which sat uneasily with Calvinist doctrine, although Afrikaner nationalism did draw upon scientific racism to bolster already existing ideas of racial difference in the 1930s.[26]

Long after these theories were brought into dispute, Penn posed the following: "The question arises as to whether black people are intellectually inferior to white people".[27] He aimed criticism at contemporary "intellectuals [such as] sociologists and anthropologists" who were disinclined to support his by now anachronistic view that intellectual ability had a racial and a biological basis. In a manner reminiscent of the racial classification and hierarchies of the nineteenth century that situated the "Bushmen" at the very bottom, Penn emphasised their incompatibility with the expectations of modern life. They were instead ideally suited to

[24] Saul Dubow, *A Commonwealth of Knowledge: Science, Sensibility and White South Africa 1820–2000* (Oxford, Oxford University Press, 2007), pp176–177.

[25] Susanne Klausen, "The Race Welfare Society: Eugenics and Birth Control in Johannesburg, 1930–40" in *Science and Society in Southern Africa*, Saul Dubow (ed) (Manchester, Manchester University Press, 2000), pp164–187.

[26] *Cf* Saul Dubow, "Afrikaner Nationalism, Apartheid and the Concept of 'Race'", *Journal of African History*, 33, 2, 209–237, 1992.

[27] Penn, *The Right to Look Human*, p249.

"the rigours of desert life" and indeed, demonstrated their superiority in this area.[28] He would expand on this when questioned by a sceptic:

> I could not survive in the Kalahari Desert, but a bushman can live there for many years, and bring up his children. He can extract water from plants and can paint beautifully on the wall of a cave with self made implements, and fashion pots for use, with great skill. But for several generations he will not be able to compete with me or my offspring in the life of a city. We are equally intelligent – but to each his own.[29]

Penn's belief, still evident as late as 1983, ignored the changing nature of these societies that were increasingly marginalised and relegated to the more inhospitable regions of southern Africa in both the precolonial and colonial eras, requiring substantial adaptation. He chose instead to see them as eternal and unchanging, continuing their "traditions" as they had for millennia, isolated from the world around them. It was also a view that implied a lack of readiness or ability to embrace modernity or "Western civilisation". While claiming theoretical intellectual equality, Penn's view of intelligence was not simply related to the "acquisition of knowledge" but to what he described as "initiative thinking"—the ability to be creative and to apply what is learned, "the breaking of boundaries either in a physical sense, such as mechanical or medical inventions, or in a philosophical sense, such as improvement of ecology generally or mankind".[30] It was a sense of intelligence drawn from a particularly Western sensibility.

Penn's views of intellectual ability were not new—the question of African intellectual ability had been debated since the era of segregation. In the 1920s, anthropologist Werner Eiselen—based at Stellenbosch University and later head of the Eiselen Commission in the 1950s responsible for investigating and recommending changes to African education—defended the system of racial segregation based on what he believed to be innate biological differences between indigenous Africans and whites. His phrasing would be echoed by Penn along with the belief that the "Bantu" was "passive", lacked the ability for "responsible undertakings". Their

[28] Ibid.

[29] Jack Penn, "The Benefits of Travel" in "Philosophy Is Fun" (Unpublished Manuscript), December 1983, File: Penn, Jack—Writings (5), AMUW.

[30] Jack Penn, "The Value of Initiative Thinking" in "Philosophy Is Fun" (Unpublished Manuscript), December 1983, File: Penn, Jack—Writings (5), AMUW.

worldview was in stark contrast to the "Nordic race", considered the apex of civilisation, who were the heirs to Greek "civilisation". The "Bantu" was thus unsuited to Western liberalism and racial mixing would instead lead to the degeneration of white civilisation rather than the upliftment of the indigenous Africans.[31]

Yet his was not the only view. Social scientist and member of the South African Bureau for Educational and Scientific Research, E.G. Malherbe—who had received his Ph.D. from Columbia University and was a proponent of the use of statistics—believed that Africans could theoretically achieve intellectual equality. As growing industrialisation made evident the desperate need for skilled workers—with an insufficient number of white workers to meet this demand—another figure, Simon Biesheuvel, argued for African ability, believing they could be trained in the skills necessary for economic growth. Whatever potential for flexibility may have existed, the apartheid state came to prioritise the ideology of racism and the maintenance of state security over economic development. At the time of Penn's writing, the successor of Malherbe's Bureau, the Human Sciences Research Council, was publishing research that—amongst other things—debated on the ability of the "black man" to understand mathematics due to his cultural inability to grasp "objective time" and "punctuality".[32] Penn's writing then, may not be as anachronistic as it appeared—the perceived incompatibility of the culture of the "black man" with mathematics is little different to the inability of the "Bushmen" to adapt to modernity.

Yet "culture" was not the only component and Penn veered close to Social Darwinism in his thinking. While acknowledging the possibility of achieving intellectual equality, this was less related to environment than it was to biology. Citing the example of the potential technological abilities of the Igbo, Penn argued that this could only have been achieved "through a process of selective breeding". He was therefore careful to distinguish genetics from race, "It is not the colour of the skin that dictates capabilities or weaknesses – it is the genetic background over thousands of years. I am a firm believer in Darwin's dictum that

[31] *Cf* Andrew Bank, "Fathering *Volkekunde*: Race and Culture in the Ethnological Writings of Werner Eiselen, Stellenbosch University, 1926–1936", *Anthropology Southern Africa*, 38, 3 and 4, 163–179, 2015.

[32] Bill Freund, *Twentieth-Century South Africa: A Developmental History* (Cambridge, Cambridge University Press, 2019), pp75, 117, 134–136.

man evolves by the survival of the fittest variation".[33] Simultaneously, the attributes of the Igbo were apparently due "to their exposure to **culture** for thousands of years", rendering them the technological equal of their white counterparts but, contradictorily, this did little to alter Penn's view of the innate influence of nature over nurture.[34] It also indicates a particular view of "culture". In the twentieth century where technology was associated with progress and had its origins in the Western Enlightenment, for Penn, genetics was destiny. And genetics was given a racial cast. He offhandedly dismissed any evidence to the contrary—any "exception" to the rule i.e., demonstration of intellectual ability that deviated from the expected capabilities of a particular racial group was attributed to a "fortuitous shake-up of the genes"—a mutation that did little to challenge the trend.[35]

Penn's various travels had simply confirmed in him the suitability of different groups for their environments, a suitability that did not translate across these environments and was embedded in their genetic make-up. This suitability was termed "competence" and was not the same as intellectual, scientific and technological capability which was a hallmark of Western civilisation.[36]

The measure of progress or superior evolution was determined by intellectual capability, creating a racial intellectual hierarchy:

> We therefore have some races that have already reached the highest form of original thought and the application of knowledge, while other groups are able to assimilate facts but find difficulty in applying them in any original fashion. It is therefore understandable that the mental flexibility and inventiveness of the Chinese should be ahead of the Australian aboriginal. It is possible of course, that the latter will catch up in evolutionary time, while the former may reach a phase of decadence, but the process is likely to take many millennia.[37]

[33] Penn, *The Right to Look Human*, p250.

[34] Jack Penn, *Reflections on Life* (Johannesburg, Ernest Stanton Publishers, 1980), p31. Emphasis added.

[35] Penn, *The Right to Look Human*, p250.

[36] Penn, *Reflections on Life*, p31.

[37] Penn, *The Right to Look Human*, p251.

Penn's views then, reflected his understanding of the ability—or lack thereof—of racial groups to govern themselves without the helping hand of their intellectual superiors. It precluded racial mixing and in a concession to social differences, Penn also added religious incompatibility. The argument was clear—the mixing of people deemed inherently different would lead only to conflict and stringent measures needed to be maintained to prevent this, especially in the context of a black majority. South African "stability" was contrasted to the civil unrest occurring in the United States due to the latter's "more liberal attitude".[38]

The Struggle for Education

Penn's conservativism makes it a challenge to assess his own attempts at training doctors in developing countries. In contrast to Albert Schweitzer who did not implement training programmes for indigenous Africans, Penn actively attempted to both provide surgical assistance and to train prospective reconstructive surgeons all over the world, across national boundaries and societies. This was in line with his own education and with the development of modern plastic surgery in general that had its origins in the collaborative effort of surgeons across the Commonwealth. Penn's belief was that there should be "equal opportunity", that the opportunities for education and training should be available even if the success rates of their adoption varied according to genetic predisposition.[39]

Again, Penn reflects the uneasy position of the apartheid state under B.J. Vorster and his successor, P.W. Botha as attempts were made at reforming the system of racial oppression and segregation to meet the challenges of the 1970s. The apartheid state was at the height of its power in the preceding decade, the strength of its economy was a demonstration of the compatibility of racial segregation with modernisation. This changed with the economic crises of the 1970s, both national and global,[40] and was compounded by the Soweto uprising in 1976 against the systemic inequalities in education. The reform response was ultimately an uneasy amalgam of the advocacy of "civilisation" and assimilation while using "culture" as a marker of difference. Education was the

[38] Ibid.

[39] Penn, *Reflections on Life*, p63.

[40] Sau Dubow, *Apartheid: 1948–1994* (Oxford, Oxford University Press, 2014), p293.

means by which black labour could be harnessed to meet the changing demands of modernisation and cognisance was taken of reform required in education as well as in labour. Reform however was limited and only applied to those living in "white" South Africa, with the ideology of separate development continuing in the Bantustans.[41] Like its earlier incarnation "civilisation", "modernisation" was itself undisputed as the ideal. This, too, is reflected in Penn's writings.

In terms of modernisation, Penn believed that Africa was faced with a number of challenges. It lacked the tradition of intellectual endeavour that characterised other non-Western civilisations such as China where setbacks such as communism and the Cultural Revolution did not preclude an eventual recovery. Africans had a different sense of culture and knowledge that did not prioritise "initiative and invention"—while not lacking in the ability to "acquire knowledge", there was little aptitude to "apply" it and no indication that anything of novel value to the rest of the world could come from sub-Saharan Africa. Special efforts had to be made, therefore, to identify indigenous Africans who could benefit from education and develop the specialised skills for the continent to become "self-viable". This could only be done with "modern expertise".[42]

At the same time, education and modernisation were pre-requisites for independence with the need for skilled and professional people to allow self-sufficiency in "commerce, industry and technology" and the creation of infrastructure to sustain a modern state.[43] For Penn, the provision of this could only be achieved with time. One could argue, however, that the lack of skills and infrastructure also serves as an indictment of the "civilising mission" of colonialism. Yet he easily sidestepped this potential criticism with the accompanying view that, should this infrastructure exist—as it did in South Africa—Africans were incapable of making full use of them, serving in one stroke to both validate apartheid policy and justify African subordination:

[41] *Cf.* D. Van Zyl-Hermann, *Privileged Precariat: White Workers and South Africa's Long Transition to Majority Rule* (Cambridge, Cambridge University Press, 2021).

[42] Penn, *Reflections on Life*, pp63–64.

[43] Jack Penn, "He Is My Younger Brother", in *White Africans Are Also People*, Sarah Gertrude Millin (ed) (Howard Timmons, Cape Town, 1966), p131, Brn. No: 14607, Call No: 323.1128 MIL, BL.

> Even in South Africa, the African population has not taken full advantage of the facilities available. For example, the Medical School of the University of Natal in South Africa is one of the best teaching units in the continent. Matriculated Africans are fully subsidized to take the medical course. There are never more than 50 applicants a year, most of which are quite unsuitable for acceptance.[44]

An important component of education and of development was medicine and in an article published in the *British Journal of Plastic Surgery*, Penn stressed that it was not just "the difficulty [of those Africans reaching for the light] to attune themselves to the philosophy of a most sophisticated and religious world", but that the lack of "social conscience" was a major factor in impeding African development in medicine—when this was critical on a continent where tropical and venereal diseases were rife and specialisations such as plastic surgery were sorely needed. Accompanying the article was a cartoon depicting a nurse representing "The West" looming over a group of African children who were using the parts in a "UN Construction Kit" as mere playthings. The caption was: "The West: Why Not Try to Make Something?" The image spoke to Penn's view of indigenous Africans as children unable to effectively engage with modernity, requiring leadership and preparation rather than simply receiving a "hand-out" from world organisations such as the UN or the Peace Corps—it would require far greater guidance and intervention "to enable medicine and civilisation to flower in the virgin soil of Africa". He pointed to the dearth of African doctors on the continent and highlighted the very few African students at the University of Natal Medical School, despite the concession of a bridging year to compensate for possible inadequate secondary education and their "tribal background".[45] It was the very model of trusteeship.

Penn's view that "the African population" was to be blamed for their failure to make full use of the opportunities available to them to study medicine discounted the challenges experienced by prospective black medical students. For African students, with a background in "Bantu education" and a corresponding lack in English language skills as well as science, the demands of medical school were formidable. They were

[44] Ibid., p133.

[45] Jack Penn, "The Challenge of Africa", *British Journal of Plastic Surgery*, 18, 238–242, 1965.

accommodated through the provision of a "bridging year" but this simply had the effect of "weeding out" those students unable to cope, many of whom fell victim to courses such as English literature that proved a challenge for those for whom English was a second or even third language.[46] Their struggles and concerns actually mirrored to some extent those experienced by Penn—even if he remained unaware of their common ground. In the early decades of the twentieth century, there was a dearth of black doctors practising in South Africa. This, however, was less due to a lack of inclination than it was to lack of opportunity. To qualify as a doctor, African, Indian and coloured doctors had to travel abroad—to the United States, Great Britain and even India. This meant that the first generation of black doctors was drawn largely from the middle class or had been funded by the mission societies.[47] They were able to engage with one another, forming bonds based on their shared experiences as South Africans abroad and studying in Scotland had a profound impact, freeing them from the racial constraints that had been such an important component of their lives, "There was no question of a colour bar. It was a democratic society – we were free to move about without being kicked or humiliated".[48]

Educated, with a sense of status and ties to the communities they served, these doctors were well-placed to lead these communities in struggles for social, political and economic equality. In the early twentieth century, Abdullah Abdurahman—a doctor born in the Cape who received his degree from the University of Glasgow—formed the African Political Organisation, dedicated to fighting for the rights of coloureds at the Cape. In 1947, the Doctor's Pact was signed pledging an Indian and African alliance against racial inequality. Its signatories were Yusuf Dadoo of the Transvaal Indian Congress, Monty Naicker of the Natal Indian Congress and A.B. Xuma of the African National Congress. Dadoo and Naicker had—like Jack Penn—studied at the University of Edinburgh; Xuma in the United States. Decades later, medical student Steve Biko would lead the Black Consciousness Movement and usher in a new age of

[46] Vanessa Noble, *A School of Struggle: Durban's Medical School and the Education of Black Doctors in South Africa* (Scottsville, University of KwaZulu-Natal Press, 2013), p189.

[47] Anne Digby, "Early Black Doctors in South Africa", *Journal of African History*, 46, 427–454, 2005, pp429–431.

[48] Ibid., p437.

radicalism in black nationalist politics. Part of an educated elite, medical practitioners also understood and encountered the repercussions of the inequalities that defined South African society, extending their sense of social responsibility to the political sphere.

From the 1940s, the number of black doctors grew when more education opportunities were afforded them at the Universities of the Witwatersrand and Cape Town. New opportunities did not however, mean equality. The maintenance of racial boundaries was rigidly extended to teaching where black medical students at the University of Cape Town were not permitted to perform or even view autopsies on white cadavers, limiting their training. Racial ideology also meant that black doctors were expected to practise medicine within their designated racial groups, thereby limiting the interactions between white and black medical professionals, interactions that were an essential perquisite to furtherance of medical knowledge and understanding.[49] The training of black doctors at these liberal English-speaking universities can also be understood by the varying ways in which they engaged with apartheid.

From 1948 to 1959, as Howard Phillips demonstrates, the University of Cape Town shifted from one end of the spectrum to the other in addressing racial distinction. Thomas Benjamin Davie became the third Principal of UCT in 1948, a position that he would hold for the next seven years. David was a medical doctor who had served as Dean of Medicine in Liverpool and was an advocate of "intellectual freedom" which not only entailed that teaching be independent from political dictates but that learning opportunities and access to laboratories be available to everyone who demonstrated an aptitude, regardless of racial distinction. He would increasingly come to uphold academic freedom against the diktats of the apartheid state. Davie's views were further supported by his successor, Acting Principal Reginald William James, Dean of Science and Fellow of the Royal Society, who led a protest march against the Separate University Education Bill—protest that was to prove unsuccessful. The new Principal of UCT, Jacobus Petrus Duminy, however was something of an anachronism—out of touch with the student body, suspicious of radicalism and with a belief in the paternalistic stewardship of English and Afrikaans-speaking white South Africans

[49] Ibid.

of "our non-White peoples". While Duminy believed in the value of inclusive education that would lead to black graduates becoming the "standard bearers of Western learning", he was also increasingly of the view that a university should remain distinct from politics and a growing conservatism characterised his leadership until his retirement in 1967.[50] The experiences of black medical students then can be understood both by apartheid policies as well as the ways in which the leadership of these universities engaged with these policies—an engagement that changed over time.

As evident from Penn's own experiences, these black doctors—particularly those from working-class backgrounds—were torn between the competing interests of their social responsibility and individual accumulation. However, being largely confined to practising within their own communities advanced their social awareness. Moreover, the discrimination they experienced in their professional lives—restricted from holding certain positions and paid a lower salary than white doctors—made them all too aware of the inequities in South African society. As members of an educated elite, then, they took on leadership roles and engaged in political activism.[51] Unlike Penn's understanding, radicalism was less a product of education than it was of an all-encompassing system of inequality.

Penn's view of genetics in relation to education and modernity belied the complex struggles that underpinned education in South Africa. The apartheid state, rather than the paternalist overseers of a system preparing indigenous Africans for the challenges of modernity, actively sought to discourage this modernity through its emphasis on tribalism. And nowhere was this more evident than in education. Prior to the rise of the apartheid state, African education was largely the prerogative of mission schools which, although few, sought to inculcate the very socio-economic and political values that defined modern Western society, what Penn would term "civilisation". Yet after 1948, these values—which had the potential to result in agitations for political equality amongst an educated African elite—threatened Afrikaner nationalist dominance. The result was the Bantu Education Act in 1953 that, although making basic levels of education available to a larger African population than could be catered for under the mission schooling system, simultaneously sought to

[50] Howard Phillips, *UCT Under Apartheid: Part 1—From Onset to Sit-in, 1948–1968* (Sunnyside, Fanele (Jacana), 2019), pp5–10.

[51] Digby, "Early Black Doctors", pp440–442.

limit African opportunity. But even a little education was sufficient and the growing population of educated Africans would become increasingly incensed by the lower standard of education that was accorded them as well as lesser economic and political opportunities. This culminated in the Soweto uprising of June 1976 that spread across the country.[52]

The second edition of his autobiography published in the year of the Soweto uprising, Penn could hardly have been unaware of the widespread unrest and its associations with radical Black Consciousness under the leadership of Steve Biko. Born in the Eastern Cape in 1946, Biko was a product of the same mission education system reviled by Afrikaner nationalists, first enrolling at Lovedale College (from which he was subsequently expelled after his first arrest) and then St Francis College in Natal. Free of Afrikaner nationalist influence, Biko nevertheless chafed under the liberalism which he perceived to be paternalistic and another manifestation of white dominance. Simultaneously, his time at the school exposed him to the pressing issues of the day and the decolonisation sweeping across the continent. Biko's understanding of black subjugation was not unrelated to education and associated with it, psychological "oppression", resulting in his famous line, "...the most potent weapon in the hands of the oppressor is the mind of the oppressed".[53]

Penn was not incorrect in his assessment of the greater opportunities available to black students. From the 1960s there was an increase in the number of black tertiary institutions, segregated according to race and/or ethnicity. There was a corresponding increase in student enrolments. The lower fees charged at these institutions were less of a financial burden to working-class and lower middle-class black families and this was complemented by bursaries made available by the state. Simultaneously, due to the control exerted by the state at these universities, there was less academic freedom and students were subject to expulsion for engaging in political activism. This was in contrast to the greater freedom at the established liberal institutions—the University of the Witwatersrand, University of Cape Town and University of Natal. And it was the University of Natal

[52] Deborah Posel, "The Apartheid Project, 1948–1970" in *The Cambridge History of South Africa, Volume 2, 1885–1994*, Robert Ross, Anne Kelk Mager and Bill Nasson (eds) (Cambridge University Press, 2012), pp339–340.

[53] Lindy Wilson, *Steve Biko* (Johannesburg, Jacana Media, 2011), pp18, 23–25, 14.

Medical School that saw increased student activism that would result in the Black Consciousness Movement.[54]

The Medical School was itself composed of diverse groups of black students, many of whom—denied access to UCT and Wits—were part of an intellectual elite with the space and freedom to come together and engage in discussion and debate.[55] It proved fertile ground for Steve Biko who formed the South African Student Organisation (SASO) that soon spread throughout the country. The movement was influenced by the civil rights and Black Power movements in the United States, anti-colonialism and the work of African philosophers such as Frantz Fanon and contextualised by the ubiquitous experience of life for black South Africans under apartheid.[56] Filling the gap left by the banned ANC and PAC, SASO became the face of black political protest in the 1970s, including a rally in support of Frelimo in 1974[57] and the Soweto uprising in 1976.

Biko later succumbed to injuries incurred while in police custody in 1977. His death drew international attention with his friend and journalist, Donald Woods, a prominent anti-apartheid activist, focusing on police brutality. For Penn, however, this was little different to events occurring in the United States and it was only "...with the advent of vengeful South African, Donald Woods, [that] unusual attention was given to South African police methods and suicides".[58] Three years later, Penn's *Reflections on Life* was published where he articulated the view of African cultural and genetic differences that were at odds with the education and skills required in a modern society.

In Penn's view of apartheid, the desire for segregation was not simply a desire on the part of whites but on the part of other racial groups as well, agitating for self-government. Where whites were "tolerated" it was only due to their superior "knowledge and skills", the flip side of which was paternalism. Citing Schweitzer's view of the African's relationship to him—"He is my younger brother"—Penn advocated the role of whites as assisting the "emergent African" to reach "his maturity",

[54] Noble, *A School of Struggle*, pp212–214.

[55] Ibid.

[56] Ibid., pp221–222.

[57] Ibid., p254.

[58] Jack Penn, "A Sentimental Journey", File: Biography—Jack Penn, AMUW.

a relationship that would continue even as said maturity was reached.[59] Simultaneously—and contradictorily—Penn's espousal of the genetic basis of intellectual ability and progress meant that this theoretical equality could potentially take centuries to achieve, subject to the slow process of evolutionary change.

Sol Plaatje's response to the 1913 Land Act with which this chapter begins was more than a poignant description of the exploitation and exclusion of Africans from the newly formed Union of South Africa. Plaatje's own life as an intellectual and writer challenged the view of African incapability as did the struggles over equal education that marked the second half of the twentieth century—and continue to this day. The notorious Land Act, however, was not simply a marker of racial discrimination and dispossession but linked to the modernisation project, affecting black sharecroppers, forcing them into the labour market to service mining, industry and agriculture. It also affected white *bywoners*,[60] creating the new workers of an industrialising economy and promoting urbanisation. It allowed for the commercialisation of agriculture, meaning that South Africans would now be able to provide the grains and meat required to feed an increasingly urban population instead of relying on imports. It went together with the process that Penn would later accredit to genetic difference—the preferential skilling of the white labour force, the reduction in competition from black labour and the favoured employment of white workers. The prevailing pre-Second World War ethos of "South Africanism" that saw the alliance of English- and Afrikaans-speaking white South Africans necessitated the marginalisation of coloureds, Indians and particularly, Africans, a marginalisation that was reflected in education and in work and one which would become even further entrenched from 1948.[61]

The complexity of this is ignored in Penn's writing in favour of a more simplified explanation of biological determinism. In the following decade Penn would play a more active role in advocating for reform as a member of the President's Council however his views of race and education were contextualised by the increasing prioritisation by the apartheid state on the preservation of its security from enemies within and without,

59 Penn, *The Right to Look Human*, p253.

60 Tenant farmers.

61 Freund, *Twentieth-Century South Africa*, pp29, 49.

even if this contradicted the requirements for effective modernisation and economic development. The importance of the security of the state was of great concern to Penn and in this context, his view of "A multitude of different genes" became just another way of saying "separate but equal".

CHAPTER 11

"He Is My Younger Brother": Nationalism, Independence and the Cold War

Penn's autobiography—containing his thoughts about African independence, nationalism and race—was contextualised by the events of the 1970s, much of which was alluded to in his work: the Cold War; the end of Portuguese colonialism in Angola and then Mozambique which would further increase South Africa's sense of isolation; the oil embargo that created an international economic crisis in 1973; and the rise of Black Consciousness in South Africa under the leadership of the charismatic Steve Biko that culminated in the Soweto uprising of 1976. The period saw increasing challenges to the power of the state, from within and without, in contrast to the self-assured dominance of the previous decade.

The 1960s had also been a decade of upheaval with successful challenges to the existing world order. Framed by Harold Macmillan's "Winds of Change" speech in 1960, just prior to South Africa's exit from the Commonwealth, and the revolutionary fervour, protest and unrest that characterised 1968, the decade had also seen the consolidation of the

---

Quote taken from Jack Penn, "He Is My Younger Brother", and accredited to Albert Schweitzer in *White Africans Are Also People*, Sarah Gertrude Millin (ed) (Howard Timmons, Cape Town, 1966).

S. Chetty, *Reconstructive Surgery and Modernisation in Twentieth-Century South Africa*, Medicine and Biomedical Sciences in Modern History, https://doi.org/10.1007/978-3-031-38673-2_11

power and confidence of the apartheid state, with relative quiescence on the part of black activists due to the banning of the ANC and PAC. Yet the growth of African independence was no small cause for concern on the part of the South African state—and was responsible to some extent for Penn's overtures to independent African states as an "ambassador" for the medical and technological prowess of South Africa—and the benefits of an alliance with it.

Penn's view of African independence was shaped by his experiences in Africa and Asia—and his perception of the role of education as spelled out in the preceding chapter. This is succinctly summarised in a chapter he contributed to *White Africans Are Also People*, a collection of essays edited by Sarah Gertrude Millin. Of the figures who contributed to Millin's compilation, it is perhaps Millin herself who had the strongest parallels with Jack Penn. Like Penn, Millin was of Jewish extraction and cognisant of the anti-Semitism that characterised South Africa in the late nineteenth and early decades of the twentieth centuries. Like Penn, she too moved steadily to the right, ultimately coming to support the policies of Afrikaner nationalists, and notions of Social Darwinism that were already anachronistic. Millin was also one of the country's most recognised literary figures, on par with another Jewish writer, Nadine Gordimer—although the political leanings of the two could not be more different.

It was Gordimer who first used the term "white African" as a means of describing her identity in the complex world of apartheid South Africa. Millin's adoption of the term was however, to assert a claim to Africa, even as black nationalism, Pan Africanism, decolonisation and international opinion were undermining this. For Millin, "white civilization [was] precious, fragile, and must at all costs – the costs, it is understood, will be paid by black people – be preserved."[1] As early as 1924, in her internationally successful novel *God's Stepchildren*, Millin articulated an early view of the inherent African incompatibility with Western education—a biological inability to effectively "compete" against their white counterparts even if they had, against all the odds, managed to study abroad and enter a profession.[2] Penn would echo this four decades

[1] Margaret Lenta, "Choosing Difference: South African Jewish Writers", *Judaism: A Quarterly Journal of Jewish Life and Thought,* 50, 1, Winter 2001.

[2] Matthew Eatough, "National Citizens, Global Economies: Sarah Gertrude Millin and the Professionalization of Envy", *Safundi: The Journal of South African and American Studies*, 14, 4, 395–424, 2013, p395.

later. The publication of *White Africans Are Also People* in 1966 coincided with the four-day visit of Robert F. Kennedy to South Africa with Millin, in a cartoon appearing in the conservative newspaper *Die Vaderland*, pointing to the hypocrisy of Kennedy's criticism of apartheid policy when civil rights figure James Meredith had just been shot in Mississippi.[3] This contrast between civil rights struggles in the United States and the apparent stability of apartheid policy was also evident in the essay contributed by Clarence B. Randall—addressed later in this chapter.

Another contributor to *White Africans Are Also People* was Roy Welensky. Like Millin and Penn, he was the son of Eastern European Jews who had immigrated to Southern Rhodesia (present-day Zimbabwe). Born into poverty, Welensky was the archetypal rags-to-riches story—working on the railways and serving as head of the Railway Workers' Trade Union which paved the way for his move into politics. Between 1955 and 1963, Welensky was Prime Minister of the Central African Federation comprising Southern Rhodesia, Northern Rhodesia (Zambia) and Nyasaland (Malawi). He also attempted unsuccessfully to mount a political opposition to Ian Smith who declared Rhodesian independence.[4] Penn painted an empathetic picture of Welensky—a man who had "desired to follow in the steps of Cecil John Rhodes and enlarge the prestige and possessions of Empire" but who had become "disillusioned" with the declaration of independence in 1965.[5] During his final year as Prime Minister, Welensky articulated the unenviable position of the white settler population during decolonisation:

> I am a white African and I have struggled for the whole of my political life against colonialism. I share a belief with many thousands on the African continent that as soon as people and young countries are able to stand on their own feet to conduct their affairs and govern themselves they should be allowed to do so but I am [an] anti colonialist with a difference. I want to see colonialism go, but to go in an orderly way and go only when it gives place to something better. And being a white African and knowing

[3] *Rand Daily Mail*, 7 June 1966.

[4] Sir Roy Welensky, https://www.oxfordreference.com/view/10.1093/oi/authority.20110803121643788, accessed 14 February 2021.

[5] Jack Penn, *The Right to Look Human: An Autobiography* (Johannesburg, Hugh Keartland Publishers, 1976), pp240–241.

> no other home but Africa, what happens when [it] doesn't go in this way is perforce of considerable personal concern to me.[6]

The extract from Welensky's talk demonstrates a deep insecurity, that was perhaps shared by his South African contemporaries such as Penn and Millin in their defence of the apartheid state—the future of white South Africans on the continent. Welensky elaborated on his anti-colonial stance, pointing out that colonialism tended towards the exploitation of Africa by the metropole, yet also suggested the chaos that would result should independence be granted prematurely, citing the Congo as an example of a state that had "slipped back into the twilight that was Africa seventy years ago".[7] In other words, the Congo returned to a state before the implementation of modernity associated with colonialism and imperialism. This was a simplistic explanation that belies the horrendous exploitation of the Congo and concomitant atrocities committed under Belgian rule as well as the involvement of the former colonial powers and the United States after independence. Like Penn, Welensky was concerned about communist influence on the African continent especially as Western influence declined with the withdrawal of the colonial powers and cited the "extremist" threat presented by an emerging African leadership that would subvert the process of democracy.[8]

The conservatism evident in *White Africans Are Also People* was strengthened—and leant an internationalist perspective—by American Clarence B. Randall. Randall, a prominent businessman, had served as an economic advisor under numerous presidential administrations, including Eisenhower, Kennedy and Johnson. At the time of his contribution to Millin's book, he headed the Department of State's Advisory Committee on International Business Problems and in this capacity, had visited South Africa on numerous occasions.[9] A prolific writer, Randall was devoted to liberalism and the free market with an attendant abhorrence of Communism—the rights of the individual were paramount, the freedom of choice of the individual to be educated, work and live as they saw fit was, for

[6] Sir Roy Welensky, Transcript of Talk Given on 12 October 1963, NYPR Archive Collections, https://www.wnyc.org/story/sir-roy-welensky/, accessed 14 February 2021.

[7] Ibid.

[8] Ibid.

[9] "Clarence B. Randall Papers", https://library.princeton.edu/special-collections/collections/clarence-b-randall-papers, accessed 15 February 2021.

Randall, the means by which society as a whole could benefit.[10] Yet Randall's view of the rights of the individual was a somewhat qualified one when applied to the South African context.

Randall's contribution, "Do We Understand the New Africa?" addressed what he believed to be American preconceptions regarding the continent—preconceptions that had been evident on the part of leading American figures such as Robert Kennedy. The latter's visit to South Africa was memorable for the snubbing of the state with representatives refusing to meet him and the belief on the part of Afrikaner nationalists that the senator had already condemned apartheid policy with insufficient understanding of its context.[11] For Randall, American misunderstanding came from equating the civil rights movement in the United States with anti-colonial and anti-apartheid struggles in Africa with an inadequate understanding of the uniquely African context.[12]

A large part of Randall's argument was based on a fundamental misunderstanding of early South African history with his articulation of the *terra nullius* narrative that privileged Afrikaner primacy in southern Africa:

> He[13] makes no inquiry as to the origin of separateness in the history of South Africa. He does not know that the whites, and not the blacks, were the indigenous race in that part of the world. This is so because the Bantu people, who are the ones involved in the controversy, were far to the north in Africa when the Boers established control over their area, then inhabited by no one but Bushmen and Hottentots – whose sparse population has long since disappeared.[14]

[10] Clarence B. Randall, "'Individualism: Human Satisfaction Is What We Seek', transcript of speech delivered at John Carroll University, Ohio, 26 January 1962", *Vital Speeches of the Day* (Pro Rhetoric LLC), pp414–416.

[11] *Cf* Suryakanthie Chetty, "Containing the Ripple of Hope: Apartheid, the Afrikaans Press and Robert F. Kennedy's Visit to South Africa, June 1966", *Southern Journal for Contemporary History*, 45, 1, 119–144, 2020. https://journals.ufs.ac.za/index.php/jch/article/view/4564; https://doi.org/10.18820/24150509/SJCH45.v1.7.

[12] Clarence B. Randall, "Do We Understand the New Africa?" in *White Africans Are Also People*, Sarah Gertrude Millin (ed) (Howard Timmons, Cape Town, 1966), p79, Brn. No: 14607, Call No: 323.1128 MIL, BL.

[13] The pronoun refers to the unnamed and generalised American who condemns apartheid policy.

[14] Randall, "Do We Understand the New Africa?", p84.

Randall's view of the South African past drew its inspiration in part from colonial and settler historiography—and this was not simply confined to history writing. As Clifton Crais shows in "The Vacant Land", there was a symbolic shift in the portrayal of indigenous Africans in visual depictions of southern Africa. Influenced by the Enlightenment, anti-slavery movements and monogenesis (or the notion of common descent), British artists in the late eighteenth and early nineteenth centuries, portrayed southern African landscapes as little different to a pre-industrial Britain with Africans depicted as "noble savages", the potential beneficiaries of the civilising mission and progress. From the late 1820s, however, after the arrival of the first contingent of British settlers, accompanied by increasing conflict with the Xhosa along the Eastern Frontier, landscapes tended to depict empty vistas, marginalising indigenous people and suggesting settler expansion and conquest. This was also evident in widely read publications such as *The Grahamstown Journal* which stressed the notion of a largely unoccupied land or one that had not been permanently settled for a great length of time but was still currently in the process of being "conquered" by "barbarian" groups such as the Xhosa—who had to be halted. Scientific racism was used to justify British dominance of these inherently "savage" races. The historian emerging from this context and most associated with the *terra nullius* mythology is George Theal.[15]

Demonstrating a marked disjuncture in his writing from the 1870s (when he was based at Lovedale seminary school) to the 1880s (after his relocation to the Cape colonial world and conversion to Social Darwinism), Theal's writings privileged white "legitimacy" in South Africa and used racial typology to promote a view not unfamiliar to Penn—the intrinsic inability of indigenous Africans to "progress", "His [the "Bantu youth"] intellect has become sluggish, and he exhibits a decided repugnance, if not incapacity, to learn anything more."[16] Theal also popularised the view that Bantu-speaking Africans had migrated to

[15] Clifton C. Crais, "The Vacant Land: The Mythology of British Expansion in the Eastern Cape, South Africa", *Journal of Social History*, 25, 2, 255–275, 1991, pp259–260, 266–267.

[16] Andrew Bank, "The Politics of Mythology: The Genealogy of the Philip Myth", *Journal of Southern African Studies*, 5, 3, 461–477, September 1999, pp465, 469–470.

South Africa at approximately the same time as Europeans, thus legitimising white conquest, expansion and settlement and providing a strong foundation for Afrikaner nationalist mythology.[17]

A historical fallacy notwithstanding, Randall highlighted the ingratitude of African nationalists who did little to "acknowledge the debt they owed to the sturdy white pioneers" who, as in the case of South Africa, were considered responsible for the provision of a relatively high quality of life and education for black South Africans that surpassed that of the rest of the continent, progress that was attributed to white guidance over the past three centuries.[18] While glossing over the conflict and complexity that underlay the colonial encounter in southern Africa, Randall's conclusion was similar to that of Jack Penn—slow and steady change that would lead to an accommodation between black and white and be a production of "evolution" rather than the dramatic upheaval of "revolution".[19]

Penn also played an active role in convincing another prominent American of the misconception held by most of his countrymen towards South African policies. Page 4 of the *Rand Daily Mail* issued on Valentine's Day 1972 was almost a *precis* of apartheid policy and black discontent—there was a demand by coloureds to be able to purchase council houses which they were already occupying; a "call to conscience" came from the Roman Catholics Bishops' Conference held in Pretoria the previous week that comdemned "detention without trial, bannings and the problems of migrant labour";[20] and criticism was aimed at state policy of dividing African schools and school boards along ethnic lines. A short column buried in the midst of this is entitled "Nixon Man Visits SA" and describes the arrival of General Matthew Ridgway, the "personal military advisor to President Nixon". Ridgway was to be hosted by Jack Penn and Jan S. Marais.[21] Marais was the chairman of Trust Bank, a prominent financier, who believed in reform to the system of apartheid that

[17] Crais, "The Vacant Land", p267.

[18] Randall, "Do We Understand the New Africa?", pp81, 84.

[19] Ibid., p98.

[20] Anthony Holiday, "Churchmen Support Bishops' 'Call to Conscience'", *Rand Daily Mail*, 14 February 1972.

[21] "Nixon Man Visits SA", *Rand Daily Mail*, 14 February 1972.

would allow representation for all South Africans, including Africans relegated to the Bantustans.[22] He represented business interests in the wake of 1973, increasingly concerned about the detrimental economic impact of apartheid and his views echoed that of the *verligte* camp within the National Party. During the course of the visit, Ridgway also met with P.W. Botha, at the time the Minister of Defence.[23] Botha would later become Prime Minister in 1978—and name Jack Penn as one of the members of his President's Council.

Ridgway was a highly decorated veteran of the Second World War, a four-star general who led the Eighth US Army during the Korean War, served as Supreme Allied Commander in both the Far East and in Europe and was Chief of Staff of the Army.[24] After his South African visit, Ridgway gave an interview where he claimed to have "obtained a totally different perspective of the Republic's racial situation than is depicted in the American media".[25] While not specific on these issues, he addressed the concerns raised by South African officials regarding the increasing Russian naval presence in the Indian Ocean and also said that he would use "whatever influence" he had in Washington, DC to make them aware of his own experiences and conclusion in South Africa—although the article carefully pointed out that Ridgway did not hold an official "advisory post".[26] Ridgway also made special mention of Penn's hospitality and was so impressed by him that he contributed the Foreword to Penn's autobiography.

The Foreword suggests that Penn made no small contribution in briefing the General on South African policies and Ridgway wrote glowingly of Penn's political astuteness:

[22] John F. Burns, "Industry Mellows in South Africa", *New York Times*, 21 November 1976, https://www.nytimes.com/1976/11/21/archives/industry-mellows-in-south-africa-south-africa.html, accessed 19 April 2021.

[23] "Nixon Man Visits SA".

[24] Billy A. Arthur, "Obituary: General Matthew Ridgway", *Independent*, 23 October 2011, https://www.independent.co.uk/news/people/obituary-general-matthew-ridgway-1460281.html, accessed 19 April 2021.

[25] Raymond Heard, "General Has New View on SA", *Rand Daily Mail*, 1 March 1972.

[26] Ibid.

> Dr Penn is an extraordinarily farseeing and broadminded internationalist and humanitarian, with a fine grasp of international relations and a profound understanding, gained through first-hand contacts of Africa's problems, particularly of those of the Continent south of the Sahara and of his native land, the Republic of South Africa.[27]

Ridgway made clear that it was Penn's logical expounding of the South African issue that contributed to his own understanding of the South African (and African) situation, an understanding that was lacking amongst many of his fellow Americans.[28] And this understanding is particularly evident in Penn's essay in *White Africans Are Also People.*

The title of Penn's chapter, "He is My Younger Brother" draws its inspiration from the paternalism of Albert Schweitzer who is quoted extensively in the chapter. Despite his occasional frustrations with the operation of Schweitzer's Lambarene hospital and the older man's reluctance to embrace modern medical practices, Penn was nevertheless not immune to the cult of personality associated with Schweitzer—and a tendency to hagiography. Penn also clearly empathised strongly with Schweitzer's political views—and these views did not envision equality:

> Why did this philosopher, this musician, this lover of civilization, spend his life among the lowest he could find? Because they were the lowest, because they were the neediest. Not because he loved Africans, but because he did not – this was what he believed to be Christianity.[29]

Serving those considered the "lowest" allowed Schweitzer the opportunity for individual redemption but this was a relationship predicated on paternalism and difference.

Penn echoed Schweitzer's views regarding African self-determination—and granting independence to the colonies in general. A point made was their inherent incompatibility with the modern nation state due to "tribalism". Ethnic and other divisions had been papered over under colonial rule which had forged a whole from disparate elements; the withdrawal

[27] Matthew Ridgway, "Foreword" in Jack Penn, *The Right to Look Human: An Autobiography* (Johannesburg, Hugh Keartland Publishers, 1976).

[28] Ibid.

[29] Jack Penn, "He Is My Younger Brother", in *White Africans Are Also People*, Sarah Gertrude Millin (ed) (Howard Timmons, Cape Town, 1966), p127, Brn. No: 14607, Call No: 323.1128 MIL, BL.

of this unifying force created the conditions for internecine conflict. India is used to provide an inkling of the future of Africa where independence and the partition of India with the creation of Pakistan led to the perpetration of atrocity. And this occurred despite the political leaders spouting the ideals of nationalism and unity.[30]

Penn drew a clear disjuncture between political leaders agitating for equality and independence and the vast majority. Enlightenment ideals of self-government and the ideal citizen had been forged in Europe over centuries, with origins as far back as the birth of Western civilisation in ancient Greece; to expect its successful implementation in Africa could only be considered folly:

> Millennia of civilized thought and philosophy cannot be telescoped into a few months or years, and the veneer supplied by the ruling intelligentsia is not an adequate covering for the raw and unsophisticated turmoil stirring beneath the surface.[31]

Faced with the impending independence of Gabon a decade earlier, Schweitzer's pessimism—and apprehension—was just as evident. The lack of "comprehension" on the part of the average African meant that they would not be able to exercise responsible citizenship in choosing their representatives. Moreover, the heady freedom of democracy would lead to the privileging of "passion" over reason, with unforeseen—but assuredly not positive—consequences.[32]

Perhaps even more telling was Penn's belief in the inherent incompatibility of Africans—whether based on race, culture or genetics—with the modern democratic process that lay at the heart of self-governance. He drew upon another medical missionary, David Livingstone, accrediting to him the view of Africans as "lazy, ungrateful, greedy and [lacking] inventiveness", with "the same deficiencies [afflicting] the emergent African now".[33] This was compounded by "a lack of social responsibility" in contrast to the self-sacrificing virtues of Albert Schweitzer and his team of volunteers in Lambarene. As Schweitzer pointed out, "To date there is

[30] Ibid., p128.

[31] Ibid., p133.

[32] Ibid., p128.

[33] Ibid., p133.

no comprehension of the concept of common humanity".[34] Schweitzer's views resonated with Penn who alluded to the lack of African medical volunteers to step into Schweitzer's shoes, "The reason may be because the Africans have not had the opportunity for training, or were not capable of being trained, or did not wish to do this type of work."[35] A lack of social consciousness was incompatible with the "imagined community",[36] the necessary pre-requisite for the nation state. According to Penn, "social conscience" went with "social responsibility" and this, compounded by the lack of tertiary educational opportunities in Africa, meant that Africans—facing poverty, disease and other ills that increased mortality—demonstrated little in the way of "foresight" and thus societal progress.[37]

Just as significant was what Penn termed the absence of "civilised evolution", related to a sense of empathy and notably absent in the examples he put forth: the Mau Mau rebellion, the depredations of the Zulu king Shaka as well as "cannibalism in Nigeria". While this "cruelty" was not unique to Africa—and Penn acknowledged the Holocaust—his vision of Africa was nevertheless one that seemed little changed from the tales of savagery and inhumanity associated with the "Dark Continent" from the early days of European exploration. Perceived African lack of empathy and common purpose explained the potential failure of African bodies proclaiming solidarity. It would only be through education, the emulation of Western civilisation and "centuries of civilized evolution" that Africans would overcome their inherent limitations and reach the "highest of human attributes" which Penn termed "sympathy".[38]

As he had in his discussion on education, Penn employed an anachronistic interpretation of evolution that conflated the genetic with the social, in line with the Social Darwinism that characterised thinking decades earlier. His view of evolution as it related to political development and self-governance could not be divorced from education and the tradition of Western "civilisation", wherein lay the origins of democracy. This social

[34] Ibid., p129.

[35] Ibid., p130.

[36] *Cf* Benedict Anderson, *Imagined Communities: Reflections on the Origin and Spread of Nationalism* (London and New York, Verso, 2006).

[37] Penn, "He Is My Younger Brother", p133.

[38] Ibid., p136.

and political evolution was linked with progress and was the prerogative of an elite with Africans by no means ready or capable of self-rule.[39]

It is difficult not to see this chapter written by Penn in 1966 as an attempt to put an intellectual spin on contemporary concerns and fears. Looming over his views of nationalism, race and racial policy is the Cold War and his strong ideas regarding race and the policies of the apartheid state indicate a sense of defensiveness, a feeling of being besieged with a particular way of life under threat. To this end, he appeared convinced that the various groups opposing apartheid were in league with communists. He drew attention to the lack of unity evident across Africa with the only unifying factor in the Organisation of African Unity (OAU) being "the desire to eliminate Western civilization wherever it may be – in the South, Rhodesia, Angola, Mozambique and South Africa; and Israel to the North." The OAU was apparently in league with and awarded funds from the World Council of Churches and some European states viz. Sweden and Holland (all of which were involved in supporting anti-apartheid activism) to arm "terrorists" with weapons obtained from communist China and the Soviet Union.[40]

For Penn, while the Soviet Union was looking to expand its sphere of influence in the Middle East—as evident in his discussion of Soviet support for Arab countries against Israel—the great threat to Africa was China. As white influence was dwindling in Mozambique and Angola and Rhodesia would eventually achieve black majority rule, it was South Africa which stood as the lone bulwark against the ambitions of the Chinese Communists, not only in defence of white minority rule but as representative of "Western civilization" itself. While international criticism of apartheid policies should not result therefore in the end of white minority rule, it had initiated a conciliatory policy of the state towards its African neighbours, united in the fight against communism.[41]

Penn was more specific about Chinese infiltration in Africa in an article published two years earlier in the *New York Times*:

> The focal line of Chinese Communist Infiltration is along the Tanzanian Zambian railway presently being built by the Chinese. This is calculated

[39] Ibid., p139.

[40] Penn, *The Right to Look Human*, p244.

[41] Ibid., p245.

> to enable tens or hundreds of thousands of Chinese to come to Africa to strengthen their hold, in the first instance across the waist of Africa all the way from Dar-es-Salaam to Lusaka, and then to spread south in order to take control of the whole of "white" Southern Africa and the sea route to Europe and the U.S.[42]

Aiding and abetting the Chinese were Makonde guerrillas:

> Along the borders of Tanzania are to be found the Makonde tribes, intelligent and artistic but primitive to a degree. Until recently they were cannibals. They still assume the habits of their past by filing their teeth and lacerating their faces, presumably to terrorize their neighbors. Many of the Makonde have been educated by mission schools and a small percentage have been granted scholarships in the U.S. and Europe where, fully educated, they have been snapped up by the Communists and trained in sabotage and guerrilla warfare in Moscow or Peking for two to three years.[43]

On their return to Africa, these members of the Makonde wrought havoc, recruiting by force villagers to swell the ranks of Frelimo (the Marxist-influenced Mozambique Liberation Front). The depredations of Frelimo were, however, countered by the majority of the Makonde in alliance with the Portuguese. The latter were especially singled out for their benevolence in providing medical aid to both sides. For Penn, it was the aim of China to wage a "third world war" against the West through its manipulation of the "black tribes". The West was not only oblivious to this threat but unwittingly aided Chinese ambitions through their support of these groups termed "freedom fighters" while simultaneously preventing arms sales to those fighting the communist threat.[44]

Penn's article reveals his ambivalence about African independence, his perception of African ability or lack thereof through the use of adjectives such as "primitive", as well as the lack of agency attributed to Africans, leaving them easily open to foreign manipulation. In contrast, medical

[42] Jack Penn, "Communist Influence in Southern Africa", *New York Times*, 4 April 1972, The New York Times Archives, https://www.nytimes.com/1972/04/04/archives/communist-influence-in-southern-africa.html?searchResultPosition=1, accessed 7 August 2020.

[43] Ibid.

[44] Ibid.

assistance (as provided by the Portuguese) was portrayed as both disinterested and symbolic of Western beneficence. Yet his views did not go unchallenged. A letter to the editor written by Professor Robert Rotberg of the Massachusetts Institute of Technology emphasised the repression experienced by Mozambicans under Portuguese rule which was little different to the measures employed by the apartheid state. He further addressed the lack of evidence to corroborate widespread Chinese influence in the region and concluded by dismissing Penn's article as "arrant, alarmist nonsense" ending with, "Whatever moved *The Times* to publish such rubbish?"[45] Another article on 17 April 1972 also portrayed a very different picture of Portuguese rule and the actions of Frelimo. Photojournalist Robert van Lierop contrasted Portuguese bombing and napalm attacks with the experiences of Mozambicans in areas liberated by Frelimo where:

> ...men, women and children are going to schools for the first time and learning how to read and write, how to add and subtract and learning about themselves and their country. For the first time people are being inoculated against disease and are receiving medical treatment. For the first time they are able to engage in agricultural production to feed themselves rather than being forced to grow cotton to feed Portugal's textile industry. For the first time, all segments of the population cooperate in governing themselves and in building a new society without reference to age, sex, religion, race or class.[46]

Van Lierop's view of the effects of independence and the aspirations of the local population is in stark contrast to that of Penn who was described by the photojournalist as an example of a "[propagandist] [issuing] outright lies in efforts to rally support for the maintenance of racism and colonialism" as an act of "desperation" at the prospect of African independence. For Van Lierop, colonialism was equated to subjugation and the benefits of modernity—educational, economic, political, and social—were only

[45] Robert I. Rotberg, "Letter to the Editor", *New York Times*, 13 April 1972, The New York Times Archives, https://www.nytimes.com/1972/04/13/archives/a-view-of-southernafrica.html?searchResultPosition=2, accessed 7 August 2020.

[46] Robert van Lierop, "Liberty in East Africa", *New York Times*, 13 April 1972, The New York Times Archives, https://www.nytimes.com/1972/04/17/archives/liberty-in-east-africa.html?searchResultPosition=3, accessed 7 August 2020.

possible with African self-rule. In this vision, Penn was therefore an "apologist" for a repressive white state trying in vain to stem the tide.[47]

Penn remained unrepentant in his views, even after the achievement of Mozambican independence, believing that the independent country under the leadership of Samora Machel was a subversion of four centuries of "European civilisation" and an act of "self immolation." While Mozambique was still a Portuguese colony, Penn had developed a close professional relationship and friendship with Alphons Paes, a surgeon who had also visited the Brenthurst Military Hospital.[48] Paes was the son of a Portuguese president who left for Mozambique after his father's assassination. While a general surgeon, he developed an interest in plastic surgery and Penn considered him one of the most talented surgeons he had ever encountered.[49]

Penn was subsequently invited by the Portuguese to travel to Mozambique to assist with treatment for leprosy as well as yaws,[50] a disease caused by a bacterium, *Treponema pertenue* and confined largely to the tropics with its most severe effects on children.[51] When the war for independence broke out, Penn returned to Mozambique, and it was this experience that further entrenched his negative views of African independence. He noted the training of the Makonde leadership by the Russians with the rank and file coerced to fight against the Portuguese by threatening their families. Once these unwilling "terrorists" were liberated by the Portuguese, they had little compunction in changing their allegiance. He also gave an unflattering portrayal of Samora Machel, apparently a former nurse under Paes, who subsequently joined Frelimo.[52] With Machel's accession to power, Paes returned to Portugal, "disillusioned by the ingratitude of the inhabitants of Mozambique after all that he had contributed to their welfare".[53]

[47] Ibid.

[48] Jack Penn "A Surgeon's Story: It Is the Divine Right of Man to Look Human" (Unpublished Manuscript), p213, Brn No 12057, 617.95 PEN, BL.

[49] Jack Penn, "Three Great Surgeons", File: Penn, Jack—Writings (3), AMUW.

[50] Penn, "A Surgeon's Story", p213.

[51] "Rare Disease Database—Yaws", *National Organization for Rare Disorders*, https://rarediseases.org/rare-diseases/yaws/, accessed 8 January 2021.

[52] Penn, "A Surgeon's Story", p214.

[53] Penn, "Three Great Surgeons".

In contrast to other African leaders as well as the perceived radicalising effects of education, it was Machel's experiences living and working amongst ordinary Mozambicans that exposed him to the inequalities inherent in colonial rule. Colonialism in Mozambique was not radically different to that in South Africa—with job reservation, iniquitous taxation policies, the expropriation of land and a system of rule that used existing African power structures. Machel was born into a world shaped by the colonial encounter with a grandfather who had been wounded fighting the Portuguese, an uncle who had enlisted in the military during the First World War and his father working as a migrant labourer in the mines in South Africa. Machel's schooling experience was mediocre in an educational system that prioritised religious instruction and manual labour. He eventually became a nurse, a profession that allowed entry to African men and women, paid relatively well and was a much sought-after alternative to unskilled labour. While nursing offered the children of the African peasantry an opportunity to improve their economic conditions, it also highlighted the unjust nature of colonialism with African students living in less-than-ideal conditions and receiving training that compared poorly to their white counterparts. Machel's espousal of Marxism came as a result of the unequal medical treatment afforded to the elite and the opportunity to engage with other students and compare their experiences of Portuguese colonialism. By 1963, he had joined Frelimo. In contrast to the racial dichotomy with which wars of liberation were often portrayed, Machel believed that race did not determine political affiliation—it was a veneer for class oppression. He understood the importance of education in emphasising a national identity and overcoming the differences of race and class that created tension within Frelimo. Ironically, just as Penn did, Machel believed that education was necessary to engage in critical thinking: "Samora's personal experiences would free Mozambicans from the shackles of illiteracy, the tyranny of superstition, and the cultural arrogance of missionary education."[54]

Machel's view of education as well as his experiences as a nurse thus paint a different picture to that of Penn in terms of the supposed benefits of colonial rule and the unpreparedness of Africans for self-government and it was the very inequality evident in both these areas that helped radicalise him. Machel eventually rose to the leadership of Frelimo, becoming

[54] Allen Isaacman, "Toward a Biography of Samora Michel: The Making of a Revolutionary, 1933–1970 ca.", *South African Historical Journal*, 72, 1, 51–79, 2020.

the first president of an independent Mozambique. He was killed in a plane crash while flying over South African airspace in October 1986—an incident that aroused suspicions regarding the complicity of the apartheid state.[55] In his autobiography, Penn gave short shrift to Machel's fate, "This leader was killed under mysterious circumstances."[56]

While Penn condemned the activities of Frelimo, he stressed the continuation of the civilising mission of Portuguese rule as symbolised by the Cahorra Bassa hydroelectric project.[57] Yet the construction of the dam and the involvement of South Africa in the project meant that it was more than a case of simple development, serving the strategic needs of the apartheid state. The dam would be a symbol of progress, allow control over an unpredictable water supply and provide the hydroelectric power that would stimulate agriculture and mining. Yet the planned construction of the dam also coincided with Frelimo insurgency and the dam became the means by which advances by Frelimo as well as the ANC could be halted. South Africa was involved in the project from investment to construction and in return, received more than 80% of the hydroelectric power generated at an incredibly favourable rate. The provision of cheap electricity was an important factor in maintaining state control so, rather than a means of benefitting indigenous Mozambicans, the dam symbolised the control of the apartheid state. The benefit it provided to South Africa meant that even after full democracy was implemented in 1994, Mozambique only regained sole control over the dam in 2007.[58]

In addition to Penn's belief in the promise of progress, he also highlighted Portuguese largesse, their willingness to provide medical treatment to both "terrorists and loyalists"—a far cry from Machel's experiences in the provision of medical care in Mozambique. Penn attributed the loss of Mozambique to Frelimo to the failure of the government of Portugal, rather than a lack of commitment on the part of the Portuguese

[55] Augusta Conchiglia, "Was Mozambique Air Crash an Assassination? The Mysterious Death of Samora Machel", *Le Monde Diplomatique* [English translation], 1 November 2017, pp1–5.

[56] Penn, "A Surgeon's Story", p214.

[57] Ibid.

[58] Allen F. Isaacman and Barbara F. Isaacman, "Extending South Africa's Tentacles of Empire: The Deterritorialisation of Cahora Bassa Dam", *Journal of Southern African Studies*, 41, 3, 541–560, 2015, pp541–544.

in Mozambique and their indigenous allies.[59] A coup in Portugal brought with it not only a change in leadership, but a different attitude towards the retention of Portuguese colonies, leading to the conclusion of the war in Mozambique and the country's independence.

With independence, Penn believed that Mozambique was much diminished, returning to a precolonial past where, "starvation now stalks the land and all the tropical diseases which were under control are now rampant."[60] For his part, Penn was gratified by his role in assisting the Portuguese, "a kindly and highly civilised community".[61] Yet he found it incomprehensible that his views were not shared—not only as they applied to Mozambique but with regards to his own country as well.

Enhancing Penn's sense of besiegement was his "bewilderment" at the opposition—both internal and external—to the South African government. He denounced their unwillingness to engage with the state while simply condemning its policies. A major culprit was the UN. Perhaps swayed by the "propaganda" of "ex-South African journalists," the UN was criticised for singling out South Africa, appointing investigators already hostile to the country's policies and not applying a universal standard in its dealings with all countries.[62] The matter that aroused Penn's ire against the international body was South West Africa (Namibia).

South Africa had had a complex relationship with Namibia for the greater part of the twentieth century. Its first military action during the First World War was to end the German threat in South West Africa. South Africa invaded the territory and defeated German forces stationed there and upon the conclusion of the War, was awarded South West Africa as a mandated territory by the League of Nations. Its mandate was to prepare South West Africa for self-government. From the outset, however, South Africa applied the discriminatory measures that were evident in the Union—the unequal distribution of land with the privileging of South African settlers as well as those of German descent and the application of a franchise extended to white settlers only. Legislation such as Pass Laws was also implemented, arousing no small amount of resentment in the territory. This contributed to the Bondelswarts Rebellion in 1922 in

59 Penn, "A Surgeon's Story", p214.

60 Ibid.

61 Ibid.

62 Penn, *The Right to Look Human*, p247.

reaction to the heavy taxation designed to force them into waged labour. The harsh measures used against the rebels led to criticism at the League of Nations but these measures were defended by Jan Smuts. For Smuts, South West Africa was a means of realising his own imperial ambitions on the continent.[63]

Smuts—a leading international statesman at the end of the First World War—was instrumental in fostering the mandate system of the League of Nations which he assumed would be implemented in the new territories arising from the break-up of the Austro-Hungarian and Ottoman Empires. He simultaneously envisaged the ideal role of "advanced civilisations" as one of assisting their less developed brethren on the road to progress. The inexorable march of progress could potentially suffer a setback should these groups make premature demands for independence. Smuts, however, was unable to prevent the granting of mandated territory status to South West Africa and as Tilman Dedering argues, American President Woodrow Wilson's vision of self-determination was a source of inspiration to the colonised. This, in combination with harsh South African policies on a population already reeling from German occupation, led to resistance on the part of indigenous South West Africans which would play out over the course of the century.[64]

From the onset of South African involvement in South West Africa, the territory provided the means and opportunity for South Africa to foster its own development. The 1922 strike—to which a young Penn had been witness—highlighted the disaffection of an impoverished white working class and the new mandate presented the prospect of both land and employment. The diamond mines were a source of wealth for Anglo-American. Reserves were created for indigenous groups and their role was manifold: the containment of resistance; the freeing up of land for white settlers; the maintenance of segregation; the prevention of competition with white farmers and the creation of a labour force for South African

[63] Reader's Digest, *Illustrated History of South Africa: The Real Story* (Cape Town, Reader's Digest, 1992), pp463–469.

[64] Tilman Dedering, "Petitioning Geneva: Transnational Aspects of Protest and Resistance in South West Africa/Namibia After the First World War", *Journal of Southern African Studies*, 35, 4, 785–801, December 2009.

agriculture, mining and industry.[65] South Africa was therefore loath to relinquish her claim on the territory.

From 1948, the South African state continued its attempt to incorporate South West Africa into South Africa—it was already considered a fifth province. The UN again rejected this yet the state was defiant, imposing the harsh legislative measures that characterised apartheid policy such as racial segregation and the implementation of forced removals. Its actions provoked rebellion on the part of indigenous inhabitants, leading to the formation of the South West African People's Organisation (SWAPO) in 1960 which began violent resistance. To compound matters, six years later the UN ended South Africa's mandate over South West Africa and acknowledged SWAPO as the representative of the disputed territory. Notwithstanding the UN decision, the South African state continued its defiance and conflict continued.[66] Sarah Gertrude Millin was even less circumspect than Penn in her condemnation of the actions of the UN, viewing its motivation as due to the influence of groups with a particular bias against South Africa and the aim of the annihilation of the existing structure of government:

> For it is both the general desire of the World Body – not unnaturally since it is controlled by Africans and Asians, against whom South Africa for her life's sake discriminates – to destroy South Africa, and the best chance seems to be through South-West Africa.[67]

By the 1970s, SWAPO was launching attacks into South Africa from Angola and the SADF responded in kind, with both sides committing atrocities. It was only in 1990 that Namibia became independent. Penn's sense of righteous indignation towards the UN then, came from the international body's support of SWAPO and the attainment of Namibian independence as well as condemnation of South Africa's repressive role in the territory.[68]

[65] Marion Wallace with John Kinahan, *A History of Namibia: From the Beginning to 1990* (New York, Columbia University Press, 2011), pp216–219.

[66] Reader's Digest, *Illustrated History of South Africa*, pp463–469.

[67] Sarah Gertrude Millin, "Africa" in *White Africans Are Also People*, Sarah Gertrude Millin (ed) (Howard Timmons, Cape Town, 1966), Brn. No: 14607, Call No: 323.1128 MIL, BL.

[68] Reader's Digest, *Illustrated History of South Africa*, pp463–469.

By 1966, independence had largely come to the former colonies, and this was grudgingly acknowledged by Penn: "Whether the rush towards freedom from colonial rule is a good or bad thing is now only of academic interest".[69] Yet the prospect still presented a source of concern to South Africa that went beyond the "academic" as it related to her immediate neighbours, Angola, Mozambique and Southern Rhodesia as well as her control over South West Africa. Over the ensuing decades, the apartheid state would be involved in numerous conflicts related to the independence of these territories within the context of the Cold War. While recognising the inevitability of African independence, Penn's writings attempted to diminish their effects by emphasising African inability to effectively govern themselves, an inability that could only be addressed through the continuing role of white paternalism and guidance: "When Schweitzer said of the African 'He is my younger brother', he summed up in one sentence the true relationship between the sophisticated European and the emergent African."[70]

[69] Penn, "He Is My Younger Brother", p130.

[70] Ibid., p138.

CHAPTER 12

A Utopian Vision: Jack Penn's Brave New World

The Idealist

The Brenthurst Library contains an unpublished manuscript by Jack Penn entitled "Towards a Modern Utopia". It consists of a series of essays that draw together the various aspects of Penn's thinking on subjects ranging from education to the home. While Penn is the main contributor, also included are essays by figures such as Ivor Edwards, South African ambassador, Kurt von Schirnding and judge and advocate for reform, especially in urban African communities,[1] Jan Steyn. The essays reflect Penn's concerns with social, political and environmental issues and by so doing, put forth an idealised vision of the world as he saw it. These philosophies were also based on his experience in medicine and war, his far-ranging travels and the contacts he made with various figures all over the globe.

Ivor Edwards, for instance, contributed an essay "Homo Sapiens Past, Present and Future" where he raised significant concerns regarding global

[1] Justice D.G. Scott, "A Tribute to Justice Jan Hendrik Steyn (1928–2013)", *Lesotho Law Journal*, 20, 1–2, January 2013, pp201–204.

S. Chetty, *Reconstructive Surgery and Modernisation in Twentieth-Century South Africa*, Medicine and Biomedical Sciences in Modern History, https://doi.org/10.1007/978-3-031-38673-2_12

warming, deforestation and the use of fossil fuels.[2] The environmental concerns raised by Edwards have taken on a new impetus in the present but are also related to Penn's encounter with physicist Edward Teller, renowned for his involvement in the Manhattan Project beginning in 1942.[3] Teller moved from his position as a professor at Columbia University to Los Alamos, New Mexico where, in collaboration with other scientists, he was responsible for the development of the atomic bomb, a weapon ultimately used with devastating effect against Japan. Teller also played a significant role in the development of the more powerful hydrogen bomb, symbolic of the Arms Race and Cold War hostility.[4] As Teller himself stated decades later, it was on his advice that the hydrogen bomb was developed, a decision stemming largely from the fear that the Soviets were planning to do the same and for the remainder of his life, Teller remained unapologetic for his actions. He also justified scientific development for its own sake, citing "free will" as responsible for its applications.[5] Simultaneously—and perhaps not contradictorily—Teller was driven by a desire to find beneficial uses for nuclear technology.[6]

In 1975 Teller presented a series of lectures in both the United States and Israel that were adapted in the form of a monograph, *Energy from Heaven and Earth*. In his monograph, he described the beginnings of energy dating from the Big Bang, its origins (often in the form of fossil fuels) on Earth and its uses throughout human history, but particularly from the beginning of the Industrial Revolution.[7] The oil crisis of 1973 demonstrated international vulnerability to a steady supply of the fossil fuel, giving the nuclear option greater feasibility. Contextualised by events in that decade, Teller paid special attention to the use of oil and gas

[2] Ivor Edwards, "Homo Sapiens Past, Present and Future" in Jack Penn, "Towards a Modern Utopia", (Unpublished Manuscript), Brn. No: 12778, Call No: PAM.1594, BL. Note that, as this is an unpublished piece of work, no page numbers are evident.

[3] Stephen B. Libby and Morton S. Weiss "Edward Teller's Scientific Life", *Physics Today*, American Institute of Physics, August 2004, pp45–46.

[4] John Maddox, "Obituary: Edward Teller (1908–2003)", *Nature*, 425, 25 September 2003, pp362–363.

[5] Edward Teller, "Science and Morality", *Science*, 280, 5367, American Association for the Advancement of Science, 22 May 1998, pp1200–1201.

[6] Libby and Weiss, "Edward Teller's Scientific Life", pp48–49.

[7] *Cf* Edward Teller, *Energy from Heaven and Earth* (San Francisco, W.H. Freeman and Company, 1979).

as essential fuels as well as the limited nature of these resources that had the potential to precipitate conflict and the exercise of power. His view was that nuclear energy was a viable alternative. Written before Chernobyl and Three Mile Island became cautionary tales, Teller was optimistic about the safe harnessing of nuclear power where the provision of abundant, environmentally friendly energy was a pre-requisite for the creation of a utopian, prosperous world and conflict would be relegated to the past.[8] Current nuclear reactors made use of fission, but Teller was confident about the development of safer, more energy efficient and cleaner fusion technology. Also considered was the use of geothermal energy, wind, water and solar power.[9] The goal was to move away from a reliance on oil as a fuel source which weakened the United States and had left it exposed to the crisis precipitated by the oil embargo. Further, if the United States led the way in the development of alternative energy resources, the country would have a competitive edge over the rest of the world.[10]

South Africa was an important consideration in Teller's thinking. In September 1973, Teller paid a visit to the country under the aegis of the Atomic Energy Board. His trip was a mix of business—with two lectures scheduled—and pleasure.[11] The last included meeting friends and acquaintances, one of whom was Jack Penn. Penn exemplified the combination of business and pleasure by "[arranging] a social evening" for Teller, giving him the opportunity to meet South African scientists working at universities, the Council for Scientific and Industrial Research (CSIR) and the Atomic Energy Board. One of the topics discussed—albeit "lightly"—was the recent energy crisis.[12]

During the visit, Teller noted that the current crisis was due to "an artificially induced shortage" but nevertheless raised real concerns about long-term oil supply. His prediction was that oil supplies would eventually be depleted and possible solutions to the looming energy crisis could be found in South Africa. The first was nuclear power with South Africa

[8] Ibid., Chapter 8.

[9] Ibid., Chapter 11.

[10] Ibid., pp275, 278.

[11] Chris Cairncross, "Father of H-Bomb is to Visit SA", *Rand Daily Mail*, 13 September 1973.

[12] Penn, *The Right to Look Human*, p198.

already exporting uranium to the United States. The second "medium-term" solution was SASOL's innovative attempt to produce liquified, synthetic oil from South Africa's plentiful coal reserves, an innovation that the United States was following with "keen" interest.[13]

Upon his return to the United States, Teller re-iterated the claim of South African importance in helping resolve the dependence on oil with the view that South Africa's coal reserves could serve as an important source of fuel for industrialised countries. Moreover, the country, engaged in its own industrialisation, was characterised by its "forward-looking industrial and scientific manpower", and was applying its progressive ethos to "educating and training the less-developed people in its midst". The combination of its coal reserves and its progressive vision made it "the only viable country in Africa" to assist in resolving the crisis.[14]

The South African response to Teller's enthusiasm was rather more circumspect with the president of South Africa's Atomic Energy Board calling Teller's optimistic view of South Africa's ability to fuel the rest of the world "a bit far-fetched". His concern about protecting the country's coal reserves was echoed by the managing director of SASOL who re-iterated that the United States was interested only in the process by which oil was obtained from coal and not in obtaining the coal reserves.[15] Penn backed Teller's views—an American alliance with South Africa had the potential to resolve the fuel crisis.[16] And in addition to coal, was the potential of nuclear technology that was only at this point, used to provide electricity in South Africa. So convinced was Teller of its efficacy that he believed that the Arab countries responsible for initiating the oil crisis would soon find it difficult to find a market for their oil exports.[17]

Both Penn and Teller reflected the early optimism regarding the use of nuclear technology in fuelling development. The project however, was never adequately developed in South Africa and the use of nuclear technology to produce power remained prohibitively expensive. Over

[13] Chris Cairncross, "H-Bomb Father Tackles the Energy Crisis", *Rand Daily Mail*, 1 October 1973.

[14] "SA Could Solve World Fuel Crisis", *Rand Daily Mail*, 8 December 1973.

[15] "Conserve SA's Coal—Dr Roux", *Rand Daily Mail*, 10 December 1973.

[16] Penn, *The Right to Look Human*, p198.

[17] "No Fuel Oil by 2000", *Rand Daily Mail*, 27 September 1973; Chris Cairncross, "Edward Teller's View: Thorium to Replace Uranium", *Rand Daily Mail*, 27 October 1973.

the course of the decade, confronted by insurgence, South Africa sacrificed development for strategic military aims and the weapons potential of nuclear technology.[18] The oil crisis nevertheless permitted Penn to advocate a vision of development that was based on South African self-sufficiency as well as the use of technology as a panacea for socio-political and economic crises. This idealistic vision is replicated in his writing.

In "Towards a Modern Utopia", Penn addressed some of the aspects already discussed in the preceding chapters—education and ability and attitudes towards race. His own position changed little and was a mixture of considerations of ability and opportunity, equality and difference.[19] There are however, three additional areas that are of interest in this chapter.

The first is the essay entitled "The Home" where Penn made a claim for both female equality in the public sphere by alluding to female political leaders but also female superiority in the home due to their greater knowledge of and familiarity with "the cost of living, schooling, clothing and the general development of their children" than their male counterparts. It was the greater equality of women that Penn saw as a hallmark of Western culture and "civilisation" in contrast to, for instance, the prevalence of polygamy that occurred in Africa and privileged patriarchal authority.[20] Penn's perception of women's roles can be seen in his support of nurses with whom he worked in various war zones. While the nursing profession for women can be seen partly as an extension of their idealised domestic and nurturing role, Penn developed a healthy respect for the women who worked arduous hours under dangerous conditions and were often compelled by the same ideological conviction as himself. His art valorised the role of women as nurse and as mother (as evident in Hiroshima)—features that transcended racial distinction.

His essay, "Military and Police", can be contextualised by the political and military situation facing South Africa in the 1970s and especially the implementation of conscription. When P.W. Botha became Minister of Defence in 1966, it was during a period of increasing militarisation and concerns regarding security that would increase exponentially over

[18] Bill Freund, *Twentieth-Century South Africa: A Developmental History* (Cambridge, Cambridge University Press, 2019), pp174–176.

[19] Penn, "Towards a Modern Utopia".

[20] Ibid.

the following decades. According to the Defence Act of 1957, the SADF comprised the Permanent Force, the Citizen Force, the Commandos and a Reserve Force. Military service could be compelled in the Citizen Force, the Commandos and their Reserve Force counterparts. At the outset, compulsory service was set at three months for the Citizen Force and 21 days for the Commandos. In the wake of Sharpeville, the three-month period of compulsory military service in the Citizen Force and the Citizen Force Reserve was increased to nine months. Those chosen to serve were selected via ballot. As South Africa became increasingly isolated internationally, there was a marked lack of enthusiasm amongst white youth for military service and an amendment to the Defence Act in 1967 made it compulsory for all white male citizens to serve in the Citizen Force for nine months. This included conscientious objectors who were expected to take on non-combatant, auxiliary roles. The period of conscription lengthened steadily as South Africa became embroiled in conflict with neighbouring states while addressing unrest on the domestic front and, in 1977, conscription was lengthened to a two-year term.[21]

The ethos of militarisation that was inherent in conscription was based on an ideological underpinning that combined masculinity, Afrikaner nationalism and a form of muscular Christianity. As such, it served to force conscripts to adopt a particular set of values while simultaneously marginalising those who did not. Conscription was therefore the means of creating the perfect citizen—obedient to authority, loyal to the state and willing to defend these values. Those marginalised were condemned as cowardly and disloyal and unsuitable for the privileges of citizenship.[22]

Penn focused largely on conscription in his essay and was firmly on the side of the apartheid state, viewing conscription as a way of creating a sense of national unity even as it offered citizens "peace of mind" by securing them from threats both within and without. Rather than an infringement on individual liberties, conscription was instead the way in which citizens could concretely demonstrate their allegiance to the state

[21] Lynn Berat, "Conscientious Objection in South Africa: Governmental Paranoia and the Law of Conscription", *Vanderbilt Journal of Transnational Law*, 22, 1, 127–186, 1989, pp136, 138, 139, 148.

[22] Daniel Conway, "'All These Long-Haired Fairies Should be Forced to Do Their Military Training. Maybe They Will Become Men': The End Conscription Campaign, Sexuality, Citizenship and Military Conscription in Apartheid South Africa", *South African Journal on Human Rights*, 20, 2, 207–229, 2004, pp208, 212.

regardless of their "politics, colour or creed". It gave them the opportunity to do their duty by their country in return for the benefits reaped from their citizenship, as well as permitted them "to take stock of their own lives".[23] He drew comparisons between the more responsible citizen produced by conscription and the "drop-outs and troublemakers" who he believed to "come from the section of the population which [had] escaped conscription".[24]

Yet Penn was aware of the resistance to conscription, especially on the grounds of pacifism, suggesting that less martial roles may be accorded to those who found "killing…morally abhorrent". Despite his own exposure to war and its effects over the course of his career, as well as his intolerance of military hierarchies and bureaucracy, he was convinced of the necessity for soldiers "to fight for their homes and the women and children in them, than [to] allow a passive slaughter by the enemy by nuclear bombs or chemical warfare".[25] On an individual level, conscription was not just important to the "welfare of the country", it was even more "beneficial for the future of the individual himself" and he advocated conscription for "**all** citizens".[26]

Penn's view on conscription—especially for black South Africans—would create some controversy as discussed later in this chapter. Yet, as a figure who did not easily follow military dictates throughout his career, he advocated a less heavy-handed approach towards the treatment of military recruits. At a conference on military medicine in 1973, Penn—at the time, a Brigadier in the SADF—stressed the importance of the "common touch" in the handling of recruits to maintain morale. This was especially true for conflicts that did not enjoy unequivocal support—and he cited the Middle East and Vietnam as pertinent examples demonstrating the importance of morale: "Discipline is essential, but arrogance is not discipline…If we are to prevent resentment – which leads to drug-taking and finally drug addiction – the men must feel they belong and like it."[27]

[23] Penn, "Towards a Modern Utopia".

[24] Jack Penn, "Military Service" in "Philosophy is Fun" (Unpublished Manuscript), File: Penn, Jack—Writings (5), AMUW.

[25] Penn, "Towards a Modern Utopia".

[26] Penn, "Military Service".

[27] "Make Trainees Feel Welcome, Says Brigadier", *Rand Daily Mail*, 26 July 1973.

This was contextualised by Penn's perception of the precarious position of a South African state, beset by communist forces and communist sympathisers with little support afforded by the country's democratic allies. A grim picture was painted of precarious land borders where neighbouring states were engaged in a life and death struggle "against communist-trained guerrillas" with the seas seething with Soviet submarines while "the Indian Ocean has become a communist playground".[28] The proper treatment of recruits—as with conscription—was to ensure the country's borders. And military medicine had a significant role to play. At the conference, Penn announced the creation of a degree in military medicine at Pretoria University—which could possibly be emulated in other tertiary institutions as well—to ensure trained military medical personnel to support the efforts of the SADF in the fight against communism and to maintain the security of the state.[29]

In his view of the state, Penn departed significantly from the multi-party democratic system with a "no party" state where individuals were accorded votes based on their ability and utility in what was clearly a qualified franchise. The following was the basis on which he envisaged the votes to be allocated:

> One vote for every literate citizen;
> One vote for any citizen who has volunteered to defend his country or serve in an equivalent fashion;
> One vote if the citizen has matriculated;
> One vote for citizens who have graduated from the tertiary level;
> One vote if the citizen is a taxpayer;
> One vote if more than a specific amount of taxes is paid.[30]

For Penn, the ideal citizen was one who was educated, financially successful (also related to profession) and had performed some form of public service as a demonstration of their patriotism and commitment to the state. While not predicated on race, it was largely based on class which, in the South African context, was linked with race. Black South Africans overwhelmingly formed a working class and were relegated to largely

[28] Ibid.

[29] Ibid.

[30] Penn, "Towards a Modern Utopia".

unskilled labour. Penn's utopian vision can thus be argued to already be partially in existence in apartheid South Africa.

His view of democracy—and indeed, of existing political systems—was ambivalent. He considered the United States to be an "oligarchy" rather than a democracy, despite proclamations to the contrary. He was less than smitten with newly independent African states that were either "dictatorships or one-party states" despite recognition by the UN as democracies. Even in South Africa, a "true democracy" was only applied to a particular racial group. For him then, democracy was more a case of rhetoric than actual practical implementation. The creation of political parties representing different interests and segments of the population, while allowing for engagement with each other to reach consensus, could also splinter unity, dividing countries along religious, class, racial or other lines. Further, the members of these parties elected to office tended to place the concept of service a distant third after personal and party considerations. It is for these reasons that Penn did not favour the existing model of democracy. Moreover, he emphasised the dangers of a potentially fragmented democracy, rent with inefficiency or "lack of expertise" within, as well as enemies beyond its borders. This could lead to groups opposing the government or those seeking insurrection—such as the communists—to mobilise the larger part of the population against the state.[31] This, of course, was the threat that underpinned the apartheid state's mobilisation against groups both within its borders and externally.

While Penn acknowledged the theoretical and aspirational nature of his political vision, it was nevertheless shaped by a context of increasing criticism and hostility to the policies of apartheid and the repressive nature of white minority rule in South Africa. His contribution to the political life of the country would ultimately move beyond the philosophical.

The Reformer

In his revised autobiography, Penn claimed, "It is impossible to live a full life in this world without having a political opinion both nationally and internationally."[32] By 1980 however, he was ostensibly retired. He had

[31] Jack Penn, *Reflections on Life* (Johannesburg, Eric Stanton Publishers, 1980), pp56–60.

[32] Jack Penn "A Surgeon's Story: It is the Divine Right of Man to Look Human" (Unpublished Manuscript), p216, Brn No 12057, 617.95 PEN, BL.

moved to Cape Town and was living in the affluent suburb of Clifton overlooking the Atlantic Ocean. After a lifetime of travel and being based largely in Johannesburg, he had returned to the province of his birth, the "womb", or, as he put it, "a womb with a view". But retirement did not mean the cessation of activity for the seventy-year-old, "I lecture once a week at the Tygerberg Hospital in Cape Town, write a column in the *Washington Weekly*, do a couple of ops to keep my hand in, give various talks to clubs and schools, sculpt a bit, and talk to my dog when we go for walks."[33] It was however, the columns for the *Washington Weekly* that would lead to a further engagement in politics and a new phase in Penn's public life.

In July 1977, in her column, "Notes from the Dragon Lady", American commentator Dorothy Faber introduced Penn to her American readers. In addition to lauding his skills as a surgeon and his work in Africa and Japan, she emphasised his hostile reception amongst various elements in the United States who refused to publish his political musings and prevented the distribution of his autobiography, *The Right to Look Human*, in the United States due to his controversial final chapter on Africa. As a friend, Faber therefore requested that he write a column on "his observations on the relationship between my country and his".[34] The column, "A South African's View" appeared regularly and was Penn's take on American and Southern African politics.

Penn set the tone in his inaugural article with his division of American society into two groups—those opposed to South Africa and Rhodesia, motivated by "guilt" based on their treatment of African Americans and unwilling to involve themselves in "another Vietnam". The second group—who Penn favoured—were those who opposed the UN as "a servant of Communism and the Third World", an organisation that had

[33] "From a Womb with a View, Jack Penn Tells His Secrets of a Very Full Life", *The Star*, 24 August 1980, File: Biography—Jack Penn, AMUW.

[34] Dorothy Faber, "Notes from the Dragon Lady", *Washington Weekly*, 21 July 1977, p4, File: Biography—Jack Penn, AMUW. Penn's manuscript, "A Surgeon's Story" was revised for an "American public, who have not appreciated my criticism of some of the Black states noted by me at the time I wrote the first book"—Jack Penn, "Profile: Jack Penn", *SA Practice Management*, 9, 3, 1988, File: Biography—Jack Penn, AMUW.

also turned a blind eye to the "savagery and murder in Black Africa" while simultaneously being wholly hostile to "White Southern Africa".[35]

Of concern to Penn in the late 1970s was the pariah-like status of Rhodesia under Ian Smith, the growing condemnation of apartheid policy as evident in the arms embargo implemented by the UN in 1977 and the hostility and vacillation of the Carter administration. He felt the UN was largely responsible for South Africa's isolation, and termed the organisation "sanctimonious" and hypocritical due to the "double standards" exercised through its support of "communist and third world countries" and simultaneous "vilification" of "anticommunist small countries like South Africa and Israel". For Penn, despite Smuts's role in composing the preamble of the charter of the UN, the organisation had departed from the ideals of the Charter.[36]

Key was a different concept of "human rights" and the contemporary interpretation which for Penn, privileged rights without responsibility, "thus encouraging a parasitic existence on the one hand a demand for privileges on the other".[37] In his interpretation of the concept of "human rights", Penn's thinking was actually not far removed from Smuts himself decades earlier. While Smuts was criticised by African nationalist leaders for the apparent hypocrisy of using "human rights" in the preamble while supporting segregation in South Africa, for Smuts "human rights" were the basic rights to life and those associated with "spiritual growth or evolutionary progress". They did not automatically translate to political rights and equality. As Dubow has argued, rights were for those believed to have attained the level of civilisation and "maturity" to effectively exercise them. They could not be divorced from their accompanying responsibilities and Smuts did not countenance political equality for either the colonies or the black majority in South Africa, none of whom in his view had the capability of adequately exercising these rights.[38] For Penn then, it was still necessary for whites in southern Africa to retain minority

[35] Jack Penn, "The Fate of South Africa", *Washington Weekly*, 21 July 1977, File: Biography—Jack Penn, AMUW.

[36] Jack Penn, "A South African's View: Is the UN Civilised?" *Washington Weekly*, 3 September 1978, File: Biography—Jack Penn, AMUW.

[37] Jack Penn, "The Tilted Halo", File: Biography—Jack Penn, AMUW.

[38] Saul Dubow, *South Africa's Struggle for Human Rights* (Auckland Park, Jacana Media, 2012), pp58–60.

rule in order to guide the rest of the population to the necessary level of civilisation where they would be able to act as responsible citizens.

While his earlier writings had been largely concerned with Mozambican independence, by the late 1970s, Southern Rhodesia (Zimbabwe) featured prominently, especially in relation to the actions of international bodies such as the UN. Smith declared Rhodesian independence in 1965, with political power in the hands of the white minority. The state, however, did not receive international recognition and became increasingly isolated, with South Africa a staunch ally. In an article on Rhodesian leader Ian Smith, Penn portrayed the story of a war "hero" who had sacrificed much as a member of the Rhodesian Squadron attached to the RAF. Smith's plane had crashed in North Africa, leaving him with severe facial damage that did little to deter him from returning to the fray in Italy once he had recovered. The international condemnation that resulted from the declaration of Rhodesian independence was therefore seen as a betrayal by his "Kith and Kin" and a support for "terrorists" masquerading as "freedom fighters". While acknowledging that Smith would ultimately not be able to maintain white minority rule, Penn portrayed him as a martyr, "If the next few months spell the end of an era and Smith is physically defeated, the moral victory will nevertheless, for all time, be his."[39]

Like South Africa, Rhodesia was portrayed as an exemplar of white civilisation that was threatened by both the activities of black "terrorists" who formed a minority and the actions of the UN and the British Commonwealth through the implementation of sanctions and refusal to recognise Smith's state:

> It is a remarkable achievement that less than a quarter of a million whites should be able to lead over 6 million blacks to prosperity and peace – that is, until terrorists from Mozambique and Zambia, armed by the East and encouraged by the West began to torture and kill innocent men, women and children – usually black.[40]

[39] Jack Penn, "Ian Smith: Twilight of an Era", 1978, File: Biography—Jack Penn, AMUW.

[40] Jack Penn, "A South African's View: Rhodesians have Shown Courage", *Washington Weekly*, File: Biography—Jack Penn, AMUW.

As with Rhodesia, there was an element of defiance in Penn's writings when it came to the increased isolation of South Africa as well. He felt that isolation—while financially inconvenient and requiring some measure of sacrifice—also permitted South Africa the opportunity to develop a sense of self-reliance that would only strengthen the country and its inhabitants.[41] Writing for an American audience, Penn argued that it would instead be countries like the United States that would bear the brunt of isolation for the Carter administration's condemnation of the white settler states in southern Africa. Carter's actions are portrayed almost as an act of racial disloyalty:

> ...without the raw materials from South Africa and Rhodesia the steel industry would crash and unemployment would be rife. But the President, who has never been to Rhodesia and South Africa has been told that White South Africans, although of the same stock as White Americans, are ghouls, and must be eliminated from governing their country because there are more blacks.[42]

In contrast to Jimmy Carter, Penn surprisingly wrote approvingly of civil rights activist Jesse Jackson for the latter's advocacy of black responsibility. Ever the plastic surgeon, Penn observed that Jackson had apparently "overcome the handicap of a healed cleft lip and possibly a cleft palate" to encourage that same level of perseverance in his followers who were expected not simply "to accept special privileges" but instead to "prove" their equality and "pull [themselves] out of the morass of the past" through their own efforts. Penn's interpretation of "human rights" was again apparent—rights were not a given but were part and parcel of responsible citizenship.[43]

For Penn, black self-sufficiency was embodied in the Bantustans. Through the beneficence of the South African state—and at "great cost"—the creation of nine Bantustans was the means by which restitution could be made after the dispossession initiated by the British Empire. The apartheid state would also undertake to assist in the modernisation of these Bantustans through the creation of transport infrastructure,

[41] Jack Penn, "A South African's View: Strength from Isolation", *Washington Weekly*, 2 March 1978, File: Biography—Jack Penn, AMUW.

[42] Jack Penn, "The Tilted Halo", File: Biography—Jack Penn, AMUW.

[43] Jack Penn, "The Philosophy of Jesse Jackson", File: Biography—Jack Penn, AMUW.

industry, schools, medical facilities and farms as the Bantustans made steady progress "towards self viability". He emphasised the progress made in these "tribal homelands", asserting that in contrast to much of the rest of Africa, "they are amongst the most qualified for independence" yet were not given due recognition by the UN.[44]

Penn's perception of the Bantustans and the benevolent and modernising role of the apartheid state harmonised with his view of the role of white South Africa in general which, throughout the history of the country, he believed, had tried to dominate southern Africa through "democracy, segregation and paternalism". Yet he was not unaware of the changing times and understood that there needed to be drastic reform implemented if white South Africans were to survive in a changing and hostile environment. He argued that while segregation was not a solely South African development, it was only in South Africa that it was integral to the constitution and as such, had to be removed so as to appease world opinion. Paternalism had been a force for good and had contributed to the "affection between average whites and average blacks" in southern Africa in contrast to the enmity elsewhere but that, too, had to be eliminated as it was injurious to black "pride". Penn's solution was instead a commonwealth system led by South Africa (which he went so far as to consider renaming the "Republic of the Good Hope") that would ally itself with its African neighbours—the Bantustan states. He was also determined that white South Africa would retain its power as "that part of Africa first settled and developed by the Whites belongs to them and they will never give it up to be controlled by a tribal group".[45] This combination of political change within specific limitations, as well as his defence of South Africa in the face of international criticism, would make Penn an ideal candidate for proposed reform to the system of apartheid. Yet Penn was also an "outsider", described as an "English-speaker" rather than an Afrikaner which allows for an interrogation of his own identity and relationship to the apartheid state.

Jack Penn's political engagement shifted over the course of the twentieth century, and was both influenced and shaped by his work and experiences as a plastic surgeon. As he wrote his autobiography in 1976,

[44] Jack Penn, "A South African's View: Double-Dealing Standards", *Washington Weekly*, 23 February 1978, File: Biography—Jack Penn, AMUW.

[45] Jack Penn, "Quo Vadis", File: Biography—Jack Penn, AMUW.

it is possible to detect these changes that highlighted the complicated position of Jewish South Africans. Penn's early enlistment in the military before the outbreak of the Second World War, for instance, demonstrated his desire to further his experience in reconstructive surgery as well as his commitment to anti-fascism. Penn would also be one of approximately ten thousand South Africans Jews—or 10% of the Jewish population—who played an active role in the Second World War.[46]

And fascism was not merely a European phenomenon but had been evident in South Africa amongst right-wing Afrikaner nationalists. Anti-Semitism too, was increasingly prevalent during the first decades of the twentieth century with a Quota Act passed in 1930 under Hertzog's National Party government that sought to restrict immigration from Eastern Europe. These anti-immigration measures were refined and became more draconian over the next decade and, on the eve of the outbreak of the Second World War, anti-Semitism continued to flourish under the Nazi-styled fascist organisations, such as the Ossewabrandwag and the Greyshirts who sought to exclude Jews from the "white" racial category.[47] Prior to 1948 then, the South African Jewry and Afrikaner nationalists existed in a state of tension. Surprisingly, however, this changed with the Afrikaner nationalists coming to power and the implementation of apartheid in 1948.

Over the early decades of the twentieth century, Afrikaner nationalists had drawn their support from working-class Afrikaners, vulnerable to competition in the labour market from black South Africans as well as increasing numbers of Eastern European Jewish immigrants. Once in power however and increasingly self-assured, the apartheid state was more conciliatory towards Jewish South Africans. Once barely considered "white" by anti-Semitists, Jews—like English-speaking white South Africans—were eventually incorporated into the apartheid state as a means of preserving white minority rule. For Jewish South Africans, there were three potential responses. The first—adopted by many—was to be compliant with the apartheid system which brought with it

[46] Milton Shain, "Jewish Cultures, Identities and Contingencies: Reflections from the South African Experience", *European Review of History*, 18, 01, 89–100, February 2011, p92.

[47] Norman Bentwich, "Jewish Life in British South Africa", *Jewish Social Studies*, 4, 1, 73–84, January 1942, p79; Franklin Hugh Adler, "South African Jews and Apartheid", *Patterns of Prejudice*, 34, 4, pp23–36, December 2010, p28.

material reward for white South Africans. At the same time, many—remembering the experience of anti-Semitism and thus identifying with marginalised and oppressed groups—took up active roles in the anti-apartheid struggle.[48] For a few however, there was support for some aspects of apartheid policy, evident in figures such as Sarah Gertrude Millin and Jack Penn.

As evident in his autobiography and writings on racial ability, intellect and development, Penn had valorised the Afrikaner in terms of the latter's ability to easily and quickly "catch up" with the apex of civilisation and Western modernity that had been the hallmarks of British imperialism.[49] Perhaps too, while Penn lambasted the British for their subservience to class structures that restricted innovation and privileged an elite, he had greater empathy for Afrikaners who were self-made, much like the Eastern European immigrants who had risen through the social hierarchy by virtue of hard work and individual achievement. And conceivably, by being incorporated into white South Africa, Penn was subject to the vulnerability and anxieties that accompanied white minority rule.

Yet, "petty apartheid" with its blatant racial discrimination without clear ideological justification was a major bone of contention for Penn, especially during his international travels. In 1968 he travelled to Taiwan at the behest of General Tang Chun-Po, the Cambridge-educated director of the Chung Shan Institute of Science and Technology.[50] The Institute is largely engaged in military technology research ranging from aeronautics to chemistry.[51] It was also associated with Taiwan's nuclear weapons development programme begun after China tested its first nuclear weapon in 1964. By the time of Penn's visit, Taiwan had already started sending scientists to Israel and had purchased a nuclear reactor from Germany.[52] Furthermore, as with the other places to which Penn had travelled and where he had advised on plastic surgery such as Israel and Japan, Taiwan

[48] Shain, "Jewish Cultures, Identities and Contingencies", p93.

[49] *Cf* Penn, *The Right to Look Human*, pp234–235.

[50] Penn, *The Right to Look Human*, p158.

[51] "Chungshan Institute of Science and Technology", *Globalsecurity.org*, https://www.globalsecurity.org/wmd/world/taiwan/csist.htm, accessed 26 April 2021.

[52] Gloria Kuang-Jung Hsu, "Control of Manipulation? Nuclear Power in Taiwan" in *Learning from Fukushima: Nuclear Power in East Asia*, Peter Van Ness and Mel Gurtov (eds) (Acton, Australian National University Press, 2017), pp157–158.

would also develop close ties with the South African state. However, the Taiwanese were very much aware of the discriminatory policies of "petty apartheid".

During his time in Taiwan, Penn was feted by the military establishment and accompanied by his son John, inspected the hospitals in the country ranging from those associated with the military to the Taiwan University Hospital. While the standards varied, Penn wrote approvingly of the well-trained medical doctors. Both Penns also demonstrated reconstructive surgical techniques and worked on cases.[53] In this way, Penn perceived himself to be an ambassador for South Africa, using science, technology and medicine to foster good relations with other countries and challenging the prevailing international and condemnatory view of South Africa. Yet petty apartheid threatened to undermine much of what he did. In a conversation with the chief of the Surgical Division of the National Defence Medical Centre, Penn asked him if he would like to visit South Africa to see Chris Barnard's by now renowned heart transplant unit. The response, "Of course I would but if I come to South Africa I will be treated like an African aboriginal, and I am not used to that."[54] Penn's realisation was that apartheid policies would have the effect of humiliating and alienating potential allies. This made him amenable to the policies of reform initiated by P.W. Botha, reform in which he would play an active role.

Upon Pieter Willem Botha's accession to power as Prime Minister in 1978, he was faced with a daunting task during a decade that had seen increasing challenges to the system of apartheid. His solution was to initiate a process of reform while still maintaining white power—no easy task when he was confronted with the competing interests of conservative Afrikaners unwilling to give an inch and radicals who demanded complete political equality. Penn was very much aware of "delicate balancing act" that Botha would need to maintain between "critical world politics" and "self respect and self preservation"; the requirement for reform while preserving minority rights in the face of a black majority.[55]

[53] Penn, *The Right to Look Human*, pp162–163.

[54] Ibid.

[55] Jack Penn, "South Africa and Its New Prime Minister—P.W. Botha", File: Biography—Jack Penn, AMUW.

Added to the mix was the unrest of the 1970s that seemed to necessitate changes in the existing structure, and the country's increasing international isolation, all of which had detrimental effects on economic growth. For Botha, apartheid had to be maintained but it had also to be adapted to serve as a means of supporting a new "phase" of modernisation.[56] Penn believed that Botha would be up to the task—his career to date where black recruits were permitted to join the army as well as the opening up of some public spaces to all races in the Cape, suggested that he was capable of carrying out reform. Simultaneously, he would not simply give in to international demands for change, "P.W. has indicated his personal approach – the gate of friendship is wide open, but although South Africa would welcome advice she will not be dictated to."[57]

Over the course of the first decade of Botha's administration, his biographer, Brian Pottinger detects three phases of reform with increasingly limited success. The first, however, from 1981 to 1984, had arguably the greatest impact with a focus on addressing "the social, economic and political crises" that were a legacy of forty years of the uneven and unequal development under apartheid. Simultaneously, as had been the case in the preceding decades and as evident in countries such as Israel and Iran, development often took second place to security concerns and in the case of South Africa, the maintenance of power.[58] Jack Penn's role was during this first phase.

On 31 May 1980, an article appeared in the *Rand Daily Mail* detailing the prospective formation of the President's Council. As evident by the title, it would fall largely under the control of the State President of South Africa and was to be comprised of a number of committees, their numbers and membership to be decided by the President. The role of the council was to "advise him on any matter, excluding draft legislation, which in its opinion is of public interest".[59]

The *Rand Daily Mail's* political correspondent Helen Zille—later to become the leader of the opposition party, the Democratic Alliance—painted a less than rosy picture of the chances of success of the President's

[56] Brian Pottinger, *The Imperial Presidency: P.W. Botha, the First 10 Years* (Johannesburg, Southern Book Publishers, 1988), pp76–77.

[57] Penn, "South Africa and Its New Prime Minister".

[58] Pottinger, *The Imperial Presidency*, p79.

[59] "The 'New-look' Parliament", *Rand Daily Mail*, 31 May 1980.

Council. The formation of the Council was seen as a last-ditch attempt by Botha to attempt reform by bypassing the hostility of the *verkrampte* or conservative elements within the National Party. Drawing upon the recommendations made by the members of the Council, Botha hoped to implement constitutional reform outside the confines of his National Party, thereby ensuring his own executive power. His desire smacked of a sense of desperation as he declared that he would "stand or fall" based on the success of the Council to create an environment conducive to change. This created a tremendous sense of expectation for the Council which was however, hampered even before its formation by several caveats. These included the exclusion of Africans on the Council as well as the nomination by Botha of the white, Indian and coloured members who would comprise the Council. Botha was in an unenviable position—the creation of the Council was necessarily a means of working outside recalcitrant elements within his own party and support base. Yet the lack of democratic process in the determination of the membership of the Council as well as significant exclusions, would alienate those segments who were sceptical of Botha's commitment to real reform of the oppressive system of apartheid.[60]

Despite numerous reservations—and increasingly vociferous opposition to the President's Council—it was given presidential approval later that year. The President's Council comprised five committees, each with fifteen members, although the Constitutional Committee was permitted sixteen. Members could also serve on different committees. The five committees were the Committee for Economic Affairs, the Planning Committee, the Constitutional Committee, the Committee for Community Relations and, finally, the Science Committee with one of its members Jack Penn.[61]

Zille's words were to be prophetic. In letters to the editor by black readers and appearing in the *Rand Daily Mail*, opposition was voiced to the exclusion of African members in the President's Council—the group forming the majority in the country and without which, any attempt at reform was toothless. Opinions ranged from pointing out this simple demographic fact which underlay racial oppression and apartheid, to the lack of adequate black leadership to challenge the exclusion. The words

[60] Helen Zille, "P.W. Botha's Alternative Strategy", *Rand Daily Mail*, 18 July 1980.

[61] "State President Approves Council", *Rand Daily Mail*, 20 November 1980.

of one writer were particularly telling: "If blacks are not included in the President's Council, nothing will come right. And if they are involved, don't let it be that the Government is using stooges and puppets to meet their ends."[62]

The perception of nominated members of the President's Council as "stooges and puppets" was a pervasive one that would shape many reactions to its formation. The members of the President's Council were varied, ranging across racial groups (excluding Africans) and including both men and women. There were scientists, politicians, newspaper editors, members of the National Party, the former United Party, various municipalities, the Coloured Representative Council and the Indian Council. Amongst the various luminaries and reflective of the ostensibly representative nature of the Council was the inclusion of Mrs E Rose who ran a creche in Durban and was a member of the "Pinetown Relations Committee". The brief description of member Jack Penn was:

> Dr J. Penn, 71, of Johannesburg, is a plastic and reconstructive surgeon. He is also visiting professor of plastic surgery at the University of Jerusalem. Dr Penn is also a consultant to the Minister of Health.[63]

On the same page of the newspaper was aired the opposition to the Council and its members. Bishop (later to be Archbishop) Desmond Tutu, spoke of its inherent weakness based on its nominated membership and lack of black African representatives. For him, rectifying this would not necessarily alienate Botha's National Party members further but instead win the state allies by signifying a real commitment to change. Political leaders were less circumspect in their wording with Frederik van Zyl Slabbert, leader of the opposition Progressive Federal Party, emphasising the dominance of National Party members in the Council and the inclusion of Indian and coloured members who did not necessarily represent their segments of the population. This was reinforced by Alan Hendrickse of the Labour Party (which represented coloureds) damning the inclusion of coloured members on the Council who he said had little "standing" amongst coloured people and could therefore not adequately

[62] Trupa Monaisa (Potchefstroom), Letter to the Editor, *Rand Daily Mail*, 1 October 1980.

[63] "Pen Pictures of All the Councillors", *Rand Daily Mail*, 3 October 1980.

represent their interests.[64] The Pretoria Chinese Association went a step further in expelling their assistant secretary, Kenneth F. Winchiu for agreeing to serve on the Council, counter to a decision adopted by the Association.[65] No punches were pulled when M.J. Naidoo of the Natal Indian Congress described Ismail Kathrada as a "sell-out" for serving on the Council, although Kathrada defended his actions with his belief that the Council would mark a step in the right direction, despite its current limitations.[66] Pat Poovalingam, attorney and writer at *The Graphic*—an Indian newspaper—stated that his role on the Council would be temporary unless Africans were included. But many black political leaders were unwilling to accept the Council as a compromise solution, unequivocally condemning those who participated.[67]

By attempting to use the President's Council as a compromise solution, Botha apparently pleased no one and in an opinion piece the following year and just prior to the first session of the Council, Zille continued her reservations with a piece entitled "1981 – the year of high expectations and low possibilities". The less than enthusiastic endorsement of the President's Council was accompanied by a cartoon depicting an unsteady-looking P.W. Botha atop a tightrope holding a wobbly pole—the one end depicting the Council and the other the National Party.[68] It was hardly an auspicious beginning to the President's Council before it had even had its first sitting. At the same time, those who were appointed to the President's Council had an idealised vision of the aims of the Council,

64 "Council Is Still-born, Say Its Opponents", *Rand Daily Mail*, 3 October 1980.

65 "Chop for Chinese Member", *Rand Daily Mail*, 3 October 1980.

66 Ameen Akhalwaya, "Kathrada a 'Sell-out' for Joining Council", *Rand Daily Mail*, 9 September 1980.

67 Ameen Akhalwaya, "More Candidates for President's Council", *Rand Daily Mail*, 13 September 1980.

68 Helen Zille, "1981: The Year of High Expectations But Low Possibilities", *Rand Daily Mail*, 17 January 1981. Botha's attempts at reforms further alienated the *verkrampte* elements within his own party, evident when Andries Treurnicht was ousted from the National Party and subsequently formed the Conservative Party which was vehemently opposed to reform. *Cf* F.A. Mouton, "'Dr No': A.P. Treurnicht and the Ultra-Conservative Quest to Maintain Afrikaner Supremacy, 1982–1993", *South African Historical Journal*, 65, 4, 577–595, 2013. Penn also alluded to the split within Afrikaner politics advocating instead the interests of "Afrikanerdom" over political ambitions to ensure that "white South African is not to be expendable."—Jack Penn, "The White South African", File: Biography—Jack Penn, AMUW.

perceiving it as a real step towards reform. Penn, in his first speech before the Council, attacked the system of racial discrimination proposing that a means of ending it would be through "decree". His views were supported by other members—many of whom appeared united in their vision of apartheid as a "curse". For the participating members who had taken on their roles despite hostility, there was indeed a sense that the multiracial formation of the President's Council presented new possibilities for the country, a way of redressing the inequalities of the past.[69]

Writing for the *Rand Daily Mail*, John Scott's irreverent—and today, breathtakingly politically incorrect—observations of the Council in session eighteen months after its fraught inception did not however inspire confidence as to its efficacy as a forum for reform. There was, undeniably, the unusual sight of seeing the various racial groups interacting and clearly forging amiable relationships with a description that relied heavily on stereotypes:

> Yet, strangely, no one appeared to have lost his identity. The whites all looked and sounded white. The Indians all looked Indian and sounded like Peter Sellars imitating an upper-class Bombay gentleman. The coloured members continued to look coloured and only sounded white if you shut your eyes when they spoke.[70]

The differences were more than skin deep. Despite the amiability between members, there was very little urgency to advocate change with the view that reform had to be incremental. A criticism by a Council member about the exclusion of black Africans was "accorded the sort of sympathy that a church congregation would reserve for one of its members who had temporarily gone astray".[71]

Jack Penn, however, was embroiled in controversy after co-writing a report which was released in August 1981.[72] The controversy came less with the report itself than with how it was portrayed in the press—a

[69] "Council Members Call for an End to Racism", *Rand Daily Mail*, 10 February 1981.

[70] John Scott, "Goodwill to All Men, But This Just Wasn't Politics", *Rand Daily Mail*, 14 May 1982.

[71] Ibid.

[72] Bev Mortimer, "'Aliens' Report Condemned as 'Ludicrous and Naïve'", *Rand Daily Mail*, 17 August 1981.

portrayal that Penn insisted was highly inaccurate. The report apparently emanating from the Science Committee suggested a concern with communist influence in academia with recommendations that the state put pressure on universities to limit their hiring of foreign academics, that university personnel be required to take an oath disavowing communism and association with "any terrorist or atheist organisation" and that black students should first undergo military service before being permitted to enrol at universities.[73]

Predictably, there was a furious response from academic institutions to proposed measures that smacked of McCarthyism and were perceived to be an attack on academic freedom. Penn however, insisted that his report (drawn up with Professor Maitland Reed) was exaggerated in the press and, moreover, was confidential and had yet to be discussed in the Science Committee. He was also unrepentant over some of the leaked information, "We feel blacks and whites should be treated the same – no privileges or charity. If it is necessary for whites to go to the army then blacks should also go."[74]

The incident and the reaction point to the tension that existed between the historically English-speaking universities and the apartheid state over university autonomy and the ideological and legislative demands stemming from the government. As early as the 1950s as the state was conceiving of separate tertiary institutions for designated racial and ethnic groups, University of Cape Town principal Davie warned against the dangers of these tertiary institutions served as sites of "indoctrination". Institutions such as UCT and Wits were particularly incensed by state policies designed to limit who could be admitted, perceiving this as an infringement of their autonomy.[75]

The points allegedly raised in the report were reflected in Penn's own writings—his belief in African incompatibility with Western education as well as its potentially corrupting influence through the radicalisation of black students; his fears of communist and especially, Chinese communist, influence and infiltration, and the use of conscription to inculcate loyalty to the state and the values and responsibilities of citizenship.

[73] Ibid.

[74] Ibid.

[75] Howard Phillips, *UCT Under Apartheid: Part 1—From Onset to Sit-in, 1948–1968* (Sunnyside, Fanele (Jacana), 2019), pp261–262.

The various committees that comprised the President's Council drew up reports that addressed the pressing socio-economic and political concerns related to Botha's vision of reform. In 1983, the Science Committee—of which Penn was a member—focused on demographics. The report flagged the potentially adverse impact of population increase on economic development, with recommendations for optimal population levels.[76] Statistics were provided on a racial basis—white, black, coloured and Asian—and it is revealing that a correlation was made between population growth and level of "Western" influence:

> If the relevant vital rates of the respective population groups in South Africa are compared with those in other parts of the world, it is evident that in the case of the Whites the rates correspond with those of countries in the developed world; the rates of the Asians and Coloureds correspond with those in the more developed areas of Asia and Latin America; while the Blacks' rates, although not quite so high, show a greater measure of correspondence with rates in the rest of Africa.[77]

Within the "black" group, distinctions were also made between various ethnicities with the Sotho-speaking people demonstrating a lower rate of fertility than their Nguni-speaking counterparts. This was attributed to the latter living in closer proximity to urban "white" areas, giving them a greater familiarity with modern values and permitting better access to methods of contraception.[78]

Particularly noteworthy was the fertility rates of migrant labourers making the transition from rural to urban, industrial areas. It was determined that the longer the time spent in an urban environment, the greater the decline in fertility—and this would be passed onto offspring. The committee predicted that while greater urbanisation of blacks would mean an initial growth in numbers due to both increasing migration as well as rural patterns of fertility, this would eventually stabilise and fertility would ultimately decline due to acculturation.[79]

[76] South Africa President's Council Science Committee, "Report of the Science Committee of the President's Council on Demographic Trends in South Africa", SP (PC 1/1983), Stellenbosch University Library Government Publications.

[77] Ibid., p20.

[78] Ibid., p47.

[79] Ibid., p56.

The education system was also cited as a means by which Western middle-class values could be imparted, with "development [resulting] in changing the traditional social and family structures" and challenging the patriarchal structure seen as an obstacle to modernisation. Education was one aspect of reform with the committee also recommending job creation as well as the provision of social security to provide a degree of financial stability that obviated the need for larger families.[80]

In the spirit of reform then, this was an acceptance of greater African urbanisation and a challenging of the racial division of labour that reserved skill employment for whites who were unable to meet the growing labour demands for economic development. The monopolisation of the high skilled job sector was highlighted in the report with the concomitant acknowledgement that, "it is not very probable that Whites will be able to constitute a much larger proportion" and the recommendation that, "Other groups should therefore be exploited as sources".[81]

In addition to servicing the growing needs of the economy however, Penn's influence can be seen in the potential solutions for the independent homelands or the "Black States", characterised by poverty and unemployment. A proposed solution was a restructuring of agriculture and the implementation of a system of "collective farming" not unlike "the *kibbutz* system in Israel".[82] Penn would no doubt have been familiar with the system during his time spent in Israel, yet the *kibbutz* relates to a particularly socialist form of Zionism that was based on class and gender equality and the redeeming feature of manual labour. It emphasised the collective rather than the individual and was a vision that was more idealised than realised.[83] Within the South African context, it sat uneasily with modernisation and urbanisation and suggested the limitations of reform. In a later essay, Penn would expand on his vision of what he termed "Self-Development Community Schemes" necessary to make the rural areas more viable for their African population. This included small settlements complete with schools, clinics and facilities for the elderly and

[80] Ibid., p82.

[81] Ibid., p185.

[82] Ibid., p153.

[83] Michael Brenner, *In Search of Israel: The History of an Idea* (Princeton and Oxford, Princeton University Press, 2018), pp76–78.

for recreation. Economic activity would be "a localised home industry or a form of decentralised industry" and these settlements would ideally be serviced by "mobile educational facilities", bringing with them all the benefits of modernisation—"formal and non-formal education, with advice and supervision, mechanically, industrially and agriculturally".[84] It suggested a compromise solution.

And the limitations were evident in another area as well. A pressing concern evident in the report was not just the negative impact of high population growth on economic development but the high fertility of some groups when compared to the lower fertility of others:

> In 1980 every 1 000 White women of reproductive age gave birth to only 963 girls who will become old enough to take part in the process of reproduction – White women are at present not producing enough girls to be able to reproduce themselves. In contrast with this, every 1 000 Asian women gave birth to 1 278 girls, Coloureds to 1 427, and Blacks to an estimated 2 500.[85]

It was redolent of the fears of white South Africans for much of the twentieth century, fears that underpinned the apartheid state and the system of racial segregation—the vulnerability of a minority. While lower fertility was equated to modernity and in effect, Western civilisation, it was ironically also a threat to Western dominance.

In a later assessment of his time on the Science Committee, Penn was particularly influenced by the findings regarding the "population explosion, particularly amongst the black, illiterate people", predicting a doubling of the population with the majority being illiterate and hence unsuited to employment. The "population explosion" was attributed by Penn to be due to the better medical care provided by white medical practitioners that thus surpassed the treatment accorded to Africans on the rest of the continent. His solution was both a reduced birth rate and better education in order to increase employment.[86]

84 "We Can't Always Win!" in "Philosophy Is Fun" (Unpublished Manuscript), December 1983, File: Penn, Jack—Writings (3), AMUW.

85 SA President's Council Science Committee, "Report on Demographic Trends in South Africa", p59.

86 "We Can't Always Win!" in "Philosophy is Fun" (Unpublished Manuscript), December 1983, File: Penn, Jack—Writings (3), AMUW.

The ambiguity of reform initiatives was further reflected in a report on education released by the Science Committee in the following year. A major part of the report was the addressing of cultural difference. From the outset, the superiority of Western culture and its equation to modernity and industrialisation (as well as a "Christian work ethic" and set of values) was taken as a given and the Report noted that different cultures existed in South Africa from the industrialised Western culture at one extreme to the rural "Black" culture at the other with the latter necessarily proving a hindrance to "development". Between the two were the "transitional" cultures.[87]

This hindrance was termed "cultural deprivation" and referred to the supposed incapacity of one culture to adequately acculturate when in another environment. Yet by 1984, "culture" was a loaded term and one used as a marker of racial and ethnic difference. While the Committee was careful to state that "cultural deprivation" did not suggest "inferiority", they believed it less "objectionable" to use "environmental disadvantage":

> A person can be considered to be environmentally disadvantaged only when he functions ineffectively in a cultural environment which is different from the one in which he was brought up...If an individual or a group of people is declared environmentally disadvantaged, this judgement is passed *in accordance with the norms and values of the environment in which they have to operate.*[88]

One would be hard pressed to find a difference in meaning between the two. It also echoed Penn's views on racial ability and suitability.

There was, however, a significant departure from Penn's earlier beliefs regarding genetic capability—the report acknowledged the interaction of environment and genes, nurture and nature, and placed particular emphasis on the former. Poverty, unemployment, lack of skills, illiteracy, social ills such as alcoholism and the breakdown of the family, a sense of "apathy" and "fatalism" were not considered to be based on "race" but on an exclusion from the narrative of progress, which was based on

[87] South Africa President's Council Science Committee, "Report of the Science Committee of the President's Council on Informal and Non-Formal Education in South Africa", SP (PC 6/1984), Stellenbosch University Library Government Publications, pp13, 17, 23.

[88] Ibid., pp39–40.

a failure of "institutions" and fell short of the aim of a democracy to promote "the development of their human goals for all people".[89]

And perhaps most telling was that this report—like its predecessor—included "Black" Africans, even if a major criticism was that this group had no actual representation on the Council itself. Yet, even in this spirit of reform, "environmental degradation" was largely applied to this majority population. Taking little account of the struggles for equal education as well as the inequalities of job reservation (although both factors were acknowledged when the Committee considered other racial groups), comparisons were made between the environment of the "white child" and that of its African counterpart. In the case of the former, the child grows up in an environment where technology is commonplace, there are stimulating toys, electronic gadgets, active parenting and a familiarity with money, consumer goods and a concept of time alien to the black child in the rural area. Here, toys are home-made, with little exposure to technology, time is based on the movement of the sun and parents apparently discuss only rural matters such as "water, cattle and food". Further, the child's language—and with it, cognitive—abilities are stifled by the "limited vocabulary [that] is required for the scant communication between parents and children". The stifling of language skills is compounded by the child's lack of familiarity with English when entering school and all contribute to a lack of preparedness for school, a high drop-out rate, high levels of illiteracy, unemployment and poverty.[90] "Environment" viz culture also played a role as well—the emphasis on the group rather than the individual stifled individual thinking and competition, and a strong sense of "acceptance" of authority was responsible for "rote learning" which limited the child in terms of educational development.[91]

The repercussions for the country were immense—not only was the individual unable to reach their full potential, it was a blow for the developmental aspirations of the nation as well.[92] It also contributed to "social pathologies" which led to "delinquent and dissident behaviour": "The signs of breakdown in the form of violence, drug addiction, sexual licence,

[89] Ibid., p45.

[90] Ibid., p49.

[91] Ibid., p50.

[92] Ibid., p51.

instability of the family, terrorism and political anarchy."[93] "Environmental degradation" was therefore linked directly both to development and the security of the state, with the portrayal of black resistance as a manifestation of antisocial behaviour.

Yet it was a theory that seemed to be undermined within the report itself. Coloureds were considered to have "no unique culture of [their] own" and were part of the dominant Western environment—which did little to explain the very high levels of poverty and illiteracy that characterised the population. The solution was a rather tentative one—the suggestion that there needed to be reform from within through initiatives by a community leadership although an apparent lack of "group identity" also made this a challenge.[94] Indians were considered to have both acculturised and to have a "culture…[compatible] with the development requirements in the South African industrial environment", strengthened by a value placed on education.[95] And as for the social pathology that was evident even in the dominant cultural group, this was vaguely attributed to "rapid change in the social structure".[96] There was clearly no coherent understanding of the way in which the Committee's view of "environmental degradation" functioned—there were entirely too many exceptions to the rule.

Yet the Committee was optimistic that these inequalities were not permanent and could be redressed through education and through the promotion of elements of other "environments" that were compatible with an industrialised society concomitant with the censure of those elements that served as an obstacle to progress. There was the belief that this could be done through education and that all children—regardless of genetic predisposition—could be taught the dominant values and embrace its ethos. Perhaps what is most optimistic of this vision—even if it is one predicated on the dominance of a particular ideology—is that the report's aim was one of incorporation and "the development of *an appropriate culture, unique to South Africa*" as "an important long-term objective".[97]

[93] Ibid., p56.

[94] Ibid., pp67, 71.

[95] Ibid., pp72–73.

[96] Ibid., p77.

[97] Ibid., pp96, 104–105, 177.

The President's Council continued to make various recommendations over the next few years. In 1982 a recommendation by the Constitutional Committee for a legislative body that would represent the interests of white, coloured and Indian South Africans (Africans were again excluded),[98] led to the formation of the Tricameral Parliament. The opinion piece by Robert Shrirer of the University of Cape Town, already foresaw the unenviable position in which Indian and coloured representatives would be placed with vague promises of reform even as entrenched inequality remained in place and the majority of the population remained excluded.[99]

The Tricameral Parliament which came into existence in May 1983 expanded the powers of the President who took on the role of both the State President and Prime Minister.[100] Significantly, Parliament was composed of three houses—the House of Assembly representing the white electorate, the House of Representatives for coloureds and the House of Deputies (later Delegates) for Asians. Fifty Members of Parliament were elected in the House of Assembly, 25 in the House of Representatives and 13 in the House of Deputies, thus giving the House of Representatives a majority.[101] The Tricameral Parliament was unsurprisingly beset with the same difficulties as the President's Council and aroused similar hostility due to the complete marginalisation of Africans and its maintenance of white minority rule regardless of the increased representation of Indians and coloureds. It was boycotted by black political groups with many refusing to participate and those who did were viewed as collaborators. It did little to suppress growing resistance to apartheid and likely heightened it, and formally ended with the advent of full democracy.

It is important to note however, that the vision of the President's Council and later, the Tricameral Parliament not only reflected P.W. Botha's dilemma as he was caught between the mutually opposing poles of reform and recalcitrance but was also a reflection of Penn's political vision. During a period of domestic turmoil, external pressure and the

[98] Robert Schrire, "Simple Proposals, Dangerous Future", *Rand Daily Mail*, 14 May 1982.

[99] Ibid.

[100] Rob Nuttall, "Total Power for New President", *Rand Daily Mail*, 6 May 1983.

[101] Rob Nuttall, "How the 3 Chambers Will be Made Up", *Rand Daily Mail*, 6 May 1983.

threat of communism, Penn's utopian vision was shaped by uncertainty and fear. At the same time, Penn's views indicated a willingness to adapt to the needs of reform to foster development. However, he put forth a vision of South Africa that attempted reform within limitations—which was ultimately not true reform at all.

The Artist

In 2018, South African plastic surgeon, Dr Laurence Anthony Chait published his autobiography, marking his 45th year as a plastic surgeon. Like Penn, Chait is also an accomplished sculptor, with a view of the complementary nature of plastic surgery and art, "I like to say that sculpting is my career and surgery is my hobby, but there are many ways in which the two overlap. Both require a vision, one that has a particular goal at its end. Art and medicine are inextricably interlinked." And it was Jack Penn, surgeon and sculptor, who had provided the inspiration for the nine-year-old Chait.[102]

Art was an important part of Penn's life. He was a prominent figure in the art world, opening exhibitions for his artist friend Ernest Ullmann, as well as Anne Glaser, an artist who worked with ceramic bricks and tended to focus on religious imagery,[103] French-Ukranian and Jewish artist, Emmanuel Mané-Katz[104]—a contemporary of Pablo Picasso who fled France after the Nazi invasion and eventually settled in Israel[105]—and Fleur Ferri.[106] Penn was himself the subject of art when a watercolour painted by Ferri and entitled simply "Jack Penn" was part of an exhibition of portraiture at the Pretoria Art Museum.[107]

For Penn, plastic surgery was an art and if a surgeon was an artist, so much the better. He went even so far as to suggest that artistic ability

[102] Jordan Moshe, "Balancing His Two Passions, Sculpture and Surgery, Oh So Deftly", *South African Jewish Report*, 3 May 2018, https://www.sajr.co.za/news-and-articles/2018/05/03/balancing-his-two-passions-sculpture-and-surgery-oh-so-deftly, accessed 17 August 2020.

[103] "From Bricks to Ceramics", *Rand Daily Mail*, 18 November 1965.

[104] "Art Shows", *Rand Daily Mail*, 19 August 1968.

[105] "Mané-Katz (French/Ukrainian, 1894–1962)", *Artnet—Artists*, http://www.artnet.com/artists/man%C3%A9-katz/, accessed 20 April 2021.

[106] Advertisement, *Rand Daily Mail*, 11 June 1969.

[107] H.E. Winder, "Portraits of Distinction", *Rand Daily Mail*, 12 October 1977.

could be an important criterion in determining the specialisation in reconstructive surgery. To be theoretically proficient was a poor second to the practical and aesthetic aspect of surgery:

> A good artist can observe keenly, he can assess size, contour, and differences, he can use his hands with delicacy and co-ordination. He is a craftsman. But his essential asset must be his good taste and sense of artistic balance.[108]

Yet the final phrase "good taste and sense of artistic balance" implies a level of arbitrariness in judgement, albeit one based on experience. If reconstructive surgery and art were almost synonymous, this was based on the idealisation of a "normal" aesthetic. This aesthetic was evident in standards of beauty and physicality that were reinforced until they became a benchmark by which all deviations were measured. It was the role of the reconstructive surgeon to correct these deviations to reduce the psychological trauma of deformity and allow the injured to be incorporated into mainstream society.

Yet if the surgeon was an artist, it was a particular vision of art and realism that had its origins in Europe during the Renaissance, itself based on the art of classical Greek and Roman antiquity. Penn's surgical work was mirrored in his art that drew upon this particularly Western tradition and evident in his re-envisioning of the Hiroshima cenotaph. His art therefore cannot be divorced from his professional life and ideological belief system—it was not only evident in terms of the artistic tradition on which he drew but also in his subject matter. His many sculptures reflected the numerous facets of his career, his travels across the globe and his encounters with major political and historical figures over the course of the twentieth century—Joseph Lister, Albert Schweitzer, Moshe Dayan, David Ben Gurion, Matthew Ridgway…For Penn however, it was less about the "political personalities" themselves than it was about how he perceived their characters. As such, sculpting was the preferred medium to the "two-dimensional" paint on canvas as it allowed for the "[capturing of] many facets of a man's character from different angles" and this was

[108] Jack Penn, *The Right to Look Human: An Autobiography* (Johannesburg, Hugh Keartland Publishers, 1976), pp19–20.

particularly important when it came to portraying South Africa's most famous statesman (before 1994).[109]

There are two examples that would serve to frame Jack Penn's career as an artist. In the decade following Jan Smuts's death in 1950, he was requested by the Smuts family to sculpt a bust of Smuts that would grace the airport, established two years later and named in his honour. The Jan Smuts Airport in Johannesburg was—and remains as OR Tambo Airport—one of the most prominent airports in sub-Saharan Africa serving as an important hub for both domestic and international flights. Penn sculpted two busts—one of which he retained—and on 6 March 1968, he and the Smuts family attended an unveiling of the bust at the airport's main concourse.[110] For Penn, his main advantage in capturing Smuts in bronze was that he had personally met him and was taken with "the penetrating gaze of his grey eyes and his imperious, dignified demeanour". It was this that influenced his portrayal of the man with a conscious decision to contrast it to the existing statues of Smuts including one in Cape Town that he described as a "Neanderthal, Rodinesque" interpretation. His bust on the other hand, was designed to capture Smuts's essence as an exemplar of modernity, "a man of culture and of this century".[111]

To cater to both sides of the political spectrum, Penn also sculpted a bust of Smuts's political opposition, J.B.M. Hertzog, former Prime Minister and founder of the National Party, which was commissioned for the Bloemfontein Airport.[112] Despite Penn's rather ambiguous encounter with Jan Smuts himself in the 1940s which left him vaguely dissatisfied when the Prime Minister referred his request to the chain of command, Penn nonetheless retained the second bust in his study. A few years later however, he donated the bust to Cambridge University to commemorate Smuts's role as chancellor of the University as well as marking the hundredth anniversary of his birth in 1870. Penn personally travelled to

[109] "His Work Is on Show at Every Airport: Johannesburg Surgeon a Sculptor Too", *Tonus* 7, 21, 13 November 1970, File: Biography—Jack Penn, AMUW.

[110] "Bust of Smuts for UK", *Rand Daily Mail*, 26 June 1970; *Rand Daily Mail*, 7 March 1968; "O.R. Tambo International Airport—Johannesburg Airport", https://johannesburg-airport.co.za/, accessed 27 March 2021.

[111] "His Work is on Show at Every Airport".

[112] *Rand Daily Mail*, 7 March 1968.

Cambridge to ensure that the bust was strategically placed to best show off its features:

> My concern was that they should position it correctly for height and light…I am happy with the site they chose. As you go upstairs to the council chamber in this old building you will find it well placed in a corner of the foyer. The university will construct a plinth for it.[113]

Penn also accepted a commission to sculpt a more ambitious statue of Smuts. In this once again, he sought to contrast his own understanding of Smuts with the public portrayal of the man, "Smuts' real personality was not that of a British Field Marshal but as a Boer guerrilla fighter, an intelligent naturalist, and a lover of the mountain…". His initial model or maquette was of Smuts "as a Boer", in informal dress, standing on a mountain, walking stick in hand, symbolic of Smuts's relationship to nature and to the land. The model was however, rejected and would grace Penn's home instead.[114]

The bust at the airport was removed as a reflection of the changing political climate. With South Africa's first democratically elected government in 1994, the name of the airport was changed to Johannesburg International Airport and in 2006 it underwent another name change. The OR Tambo Airport was named after Oliver Tambo who became the president of the ANC in 1967, a position he would hold for subsequent decades while he remained in exile.[115]

Art has never been neutral and some of the artwork commissioned for the airport in the 1970s—sculptures, mosaics, murals—was removed, destroyed or lost. The position of the Jan Smuts Airport as a central hub on the African continent, linking it with the wider world, was also a symbol of modernity and this was emphasised through the extensive use of modern, abstract art. Danie de Jager created an imposing sculpture termed "Flight in Space" in 1971. Constructed in bronze at a

[113] "Bust of Smuts for UK".

[114] "We Can't Always Win!" in "Philosophy is Fun" (Unpublished Manuscript), December 1983, File: Penn, Jack—Writings (5), AMUW. Interestingly, a statue of Smuts in Parliament Lane, Cape Town, unveiled a decade earlier, bears some similarity to Penn's description, although it is of Smuts in his role as Field Marshal.

[115] "O.R. Tambo International Airport—Johannesburg Airport".

height of 3.5 metres, it dominated the first floor of the Public Departure Concourse. Designed to rotate once every minute, the sculpture was a swirling whorl of polished metal that epitomised the space age. In 1998, as the airport underwent an extensive upgrade that was concomitant with its name change, the sculpture was placed in a warehouse where parts of it were stolen. It was subsequently returned to De Jager and was restored. It would later be housed at the Voortrekker Monument in Pretoria in 2013 where it underwent its own name change, "Quo Vadis?", a symbolic marking of the move from the sense of technological triumphalism under apartheid to an uncertain future held by a sector of the South African population in the wake of 1994.[116]

While the political influences on the airport changed, it nonetheless continued to represent a view of modern and of technological innovation but within a specifically African context. In 2010 when South Africa was given the opportunity to demonstrate the country's technological and industrial might through the construction of stadia and infrastructure to host the Soccer World Cup, South African expatriate Richard Poplak's first introduction to the country was the "the spectacularly reconstituted Oliver Tambo International Airport" that he described as having "been scrubbed of every last vestige of the grim, imposing apartheid-era Jan Smuts airport circa my youth."[117]

While Jack Penn's bust of Jan Smuts at Johannesburg International Airport may have been a relic of the apartheid past and so destined for an indifferent fate, his work defies simple ideological categorisation.

In 1982, the South African Post Office issued an 8 cents stamp featuring a portrait of Cecilia Makiwane[118]; in 2002 the South African government instituted the Cecilia Makiwane Nurse's Recognition Award awarded to health care professionals; and the South African Nursing Council's building was renamed the Cecilia Makiwane Building ten years

[116] "Jan Smuts Airport—South Africa", *Art Archives—South Africa*, https://art-archives-southafrica.com/jan-smuts-airport-johannesburg-artworks, accessed 27 March 2021.

[117] Richard Poplak, "Good Times in Africa", *National Post*, 24 June 2010, CanWest Digital Media.

[118] KwaZulu-Natal Museum, https://www.nmsa.org.za/news/10-news/210-2020-05-12-06-50-13.html, accessed 28 March 2021.

later.[119] In 2017, then Deputy President Cyril Ramaphosa dedicated a new wing at the Cecilia Makiwane Hospital based in the Eastern Cape, the site of her birth, describing the "state of the art health facility [as] a victory in our people's cause to build a united, equal, non-racial, non-sexist and prosperous society".[120] The slew of accolades came after a period when very little was known about the first black African woman to qualify as a nurse in South Africa in 1908.[121]

At the dawn of the twentieth century, there was little educational opportunity for indigenous South Africans. Education was largely confined to the mission schools which could not serve the bulk of the population and the situation was particularly acute for African women, just 6% of whom had acquired basic literacy skills. This made Makiwane's achievements all the more remarkable. She was one of the products of an early mission education, her father was both teacher and Presbyterian minister and she was born at the MarFarlane Mission in Alice in the Eastern Cape in 1880. First taught at home, she eventually went to the Lovedale Girls' School, obtaining her teaching certificate.[122]

In contrast to the provision of training for black doctors in the country—which only took place towards the mid-twentieth century—there was a greater tolerance for black nurses who could provide medical care in their respective communities, due to their similar linguistic and cultural backgrounds. As a result, Lovedale Mission Hospital initiated a training school for nurses in 1898, with a three-year nursing course at Lovedale College in 1902. Yet it was not easy to enter the programme, especially due to the dearth of basic educationprospective nursing candidates were expected to already have nine to ten years of prior schooling and needed to pass an exam that had to be written in either English or

[119] "Born to be a Nurse: Cecilia Makiwane" in *#SANC News*, South African Nursing Council, Vol 3, March 2019, p4, https://sanc.co.za/archive/archive2019/linked_files/Newsletters/Newsletter%20Mar2019.pdf, accessed 28 March 2021.

[120] Cyril Ramaphosa, "Deputy President Cyril Ramaphosa: Unveiling of New Wing at Cecilia Makiwane Hospital in Mdantsane", South African Government, https://www.gov.za/speeches/remarks-deputy-president-cyril-ramaphosa-during-unveiling-new-wing-cecilia-makiwane#, accessed 28 March 2021.

[121] It should be noted that South Africa was officially inaugurated as the Union of South Africa in 1910, becoming a distinct geopolitical entity.

[122] "Born to be a Nurse: Cecilia Makiwane".

Afrikaans. The arduous requirements meant that by 1940, there would be fewer than a thousand registered black nurses in the country.[123]

In 1903, with her teaching certificate, Makiwane was able to meet the basic requirements and trained at Butterworth College, before writing the Colonial Medical Council examination in late 1907. Upon passing, she became the first black registered nurse in South Africa, working at Lovedale Hospital. Makiwane also engaged in political activism—1912 had seen the formation of the South African Native National Congress (later to be renamed the African National Congress) and it was also the year that Makiwane was involved in what was believed to the first anti-pass protest by women. She was one of five thousand signatories, comprising African and coloured women, to a petition requesting the abolition of the pass laws. Following a period of ill health, Makiwane died in 1919, aged just 39.[124]

In 1972, more than fifty years after her passing, plans were underfoot by the South African Nursing Association to erect a memorial in her honour at Lovedale Hospital in Alice, the site where she both qualified and worked as a nurse. The memorial was to comprise a sculpture of Makiwane in nursing uniform and the initial hope was that an African sculptor would be contracted to create the memorial. This did not pan out and Jack Penn volunteered for the task, for which he refused compensation.[125] Funds for the bronzing, transport and unveiling of the statue were contributed by nurses from all over the country[126] and the unveiling of the statue took place in May 1977, pre-empting the later accolades that would come Makiwane's way. The statue was unveiled by Alina Lekgetha, the chairperson of the Bantu Advisory Committee to the South African Nursing Association and one of the more than seventeen thousand black nurses who had qualified by 1977. Attending the event was the Chief Minister of the Ciskei – one of the Bantustans created by the apartheid state – L. L. Sebe, the head of the South African Nursing Association, Charlotte Searle, and of course, Penn who described the statue as his "tribute to the nurses of Southern Africa".[127]

[123] Ibid.

[124] Ibid.

[125] "E. Cape Will Get Memorial to Black Nurse", *Rand Daily Mail*, 4 July 1972.

[126] "Solid First for Cecilia", *Rand Daily Mail*, 26 September 1974.

[127] "Statue to Black Nursing Pioneer", *Rand Daily Mail*, 17 March 1977.

Conclusion

The three segments that make up this chapter appear to the general reader to be disparate yet, at the same time—along with plastic and reconstructive surgery—art and politics were an integral part of Penn's engagement with the world. They reflected ideas of progress and inequality as well as the contradictions, inconsistencies and predicaments that faced South Africans in the twentieth century. As a public and influential figure, Penn sought to resolve these through surgery, politics and art which, at their core, were his attempt to remake the world as he believed it should be. His work however can be understood as a reflection of the tension between modernisation and racial discrimination, between the humanitarian aspirations of medicine and its ideological role in apartheid South Africa.

Conclusion: "A Man's Worth"[1]

In October 1990, in the wake of the unbanning of the ANC and other political parties and the release of Nelson Mandela from prison, the now 81-year-old Penn wrote an essay entitled, "South Africa – Quo Vadis" in which he praised President F.W. de Klerk's efforts "in inspiring uniformity between all races" as this was the first step in ensuring an equal and "first world" standard of living for all. He simultaneously counselled against the "sudden emancipation of the underprivileged" which, as had been demonstrated in the rest of Africa, would lead to "a decline of standards" for all. The solution was the slow and gradual move to "Black majority rule" as a means of "[preventing] deterioration and destruction". The process was envisioned to take many years.[2]

Penn was 87 when he died on 27 November 1996. Ten months later, an obituary written by his son, John, appeared in *Plastic and Reconstructive Surgery*. The younger Penn focused largely on his father's lengthy and distinguished career as a plastic surgeon while also acknowledging

[1] Quote taken from Jack Penn "A Surgeon's Story: It is the Divine Right of Man to Look Human" (Unpublished manuscript), p217, Brn No 12057, 617.95 PEN, BL.

[2] Jack Penn, "South Africa—Quo Vadis", October 1990, File: Penn, Jack—Writings (5), AMUW.

S. Chetty, *Reconstructive Surgery and Modernisation in Twentieth-Century South Africa*, Medicine and Biomedical Sciences in Modern History, https://doi.org/10.1007/978-3-031-38673-2

his artistic accomplishments.[3] He had worked alongside his father and the two had collaborated on research published in the same journal.[4] It is however, in an earlier obituary, also written by John Penn, where the reader gains insight into Penn's character. By following the adage, "Full speed ahead and damn the torpedoes", Jack Penn was able to forge ahead in establishing a new field of surgery in South Africa and to work towards improving reconstructive surgical practices both in South Africa and further afield. John related an incident where he indicated his misgivings about the efficacy of a procedure about to be performed by his father. Jack's reply was telling:

> He responded by telling me the story of the bumblebee. The bumblebee was studied by a group of scientists, who, after calculating the bee's size, wing span, and speed of wing oscillation, concluded that bumblebees cannot fly. "However," said Jack, "the bumblebee doesn't know that, so it flies!"

Penn senior then went on to perform the procedure successfully.[5] The analogy of the bumblebee reflected his attitude of determination and optimism, a refusal to acknowledge limitation as well as an almost headstrong assertiveness that led to clashes with authority, impatience with bureaucratic procedures and a strong sense of self belief.

John Penn's obituaries are important in adding a sense of complexity and nuance to the character of the pioneering plastic surgeon whose career was controversial, to say the least. Yet, any assessment of his life should start with his own words as evident in *Reflections on Life*, that one's role in life revolved around "a sense of responsibility to oneself and the rest of the world."[6] On a more personal level, in a review of *Letters to My Son*, Penn was accredited with a "deep sense of responsibility to his son" as he set forth his various thoughts on life and duty, including his thinking on "colour prejudice" for which he was lauded in the review,

[3] John G. Penn, "Obituary: Jack Penn", *Plastic and Reconstructive Surgery*, 100, 4, 1077–1078, September 1997.

[4] *Cf* Jack Penn and John G. Penn, "Two Generations in Plastic Surgery", *Plastic and Reconstructive Surgery*, 91, 4, 718–719, April 1993.

[5] John G. Penn, "Obituary: Jack Penn", *Aesthetic Surgery Journal*, 17, 1, January–February 1997.

[6] Jack Penn, *Reflections on Life* (Johannesburg, Eric Stanton Publishers, 1980), p3.

even if his musings may have raised the hackles of some.[7] The publication of *Letters to My Son*—based on private correspondence with John—also suggested Penn's belief in the relevance and value of his philosophy—it needed to be shared in a public forum. This was based on a self-assurance and certainty which, as the reviewer wryly observed, gave the book "a hint of the pomposity of Polonius".[8] For good or bad, Penn's belief in his personal sense of responsibility underpinned a career that encompassed war service, private practice, humanitarian aid and politics.

The practice of medicine is indelibly woven into the fabric of society. While the efficacy of medicine has altered over the centuries, the need for medical specialists to ease suffering has remained undiminished. Tracing the inception of Western medicine to ancient Greece, the Hippocratic Oath taken by doctors affirms their social responsibility—and in South Africa, that sense of social responsibility exceeded the practice of medicine.

As a pioneering plastic and reconstructive surgeon at a time when the specialisation had yet to be accorded full recognition, Penn's work straddled the local and the international. His expertise built on that established by forerunners such as Harold Gillies and Archie McIndoe and was entrenched by the experiences of war. The relatively new field allowed Penn the opportunity to contribute to the specialisation through the development and refinement of technology and methods and he demonstrated a willingness to not only embrace—but to encourage—change and improvement. Like art, plastic surgery demanded a creative outlook and necessitated adaptation in the face of new forms of injury and changing circumstances.

Key to his career was not just the practice of surgery but research and the dissemination of his knowledge and skills. As such, he engaged in humanitarian work in Africa, Asia and the Middle East and was instrumental in fostering the international development of plastic and reconstructive surgery. Not neglected was his role in South Africa where he was a key figure in the formalisation of the specialisation that would ensure that professional standards were met. In this, he followed the processes that had already occurred in the United States and Britain. The field

[7] "My Son, My Son...", *Rand Daily Mail*, 23 June 1975.

[8] Ibid.

itself—initiated during a World War—exemplified global co-operation and interaction between medical professionals.

The practice of medicine was permeated with the ethos of the ease of suffering—which, in plastic surgery, was both physical and psychological. It was just as imbued with a value system that had its origins in the West. In the era of high imperialism, Western medicine was both a demonstration of intellectual superiority and colonial beneficence. Associated with health and hygiene, medicine became part of the "civilising mission". In the mid-twentieth century, as empires were broken up and as the Cold War polarised much of the world, medicine—like other areas of science and technology—was a means of asserting the importance and even dominance of the West. In the South African context, this was further complicated by the practice of apartheid with its overt policies of racial segregation and discrimination.

The importance of race in Penn's thinking is borne out in his autobiography which is literally framed by his views on race. It begins with a series of vignettes, the first of which is "The Width of a Nostril". Penn relates the case of a 22-year-old woman on the verge of marrying who had recently discovered that her mother was "coloured". Her alcoholic and abusive father had bluntly stated that, "…no white man would marry a coloured girl".[9] Her mother had never told her of her racial origins in the hopes that her daughter would assimilate into white society. On learning of her mixed-race heritage, the young woman's white fiancé was supportive, however the couple decided that she needed plastic surgery to correct her nose, a physical reminder of her ancestry. The surgery would permit them "to put the past behind them entirely". Penn duly performed the operation, the couple was married and by all accounts, went on to live happy and fulfilled lives.[10] The vignette demonstrates Penn's own complex feelings regarding race—on the one hand he was complicit in thwarting the racial categorisation and segregation of the apartheid state by enabling his patient to "pass" as white. Penn understood the limitations and discrimination that was associated with racial categorisation. By enabling the couple to marry and presumably reproduce, he was party to the miscegenation that was *verboten* under apartheid. Yet he also adhered to the physical "norms" of racial appearance initially describing

[9] Penn, *The Right to Look Human*, p5.

[10] Ibid., pp 4–5.

her "slightly flared" nostrils as a "deformity", albeit a "minor" one.[11] The corrective surgery was a means of both establishing "white" physical features as the norm and of silencing a particular history and identity that was presented as an obstacle to fulfilment. It is also indicative of the unique and complex nature of practising plastic and reconstructive surgery within the South African context.

In South Africa, the practice of medicine was intertwined with politics with black leaders—Abdullah Abdurahman, Monty Naicker, Yusuf Dadoo, A.B. Xuma and Steve Biko—who, by virtue of their education and interaction with the communities of which they were part, were ideally positioned to become political activists opposing racial policies of discrimination. Doctors working within black communities such as Sydney and Emily Kark and Mervyn Susser were cognisant of and sought to ameliorate the health effects resulting from the economic and social inequalities associated with apartheid. As a surgeon, Penn was just as convinced of the social and ideological role of medicine and he was a spirited foe of Communism, a proponent of modernisation and a paternalist.

Penn felt a keen sense of social responsibility—although it was one that was complicated by his position in the racial hierarchy. While he claimed a sense of distance from the policies of apartheid along with a sense of alienation from Afrikaner nationalism, his defence of the state and its policies tend to overpower his criticism of "petty" apartheid. Yet his vacillation and inconsistency demonstrate his own uncertainty about the absolute categorisation of race and hierarchies of power. In his later role as a member of the President's Council, his views reflected the apartheid state's attempt at reform to meet the changing demands of modernisation while nevertheless maintaining white minority rule. It would ultimately be an effort doomed to failure.

Jack Penn is remembered for his skill in shaping the human form through flesh and bone, clay and bronze. Less known is his attempt to refashion the world in which he lived through his role as a surgeon, writer and political figure. Yet the two aspects of his life are not inseparable and his public and professional life serves as the lens through which the relationship between medicine and the modernising state are exposed,

[11] Ibid., p4.

modernisation that was intricately tied to racial segregation and hierarchy, that both belied the universalism of medical humanitarianism while simultaneously upholding it.

Bibliography

Archival and Newspaper Sources

WO 373/18—21 October 1941–24 February 1942 (DCM) and WO 373/72—Italy: 21 December 1944–19 April; 1945, War Office and Ministry of Defence, National Archives, https://discovery.nationalarchives.gov.uk/results/r?_q=lionel+melzer, accessed 28 April 2021.

Adler Museum—University of the Witwatersrand (hereafter AMUW)

File: Biography—Jack Penn

- Carter-Johnson, V., "SA Plastic Surgeon Relives A-Bomb Horrors", *Sunday Times*, 10 August 1980.
- Faber, D., "Notes from the Dragon Lady", *Washington Weekly*, 21 July 1977.
- "From a Womb with a View, Jack Penn Tells His Secrets of a Very Full Life", *The Star*, 24 August 1980.
- "His Work Is on Show at Every Airport: Johannesburg Surgeon a Sculptor Too", *Tonus* 7, 21, 13 November 1970.
- Penn, J., "Ian Smith: Twilight of an Era"
- Penn, J., "The Philosophy of Jesse Jackson"
- Penn, J., "Quo Vadis"
- Penn, J., "A Sentimental Journey"
- Penn, J., "South Africa and Its New Prime Minister—P.W. Botha"
- Penn, J., "The Tilted Halo"
- Penn, J., "The White South African"

File: Penn, Jack—Writings (3)

S. Chetty, *Reconstructive Surgery and Modernisation in Twentieth-Century South Africa*, Medicine and Biomedical Sciences in Modern History, https://doi.org/10.1007/978-3-031-38673-2

- Penn, J., "Philosophy is Fun" (Unpublished Manuscript), December 1983.
- Penn, J., "Three Great Surgeons"

File: Penn, Jack—Writings (4)

- Penn, J., "Palestinian Diary"

File" Penn, Jack – Writings (5)

- Penn, J., "South Africa – Quo Vadis", October 1990.

Brenthurst Library (hereafter BL)

Brenthurst Papers, Penn, J., ed, Johannesburg, Witwatersrand University Press, 1944, Brn. No: 3297, Call No: 617.95 BRE, BL.

"Towards a Modern Utopia" (Unpublished Manuscript), Penn, J., ed, Brn. No: 12778, Call No: PAM.1594, BL.

White Africans are Also People, Millin, S.G., ed, Howard Timmons, Cape Town, 1966, Brn. No: 14607, Call No: 323.1128 MIL, BL.

Department of Defence Archives

Solomon Penchansky service record.

Jack Penn Service File, W.R. 12/6640.

Director General Medical Services, Box 26, File MD129/204.

Director General Medical Services, Box 92, File MD129/390: 17th Field Ambulance.

Director General Medical Services, Box 92, File 129/376: Plastic Surgery: MOs Studying in England.

Surgeon General, Group 2, Box 1136, File MD 580/2: Tara: Red Cross Hospital for Plastic Surgery—General.

Surgeon General, Group 2, Box 1137, File MD 580/2/5: Red Cross Hospital for Plastic Surgery (Tara): Establishment and Staff Matters.

Surgeon General, Group 2, Box 1138, File MD 580/2/1 (Vol 1): Red Cross Hospital for Plastic Surgery (Tara): Buildings and Accommodation.

Stellenbosch University Library Government Publications

South Africa President's Council Science Committee, "Report of the Science Committee of the President's Council on Demographic Trends in South Africa", SP (PC 1/1983).

South Africa President's Council Science Committee, "Report of the Science Committee of the President's Council on Informal and Non-Formal Education in South Africa", SP (PC 6/1984).

Stimson Library Collections

Historical Division, Army Medical Library, "Developments in Military Medicine During the Administration of Surgeon General Norman T. Kirk", *Army Medical Bulletin*, 7, 7, July 1947, United States Army Academy of Health Sciences.

"Army Develops Superior Artificial Eyes", *Army Medical Bulletin*, 86, March 1945, United States Army Academy of Health Sciences.

University of Cape Town Libraries—Jagger Library

A1.1—A1.81, Correspondence between Dr Jack Penn and Albert Schweitzer and Others, Mainly at Lambarene, 1956–1957.

The Rand Daily Mail

- 7 June 1966.
- 7 March 1968.
- Advertisement, 26 July 1947.
- Advertisement, 31 August 1957.
- Advertisement, 11 June 1969.
- Akhalwaya, A., "Kathrada a 'Sell-out' for Joining Council", 9 September 1980.
- Akhalwaya, A., "More Candidates for President's Council", 13 September 1980.
- "Amazing Drawings from Lambarene", 10 April 1959.
- "Art Shows", 19 August 1968.
- "Broadcasting Programmes", 19 April 1943.
- "Builder Who Never Saw His 'Plum' Contracts", 20 October 1967.
- "Bust of Smuts for UK", 26 June 1970.
- Cairncross, C., "Edward Teller's View: Thorium to Replace Uranium", 27 October 1973.
- Cairncross, C., "Father of H-Bomb Is to Visit SA", 13 September 1973.
- Cairncross, C., "H-Bomb Father Tackles the Energy Crisis", 1 October 1973.
- "Chop for Chinese Member", 3 October 1980.
- "City Dentists Invent Revolutionary Surgical Appliance", 1 April 1943.
- "Clinic is Silent on Prince", 31 September 1971.
- "Conserve SA's Coal—Dr Roux", 10 December 1973.
- "Council Is Still-born, Say Its Opponents", 3 October 1980.
- "Council Members Call for an End to Racism", 10 February 1981.
- Cummins, P., "Why the Gap?", 4 August 1977.
- "Dayan Meets Eye Surgeon", 19 April 1958.
- "Death of Sir Edward Thornton; Long Service in Public Health", 28 October 1946.
- Death Notice – Solomon Penn, 2 June 1947.
- "Dr Hymie Penn Dies in Bus Accident", 19 September 1975.
- "E. Cape will Get Memorial to Black Nurse", 4 July 1972.
- "Famous Doctor Scourges His Own Profession", 10 May 1935.
- "From Bricks to Ceramics", 18 November 1965.
- "Gabon Is Ready to Co-operate with S.A.", 26 April 1969.
- "General Dayan Given Great Welcome at Jan Smuts Airport", 30 August 1957.

- Heard, R., “General Has New View on SA”, 1 March 1972.
- “Hebrew University Anniversary Banquet”, 9 June 1955.
- H.E.W., “Why Must They be Sent Away?”, 3 April 1964.
- Hitchcock, B., “Dayan’s Big Regret”, 3 September 1974.
- Holiday, A., “Churchmen Support Bishops’ ‘Call to Conscience’”, 14 February 1972.
- “Jewish Wedding: Penn—Cartoon”, 6 July 1928.
- “Live in Israel—Dayan”, 3 September 1974.
- “Luxury Clinic Has Executive Wing”, 31 March 1964.
- “Make Trainees Feel Welcome, Says Brigadier”, 26 July 1973.
- “Men Happy in City Military Hospitals”, 10 November 1941.
- “Mid-East War ‘has lessons for S. Africa’”, 3 July 1967.
- Monaisa, T., Letter to the Editor, 1 October 1980.
- Mortimer, B., “‘Aliens’ Report condemned as ‘ludicrous and naïve’”, 17 August 1981.
- “Mrs Dayan Has Plastic Surgery”, 26 August 1974.
- “My Son, My Son…”, 23 June 1975.
- “The ‘New-look’ Parliament”, 31 May 1980.
- “New Posts for Brigadiers Orenstein and Thornton”, 2 March 1943.
- “Nixon Man Visits SA”, 14 February 1972.
- “No Fuel Oil by 2000”, 27 September 1973.
- “Nurse and Patient Married”, 22 November 1943.
- “Nurse Is Cleared of Death”, 8 May 1968.
- “Nurses Pay Tribute to Specialist”, 7 January 1969.
- “Nurse Wept as She Told of Injection”, 29 March 1968.
- Nuttall, R., “How the 3 Chambers Will be Made Up”, 6 May 1983.
- Nuttall, R., “Total Power for New President”, 6 May 1983.
- O’Connor, H., “A Pen Picture of Dayan, Israel’s Army Chief: Boy Farmer Who Became a Soldier”, 30 August 1957.
- “Part of Brenthurst Destroyed by Fire: Four Firemen Hurt”, 29 August 1944.
- “Pen Pictures of All the Councillors”, 3 October 1980.
- “Rand University to Have Chair of Plastic Surgery”, 16 September 1944.
- “Red Cross Will Care for Soldiers Long after the War”, 19 July 1944.
- “SA Could Solve World Fuel Crisis”, 8 December 1973.
- “Sir Edward Thornton’s New Appointment”, 10 August 1940.
- “State President Approves Council”, 20 November 1980.
- Schrire, R., “Simple Proposals, Dangerous Future”, 14 May 1982.
- Scott, J., “Goodwill to All Men, But This Just Wasn’t Politics”, 14 May 1982.
- “Solid First for Cecilia”, 26 September 1974.
- “Statue to Black Nursing Pioneer”, 17 March 1977.

- "Towards a Climax", 28 April 1969.
- "Transvaal Raised £543 000", 17 May 1944.
- "Union Needs Fewer, Better Doctors", 24 November 1943.
- "Vanity Fair", 1 May, 5 July, 24 July 1941.
- Winder, H.E. "Portraits of Distinction", 12 October 1977.
- Winder, H.E., "Tribute to the Late Elizabeth Macadam", 21 January 1976.
- "Women in War-Time", 28 February 1942.
- "Wrong to Pay by Colour—Barnard", 22 April 1969.
- Zille, H., "1981: The Year of High Expectations But Low Possibilities", 17 January 1981.
- Zille, H., "P.W. Botha's Alternative Strategy", 18 July 1980.

Miscellaneous Newspapers

Arthur, B.A., "Obituary: General Matthew Ridgway", *Independent*, 23 October 2011, https://www.independent.co.uk/news/people/obituary-general-matthew-ridgway-1460281.html, accessed 19 April 2021.

Burns, J.F., "Industry Mellows in South Africa", *New York Times*, 21 November 1976, https://www.nytimes.com/1976/11/21/archives/industry-mellows-in-south-africa-south-africa.html, accessed 19 April 2021.

Hamilton, T.J., "5 000 Children Evacuated from Biafra in Civil War will be Repatriated from Gabon and Ivory Coast", *New York Times*, 11 October 1970, https://www.nytimes.com/1970/10/11/archives/5000-children-evacuated-from-biafra-in-civil-war-will-be.html, accessed 6 August 2020.

Hoffman, M., "Growing with Israel: 70 Years of Sheba Success", *The Jerusalem Post*, 17 April 2018, https://www.jpost.com/israels-70th-anniversary/growing-with-israel-70-years-of-sheba-success-550038, accessed 21 March 2021.

Honan, W.H., "B. E. Simon, 'Hiroshima Maidens' Surgeon, 87", *New York Times*, 5 August 1991, The New York Times Archives, https://www.nytimes.com/1999/08/05/nyregion/b-e-simon-hiroshima-maidens-surgeon-87.html?searchResultPosition=2, accessed 10 August 2020.

Kamm, H., "A 'Hiroshima Maiden' Conquers Bitterness", *New York Times*, 22 May 1977, The New York Times Archives, https://www.nytimes.com/1977/05/22/archives/a-hiroshima-maiden-conquers-bitterness-a-hiroshima-maiden-overcomes.html?searchResultPosition=1, accessed 10 August 2020.

"The Late Robert Gillies", *Bruce Herald*, Vol 17, Issue 1759, 18 June 1886, https://paperspast.natlib.govt.nz/newspapers/BH18860618.2.12, accessed 3 May 2021.

"Letters Describing Dayan Losing His Eye to be Auctioned", *The Times of Israel*, 27 July 2015, https://www.timesofisrael.com/letters-describing-dayan-losing-eye-to-be-auctioned/, accessed 25 June 2021.

McCurry, J., "'Like Entering a Prison': Japan's Leprosy Sufferers Reflect on Decades of Pain", *The Guardian*, 13 April 2016, https://www.theguardian.com/world/2016/apr/14/like-entering-a-prison-japans-leprosy-sufferers-sue-government-for-decades-of-pain, accessed 24 August 2020.

Moshe, J., "Balancing His Two Passions, Sculpture and Surgery, Oh So Deftly", *South African Jewish Report*, 3 May 2018, https://www.sajr.co.za/news-and-articles/2018/05/03/balancing-his-two-passions-sculpture-and-surgery-oh-so-deftly, accessed 17 August 2020.

Poplak, R., "Good Times in Africa", *National Post*, 24 June 2010, CanWest Digital Media.

Rotberg, R.I., "Letter to the Editor", *New York Times*, 13 April 1972, The New York Times Archives, https://www.nytimes.com/1972/04/13/archives/a-view-of-southern africa.html?searchResultPosition=2, accessed 7 August 2020.

Siegel-Itzkovich, J., "Rambam: From Hospital for British Wounded in WWII to Most Developed Medical Center in North", *The Jerusalem Post*, 22 December 2013, https://www.jpost.com/Health-and-Science/Rambam-From-hospital-for-British-wounded-in-WWII-to-most-developed-medical-center-in-North-335762, accessed 11 March 2021.

Siegel-Itzkovich, J., "Victims of Hassadah Massacre to be Memorialized", *The Jerusalem Post*, 7 April 2008, https://www.jpost.com/Jewish-World/Jewish-News/Victims-of-Hadassah-massacre-to-be-memorialized, accessed 20 March 2021.

Van Lierop, R., "Liberty in East Africa", *New York Times*, 13 April 1972, The New York Times Archives, https://www.nytimes.com/1972/04/17/archives/liberty-in-east-africa.html?searchResultPosition=3, accessed 7 August 2020.

Webber, C., "Son's Emotional Journey to Site Where "hero" RAF Father Crashed in the Second World War", *The Northern Echo*, 20 July 2015, https://www.thenorthernecho.co.uk/news/13464833.sons-emotional-journey-site-hero-raf-father-crashed-second-world-war/, accessed 6 May 2021.

Yardley, W., "Mervyn Susser, 92, Dies; Studied Illness and Society", *The New York Times*, 26 August 2014, https://www.nytimes.com/2014/08/27/us/mervyn-susser-92-dies-studied-illness-and-society.html, accessed 22 March 2021.

Jack Penn Books and Articles (Published)

"Advances in Plastic and Reconstructive Surgery", *S.A. Medical Journal*, 26 March 1966.

"Aspects of Civilian Plastic Surgery", *South African Medical Journal*, 14 September 1940.

"The Brenthurst Clinic Tapestry", *British Journal of Plastic Surgery*, 20 January 1967.
Brenthurst Papers, Penn, J., ed, Johannesburg, Witwatersrand University Press, 1944, Brn. No: 3297, Call No: 617.95 BRE, BL.
"The Challenge of Africa", *British Journal of Plastic Surgery*, 18, 1965.
"Closure of Wounds and Incisions with Adhesive Tape", *The Lancet*, 5 November 1955.
"Communist Influence in Southern Africa", *New York Times*, 4 April 1972, The New York Times Archives, https://www.nytimes.com/1972/04/04/archives/communist-influence-in-southern-africa.html?searchResultPosition=1 accessed 7 August 2020.
"He Is My Younger Brother", *White Africans Are Also People*, Millin, S.G., ed, Howard Timmons, Cape Town, 1966, Brn. No: 14607, Call No: 323.1128 MIL, BL.
"Hiroshima and After", *Transactions of the Association of Plastic Surgeons of Southern Africa*, 3, 21, October 1957, AMUW.
"Impressions of Plastic and Maxillo-Facial Surgery in the Palestine War", *Plastic and Reconstructive Surgery*, 6, 4, October 1950.
"In the Steps of the 'Maestro'", *American Journal of Surgery*, Vol 95, February 1958.
"Plastic Surgery in Perspective", *The Lancet*, 13 October 1962.
"Plastic Surgery in the USA", *S.A. Medical Journal*, 9 November 1946.
"Profile: Jack Penn", *SA Practice Management*, 9, 3, 1988, File: Biography—Jack Penn, AMUW.
Reflections on Life, Johannesburg, Eric Stanton Publishers, 1980.
"The Removal of 'Cross-Hatch' Scars", *Plastic and Reconstructive Surgery*, 25, 1, January 1960.
The Right to Look Human: An Autobiography, Johannesburg, Hugh Keartland Publishers, 1976.
"A Surgeon's Story: It Is the Divine Right of Man to Look Human" (Unpublished Manuscript), Brn No 12057, 617.95 PEN, BL.
"Towards a Modern Utopia" (Unpublished Manuscript), Brn. No: 12778, Call No: PAM.1594, BL.
"Treatment of Hair-Lip and Cleft-Palate", *South African Medical Journal*, 25 June 1938.
"A Visit to Albert Schweitzer", *Plastic and Reconstructive Surgery*, 18, 3, September 1956.
With Bental, H., "Hypotensive Anaesthesia in Plastic Surgery: A Report on 500 Cases", *South African Medical Journal*, 9 May 1953.
With Brown, L., "A New Conception in Extra-Oral Splintage", Brenthurst Papers, Jack Penn, ed, Johannesburg, Witwatersrand University Press, 1944, Brn. No: 3297, Call No: 617.95 BRE, BL.

With Epstein, E., "Notes on a Case of Carcinoma Following Shell-Wound of the Face", *Plastic and Reconstructive Surgery*, 12, 2, August 1953.

With Gillman, T., Summary of "Plastic Surgery in the Service of the Leper with Some Comments on the Clinical and Microscopic Features of the Skin of 'Healed' Lepers", Presented at Congresso Internazionale per la Difesa e la Rehabilitazione Sociale del "Lebbroso", Rome, April 1956, *Plastic and Reconstructive Surgery*, 18, 6, December 1956.

With Gillman, T., Bronks, D. and Roux, M., "Reactions of Healing Wounds and Granulation Tissue in Man to Auto-Thiersch, Autodermal, and Homodermal Grafts", *British Journal of Plastic Surgery*, 6, 1953–1954.

With Gillman, T., and Hathorne, M., "Is Skin Homografting Necessary? A Re-examination for the Rationale for Auto- or Homo-Grafting of Cutaneous Injuries and a Preliminary Report on the Action of Plastic Dressings", *Plastic and Reconstructive Surgery*, 18, 4, October 1956.

With Penn, J.G., "Two Generations in Plastic Surgery", *Plastic and Reconstructive Surgery*, 91, 4, April 1993.

Washington Weekly, File: Biography—Jack Penn, AMUW

- "The Fate of South Africa", 21 July 1977.
- "A South African's View: Double-Dealing Standards", 23 February 1978.
- "A South African's View: Is the UN Civilised?", 3 September 1978
- "A South African's View: Rhodesians have Shown Courage",
- "A South African's View: Strength from Isolation", 2 March 1978.

Secondary Sources: Books, Book Chapters, Journal Articles and Online Sources

Abrahamian, E., *A History of Modern Iran*, New York, Cambridge University Press, 2008.

AD Editorial Team, "Spotlight: Kenzō Tange", 4 September 2019, https://www.archdaily.com/270043/happy-birthday-kenzo-tange, accessed 13 August 2020.

Adler, F.H., "South African Jews and Apartheid", *Patterns of Prejudice*, 34, 4, December 2010.

Alden, C., "The Chrysanthemum and the Protea: Reinventing Japanese-South African Relations after Apartheid", *African Affairs*, 101, 2002.

Allsobrook, C., and Boisen, C., "Two Types of Trusteeship in South Africa: From Subjugation to Separate Development", *Politikon*, 44, 2, 2017.

Anderson, B., *Imagined Communities: Reflections on the Origin and Spread of Nationalism*, London and New York, Verso, 2006.

Anson, T.V., "The New Zealand Dental Services" (Wellington, Historical Publications Branch, 1960), http://nzetc.victoria.ac.nz/tm/scholarly/tei-WH2Dent-c1.html#name-023303-mention, accessed 10 February 2021.

Anthony, D., "'Ours Is a War of Survival': Biafra, Nigeria and Arguments about Genocide, 1966-70", *Journal of Genocide Research*, 16, 2-3, August 2014.

Auslin, M., "Japan's Endless Search for Modernity: What the Anniversary of the Meiji Restoration Tells Us About the Country's Uncertain Future", *The Atlantic*, 3 January 2018, https://www.theatlantic.com/international/archive/2018/01/japan-abe-meiji-restoration-china/549536/, accessed 25 August 2020.

Baldwin-Ragaven, L., De Gruchy, J and London, L., *An Ambulance of the Wrong Colour: Health Professionals, Human Rights and Ethics in South Africa*, Cape Town, University of Cape Town Press, 1999.

Bamji, A., *Faces from the Front: Harold Gillies, the Queen's Hospital, Sidcup and the Origins of Modern Plastic Surgery*, Solihull, Helion and Company, 2017.

Bank, A., "Fathering *Volkekunde*: Race and Culture in the Ethnological Writings of Werner Eiselen, Stellenbosch University, 1926–1936", *Anthropology Southern Africa*, 38, 3 and 4, 2015.

– "The Politics of Mythology: The Genealogy of the Philip Myth", *Journal of Southern African Studies*, 5, 3, September 1999.

Barak, A. and Har-Shai, Y., "The Israel Society for Plastic Surgeons: A Brief Introduction", *Aesthetic Surgery Journal*, September/October 2004.

Barber, J. and Barrett, J., *South Africa's Foreign Policy: The Search for Status and Security, 1945–1988*, Cambridge University Press, 1990.

Battle, R., "Plastic Surgery in the Two World Wars and in the Years Between", *Journal of the Royal Society of Medicine*, 71, November 1978.

Beasley, W.G., *The Rise of Modern Japan: Political, Economic and Social Change Since 1850*, New York, St Martin's Press, 1990.

Bentwich, N., "Jewish Life in British South Africa", *Jewish Social Studies*, 4, 1, January 1942.

Berat, L., "Conscientious Objection in South Africa: Governmental Paranoia and the Law of Conscription", *Vanderbilt Journal of Transnational Law*, 22, 1, 1989.

Biernoff, S., "Flesh Poems: Henry Tonks and the Art of Surgery", *Visual Culture in Britain*, 11, 1, 2010.

Blanco, R.L., "American Army Hospitals in Pennsylvania during the Revolutionary War", *Pennsylvania History: A Journal of Mid-Atlantic Studies*, 48, 4, October 1981.

Blistein, D. and Burns, K., *The Mayo Clinic: Faith, Hope, Science*, New York, RosettaBooks, 2018.

"Born to be a Nurse: Cecilia Makiwane" in #SANC News, South African Nursing Council, Vol 3, March 2019, https://sanc.co.za/archive/archive2019/linked_files/Newsletters/Newsletter%20Mar2019.pdf, accessed 28 March 2021.

Brand, R.A., "Sir William Arbuthnot Lane, 1856–1943", *Clinical Orthopaedics and Related Research*, 467, 8, August 2009, https://www.ncbi.nlm.nih.gov/pmc/articles/PMC2706364/, accessed 9 December 2020.

Bremner, C. and Keene, R., "Archibald Sutherland Strachan 23 November 1891, Glasgow—20 February 1949, Johannesburg", *Pioneers in African Occupational Health*, 26, 2, March/April 2020.

Brenner, M., *In Search of Israel: The History of an Idea*, Princeton and Oxford, Princeton University Press, 2018.

"A Brief History of Valley Forge General Hospital", http://www.hspa-pa.org/History%20of%20Valley%20Forge%20Army%20Hospital.pdf, accessed 25 January 2021.

Brown, T.M. and Fee, E., "Sidney Kark and John Cassel: Social Medicine Pioneers and South African Emigres", *American Journal of Public Health*, 92, 11, November 2002.

Burger, M. and Gould, C., *Secrets and Lies: Wouter Basson and South Africa's Chemical and Biological Warfare Programme*, Cape Town, Zebra Press, 2002.

Chakrabarti, P., *Medicine and Empire, 1600-1960*, Basingstoke, Palgrave Macmillan, 2014.

Chetty, S., "Containing the Ripple of Hope: Apartheid, the Afrikaans Press and Robert F. Kennedy's Visit to South Africa, June 1966", *Southern Journal for Contemporary History*, 45, 1, 2020.

– "'Subjects or Citizens?' Black Soldiers and the Dilemma of the Second World War", *Journal of Natal and Zulu History*, 30, 1, 2012.

"Chungshan Institute of Science and Technology", *Globalsecurity.org*, https://www.globalsecurity.org/wmd/world/taiwan/csist.htm, accessed 26 April 2021.

"Citation Delivered by Deputy Vice-Chancellor, Professor S.P. Jackson, on the Occasion of the Conferment of the Degree of Doctor of Science, Honoris Causa, on Sydney Brenner", https://www.wits.ac.za/media/wits-university/alumni/documents/honorary-degree-citations, accessed 15 April 2021.

Claassen, J.M., "'Yonder Lies Your Hinterland': Rhodes, Baker and the Twisted Strands of the South African Architectural Tradition", *Akroterion*, 54, 2009.

Clarence B. Randall, "Individualism: Human Satisfaction Is What We Seek", Transcript of Speech Delivered at John Carroll University, Ohio, 26 January 1962", *Vital Speeches of the Day*, Pro Rhetoric LLC.

"Clarence B. Randall Papers", https://library.princeton.edu/special-collections/collections/clarence-b-randall-papers, accessed 15 February 2021.

Clarfield, A.M., Manor, O., Nun, G.B., Shvarts, S., Azzam, Z.S., Afek, A., Basis, F. and Israeli, A., "Health and Health Care in Israel: An Introduction", *Lancet*, 389, 24 June 2017.

Conchiglia, A., "Was Mozambique Air Crash an Assassination? The Mysterious Death of Samora Machel", *Le Monde Diplomatique* [English translation], 1 November 2017.

Conway, D., "'All These Long-haired Fairies Should be Forced to Do Their Military Training. Maybe They Will Become Men': The End Conscription Campaign, Sexuality, Citizenship and Military Conscription in Apartheid South Africa", *South African Journal on Human Rights*, 20, 2, 2004.

Conway, H., Reid, W.H., Beaton, J.J. and McGrouther, D.A., "Thomas Gibson, Plastic Surgeon (1915–93): Allograft Rejection by the Immune System and Prediction of Free Tissue Transplantation", *Journal of Plastic, Reconstructive and Aesthetic Surgery*, 65, 2012.

"Cope, John Patrick", Brief Biographical History as Part of Archival Note at *Archive Hub*, https://archiveshub.jisc.ac.uk/search/archives/f281acd6-0589-3943-ac90-67bdd9eaf4e2, accessed 19 April 2021.

Cousins, N., "Modern Man Is Obsolete", Editorial Obtained from https://rachelcarsoncouncil.org/wp-content/uploads/2018/01/RCC.Cousins.-SatRev.ModernMan.pdf, accessed 14 August 2020.

Crais, C.C., "The Vacant Land: The Mythology of British Expansion in the Eastern Cape, South Africa", *Journal of Social History*, 25, 2, 1991.

Davenport, J., *Digging Deep: A History of Mining in South Africa*, Johannesburg, Jonathan Ball Publishers, 2013.

Davidovitch, N. and Zalashik, R., "Pasteur in Palestine: The Politics of the Laboratory", *Science in Context*, 23, 4, 2010.

Davie, L., "The Great Synagogue in Hillbrow", March 2020, http://www.theheritageportal.co.za/article/great-synagogue-hillbrow, accessed 26 March 2021.

Davis, J.S., "Plastic Surgery in World War I and in World War II", *Plastic and Reconstructive Surgery*, 1, 3, November 1946.

Davis, W.B., "The Life of John Staige Davis, M.D.", *Plastic and Reconstructive Surgery*, 62, 3, September 1978.

Dedering, T., "Petitioning Geneva: Transnational Aspects of Protest and Resistance in South West Africa/Namibia After the First World War", *Journal of Southern African Studies*, 35, 4, December 2009.

Digby, A., "Early Black Doctors in South Africa", *Journal of African History*, 46, 2005.

"Discipline of Plastic Surgery: More About Plastic Surgery", University of KwaZulu-Natal, https://plasticsurg.ukzn.ac.za/aboutus/, accessed 20 April 2021.

Domson-Lindsay, A., "South African-Swazi Relations: A Constructivist Reading", *South African Journal of International Affairs*, 21, 3, 2014.

Dorning, W.A., "A Concise History of the South African Defence Force (1912–1987)", *Scientia Militaria, South African Journal of Military Studies*, 17, 2, 1987, http://scientiamilitaria.journals.ac.za, accessed 26 November 2020.

Douglas, L.G., "History of the Canadian Society of Plastic Surgeons", The Canadian Society of Plastic Surgeons, 1983. http://plasticsurgery.ca/wp-content-csps/uploads/2016/05/HISTORY.pdf, accessed 13 December 2020.

"Dr Lionel Melzer", http://www.machal.org.il/index.php?option=com_content&view=article&id=533&Itemid=879&lang=en, accessed 29 August 2020

Dubow, S., "Afrikaner Nationalism, Apartheid and the Concept of 'Race'", *Journal of African History*, 33, 2, 1992.

– *Apartheid 1948–1994*, Oxford, Oxford University Press, 2014.

– *A Commonwealth of Knowledge: Science, Sensibility, and White South Africa, 1820–2000*, Oxford, Oxford University Press, 2007.

– *Scientific Racism in Modern South Africa*, Cambridge, Cambridge University Press, 1995.

– *South Africa's Struggle for Human Rights*, Auckland Park, Jacana Media, 2012.

Eatough, M., "National Citizens, Global Economies: Sarah Gertrude Millin and the Professionalization of Envy", *Safundi: The Journal of South African and American Studies*, 14, 4, 2013.

Edgerton, D., *The Shock of the Old: Technology and Global History Since 1900*, London, Profile Books Ltd, 2008.

"Famous Medical Alumni", https://www.wits.ac.za/media/wits-university/alumni..., accessed 15 April 2021.

Fisher, D., "The Rockefeller Foundation and the Development of Scientific Medicine in Great Britain", *Minerva*, 16, 1, 1978.

Fisher, J.D., "Stephenson, Sir Arthur George (1890–1967)", *Australian Dictionary of Biography*, https://adb.anu.edu.au/biography/stephenson-sir-arthur-george-8646, accessed 16 April 2021.

"Follow the Drum: South African Military Hospital", *The Library Blog*, 8 November 2017, https://libraryblog.lbrut.org.uk/2017/11/south-african-military-hospital/, accessed 25 November 2020.

Fraser, J.F. and Hultman, C.S., "America's Fertile Frontier: How America Surpassed Britain in the Development and Growth of Plastic Surgery During the Interwar Years of 1920-1940", *Annals of Plastic Surgery*, 64, 5, May 2010.

Freinkel, S., "A Brief History of Plastic's Conquest of the World: Cheap Plastic Has Unleashed a Flood of Consumer Goods", *Scientific American*, 29 May 2011, https://www.scientificamerican.com/article/a-brief-history-of-plastic-world-conquest/, accessed 1 February 2021.

Freshwater, M.F., "A Critical Comparison of Davis' Principles of Plastic Surgery with Gillies' Plastic Surgery of the Face", *Journal of Plastic, Reconstructive and Aesthetic Surgery*, 64, 2011.

– "Denis F. Keegan: Forgotten Pioneer of Plastic Surgery", *Journal of Plastic, Reconstructive and Aesthetic Surgery*, 65, 8, March 2012.

Freund, B., *Twentieth-Century South Africa: A Developmental History*, Cambridge, Cambridge University Press, 2019.

Gabriel, R.A., *Between Flesh and Steel: A History of Military Medicine from the Middle Ages to the War in Afghanistan*, Lincoln, Potomac Books, 2016.

Garon, S., "Rethinking Modernization and Modernity in Japanese History: A Focus on State-Society Relations", *The Journal of Asian Studies*, 53, 2, May 1994.

"George Edward Hale Enderby: Pioneer and Architect of Modern Anaesthesia", *The BMJ*, https://www.bmj.com/content/suppl/2004/05/20/328.7450.1263.DC1, accessed 4 February 2020.

George, J.F. and Pinderski, L.J., "Peter Medawar and the Science of Transplantation: A Parable", *Journal of Heart Lung Transplant*, International Society for Heart and Lung Transplantation, 20, 2001.

Gillies, H.D., *Plastic Surgery of the Face*, London, Henry Frowde and Hodder and Stoughton, 1920.

Gillon, P., *Seventy Years of Southern African Aliyah: A Story of Achievement*, Israel, Adar Productions, 1992.

Greenblatt, S.S., "'To a Golden Land': The Circle of Immigration of South African Jews", Unpublished MA Thesis, University of the Witwatersrand, 2004.

Griffith, S., "Two Weeks in September, 1958: Atoms For Peace Conference in Geneva", *Iter Newsline*, 47, September 2008, https://www.iter.org/newsline/47/680, accessed 19 April 2021.

Harris, R., "The Allure of Albert Schweitzer", *History of European Ideas*, 40, 6, 2014.

Hachiya, M., *Hiroshima Diary: The Journal of a Japanese Physician, August 6—September 30, 1945*, Well, W., translator and editor, Chapel Hill and London, The University of North Carolina Press, 1955.

Harris, V., Hatang, S. and Liberman, P., "Unveiling South Africa's Nuclear Past", *Journal of Southern African Studies*, 30, 3, 2004.

Hedley-Whyte, J. and Milamed, D.R., "Severe Burns in World War II", *Ulster Medical Journal*, 86, 2, 2017.

– "Surgical Travellers: Tapestry to Bayeux", *Ulster Medical Journal*, 83, 3, 2014.

"Helfet, Arthur Jacob (1907–1989)", *Plarr's Lives of the Fellows*, Royal College of Surgeons of England, https://livesonline.rcseng.ac.uk/client/en_GB/lives/search/detailnonmodal/ent:$002f$002fSD_ASSET$002f0$002fSD_ASSET:379507/one, accessed 20 March 2021

Herbert, R.K., "Contextualising a Missionary's Trek" in *Clement M. Doke, Trekking in South Central Africa, 1913–1919*, Robert K. Herbert (ed) (Johannesburg, University of the Witwatersrand Press, 1993), pp xi–xv, http://pzacad.pitzer.edu/NAM/newafrre/writers/dokec/17memoir/part1.pdf, accessed 31 August 2020.

Hillary, R., *The Last Enemy*, London, Penguin Books, 2018.

"Hiroshima Peace Memorial (Genbaku Dome)", https://whc.unesco.org/en/list/775/, accessed 13 August 2020.

"History", APRASSA, https://aprassa.co.za/history/, accessed 20 April 2021.

"History of APRASSA", https://aprassa.co.za/history-of-the-association.php, accessed 3 May 2021.

Hocking, A., *Oppenheimer and Son*, Johannesburg, McGraw-Hill Book Company, 1973.

Horwitz, S., "'Black Nurses in White': Exploring Young Women's Entry into the Nursing Profession at Baragwanath Hospital, Soweto, 1948 –1980", *Social History of Medicine*, 20, 1, 2007.

Howell, J.D., "Early Clinical Use of the X-Ray", *Transactions of the American Clinical and Climatological Association*, 127, 2016, https://www.ncbi.nlm.nih.gov/pmc/articles/PMC5216491/, accessed 21 December 2020.

Howie, W.B., "The Administration of an Eighteenth-Century Provincial Hospital: The Royal Salop Infirmary, 1747-1830", *Medical History*, 5, 1, 1961.

https://biography.yourdictionary.com/norman-cousins, accessed 14 August 2020.

https://www.britannica.com/place/Hiroshima-Japan#ref289199, accessed 13 August 2020.

https://www.geni.com/people/Solomon-Penn/6000000084338103860, accessed 26 March 2021.

https://www.imdb.com/title/tt0050109/, accessed 25 June 2021.

Hsu, G.K., "Control of Manipulation? Nuclear Power in Taiwan" in *Learning from Fukushima: Nuclear Power in East Asia*, Van Ness, P. and Gurtov, M. (eds) Acton, Australian National University Press, 2017.

"International Confederation for Plastic, Reconstructive and Aesthetic Surgery (IPRAS)", *Yearbook of International Organizations Online*, https://uia.org/s/or/en/1100065003, accessed 24 May 2021.

Isaacman, A., "Toward a Biography of Samora Michel: The Making of a Revolutionary, 1933-1970 ca.", *South African Historical Journal*, 72, 1, 2020.

Isaacman, A.F. and Isaacman, B.F., "Extending South Africa's Tentacles of Empire: The Deterritorialisation of Cahora Bassa Dam", *Journal of Southern African Studies*, 41, 3, 2015.

"Israelis You Should Know: Dr Chaim Sheba", *International Fellowship of Christians and Jews*, https://www.ifcj.org/news/fellowship-blog/israelis-you-should-know-chaim-sheba-2/, accessed 25 May 2021.

"Japanese Society of Plastic and Reconstructive Surgery", https://jsprs.or.jp/english/background/, accessed 25 August 2020.

"Jan Smuts Airport – South Africa", *Art Archives—South Africa*, https://art-archives-southafrica.com/jan-smuts-airport-johannesburg-artworks, accessed 27 March 2021.

Jooste, D., "The Life of Iconic Artist, Sculptor and Designer Ernest Ullmann", *The Heritage Portal*, August 2016, http://www.theheritageportal.co.za/article/life-iconic-artist-sculptor-and-designer-ernest-ullmann, accessed 19 April 2021.

Joshi, J.S. and Kumar, K., "The Dutch Physicians at Dejima or Deshima and the Rise of Western Medicine in Japan", *Proceedings of the Indian History Congress*, 63, 2002.

Justice Scott, D.G., "A Tribute to Justice Jan Hendrik Steyn (1928-2013)", *Lesotho Law Journal*, 20, 1–2, January 2013.

Kark, J.D., and Abramson, J.H., "Sidney Kark's Contributions to Epidemiology and Community Medicine", *International Journal of Epidemiology*, 32, 5, October 2003.

Katzew, H., *South Africa's 800: The Story of South Africa's Volunteers in Israel's War of Birth*, Woolf, J., ed, South African Zionist Federation, 2003.

Keene, R., "Our Graduates: 1924-2012", Johannesburg, Faculty of Health Sciences, University of the Witwatersrand, 2013.

Kershaw, I., *Making Friends with Hitler: Lord Londonderry, The Nazis and the Road to War*, Penguin Books, 2005.

King, C., *The Reinvention of Humanity: A Story of Race, Sex, Gender and the Discovery of Culture*, London, The Bodley Head, 2019.

Klausen, S., "The Race Welfare Society: Eugenics and Birth Control in Johannesburg, 1930–1940" in *Science and Society in Southern Africa*, Dubow, S., ed, Manchester and New York, Manchester University Press, 2000.

Kohler, S., "Case 1: Rockefeller University (Formerly the Rockefeller Institute for Medical Research), 1901", Center for Strategic Philanthropy and Civil Society (Duke), 2007, https://cspcs.sanford.duke.edu/sites/default/files/descriptive/rockefeller_university.pdf, accessed 10 February 2021.

Kuljian, C., *Darwin's Hunch: Science, Race and the Search for Human Origins*, Johannesburg, Jacana Media, 2016.

KwaZulu-Natal Museum, https://www.nmsa.org.za/news/10-news/210-2020-05-12-06-50-13.html, accessed 28 March 2021.

Lenta, M., "Choosing Difference: South African Jewish Writers", *Judaism: A Quarterly Journal of Jewish Life and Thought*, 50, 1, Winter 2001.

Levin, A., "South African 'know-how' and Israeli 'facts of life': the planning of Afridar, Ashkelon, 1949-1956", *Planning Perspectives*, 34, 2, 2019.

Libby, S.B. and Weiss, M.S., "Edward Teller's Scientific Life", *Physics Today*, American Institute of Physics, August 2004.

Mabin, A., "Varied Legacies of Modernism in Urban Planning" in Bridge, G. and Watson, S., eds, *A Companion to the City*, Oxford and Malden, Blackwell, 2000.

Macintyre, I., "Sir David Wilkie (1882–1938): Surgeon, Scientist and Philanthropist", *Journal of Medical Biography*, 5, November 2007.

MacLaren, I., "A Brief History of the Royal College of Surgeons of Edinburgh", *Res Medica*, 268, 2, 2005.

Maddox, J., "Obituary: Edward Teller (1908-2003)", *Nature*, 425, 25 September 2003.

Marks, S., "Apartheid and the Jewish Question", *Journal of Southern African Studies*, 30, 4, December 2004.

– *Divided Sisterhood: Race, Class and Gender in the South African Nursing Profession*, Johannesburg, Witwatersrand University Press, 1994.

– "Reflections on the 1944 National Health Services Commission: A Response to Bill Freund and Anne Digby on the Gluckman Commission", *South African Historical Journal*, 66, 1, 2014.

Martin, N.L., "Radiology at Base Hospital #28 in France during WW1", University of Kansas Medical Center, http://www.kumc.edu/wwi/base-hospital-28/clinical-services/radiology.html, accessed 21 December 2020.

Mayhew, E., *Guinea Pig Club: Archibald McIndoe and the RAF in World War II*, Barnsley, Pen and Sword Books, 2018.

McGeal, C., "Revealed: How Israel Offered to Sell South Africa Nuclear Weapons", *A Supplement to the Washington Report on Middle East Affairs*, August 2010, Reprinted in https://www.theguardian.com/world/2010/may/23/israel-south-africa-nuclear-weapons, accessed 28 April 2021.

"Mané-Katz (French/Ukrainian, 1894–1962)", Artnet—Artists, http://www.artnet.com/artists/man%C3%A9-katz/, accessed 20 April 2021.

McLeave, H., *McIndoe: Plastic Surgeon*, London, Frederick Muller Limited, 1961.

Meikle, M.C., "The Evolution of Plastic and Maxillofacial Surgery in the Twentieth Century: The Dunedin Connection", The Surgeon, 4, 5, October 2006.

– *Reconstructing Faces: The Art and Wartime Surgery of Gillies, Pickerill, McIndoe and Mowlem*, Otago University Press, 2015.

Meir-Glitzenstein, E., "Operation Magic Carpet: Constructing the Myth of the Magical Immigration of Yemenite Jews to Israel", *Israel Studies*, 16, 3, 2011.

Millar, S.R., "Rooksdown House and the Rooksdown Club: A Study into the Rehabilitation of Facially Disfigured Servicemen and Civilians Following the Second World War", Unpublished PhD Dissertation, University of London, 2015.

Mitchell, T., "The Resources of Economics: Making the 1973 Oil Crisis", *Journal of Cultural Economy*, 3, 2, 2010.

Morris, M., Price, T., Cowan, S.W., Yeo, C.J. and Phillips, B., "William Arbuthnot Lane (1856–1943): Surgical Innovator and His Theory of Autointoxication," *Department of Surgery Gibbon Society Historical Profiles*, Paper 48, 2017, https://jdc.jefferson.edu/gibbonsocietyprofiles/48, accessed 9 December 2020.

Morris, W., "The Plastic Surgeons of Southern Africa and the History of APRASSA", APRASSA.

Mouton, F.A., "'Dr No': A.P. Treurnicht and the Ultra-Conservative Quest to Maintain Afrikaner Supremacy, 1982-1993", *South African Historical Journal*, 65, 4, 2013.

Murphy, R.T., *Japan and the Shackles of the Past*, Oxford, Oxford University Press, 2014.

"Nagashima (Japan)", https://leprosyhistory.org/geographical_region/site/nagashima, accessed 24 August 2020.

Noble, V., *A School of Struggle: Durban's Medical School and the Education of Black Doctors in South Africa*, Scottsville, University of KwaZulu-Natal Press, 2013.

Nye, J.S., "Public Diplomacy and Soft Power", *The Annals of the American Academy of Public and Social Science*, Vol 616, "Public Diplomacy in a Changing World", March 2008.

Oakley, A., "Keloid and Hypertrophic Scar", *Dermnet NZ*, https://dermnetnz.org/topics/keloids-and-hypertrophic-scar/, accessed 24 August 2020.

"Obituary: George Grey Turner", *Plarr's Lives of the Fellows*, Royal College of Surgeons, https://livesonline.rcseng.ac.uk/client/en_GB/lives/search/detail nonmodal/ent:$002f$002fSD_ASSET$002f0$002fSD_ASSET:376907/one, accessed 7 September 2020.

"Obituary: John Marquis Converse, Surgeon", *The New York Times*, 1 February 1981, p32, New York Times Archive, https://www.nytimes.com/1981/02/01/obituaries/john-marquis-converse-surgeon.html, accessed 13 December 2020.

"Obituary: Sir John Fraser", *British Medical Journal*, 2, 978, 1947, https://www.bmj.com/content/2/4536/978.1, accessed 1 September 2020.

"Obituary: Theodore Gillman", *The Lancet*, 31 July 1971.

"Obituary Notices: T Pomfret Kilner", *British Medical Journal*, 2, 127, 11 July 1964, https://www.bmj.com/content/2/5401/127, accessed 10 December 2020.

Offiler, B., *U.S. Foreign Policy and the Modernization of Iran: Kennedy, Johnson, Nixon and the Shah*, Basingstoke, Palgrave Macmillan, 2015.

O'Malley, G.F., "The Grave Is Wide: The Hibakusha of Hiroshima and Nagasaki and the Legacy of the Atomic Bomb Casualty Commission and the Radiation Effects Research Foundation", *Clinical Toxicology*, 54, 6, 2016.

"O.R. Tambo International Airport—Johannesburg Airport", https://johannesburg-airport.co.za/, accessed 27 March 2021.

O'Sullivan, K., "Humanitarian Encounters: Biafras, NGOs and Imaginings of the Third World in Britain and Ireland, 1967-70", *Journal of Genocide Research*, 16, 2–3, 2014.

Paget, J.C., "Albert Schweitzer and Africa", *Journal of Religion in Africa*, 42, 2012.

Parle, J., *States of Mind: Searching for Mental Health in Natal & Zululand, 1868-1918*, Scottsville, UKZN Press, 2007.

Payne, R.T., "Japan's South Africa Policy: Political Rhetoric and Economic Realities", *African Affairs*, 86, 343, April 1987.

Penn, J.G., "Obituary: Jack Penn", *Aesthetic Surgery Journal*, 17, 1, January-February 1997.

Penn, J.G., "Obituary: Jack Penn", *Plastic and Reconstructive Surgery*, 100, 4, September 1997.

"Petersen, Norman August Marais", *Plarr's Lives of the Fellows*, Royal College of Surgeons of England, https://livesonline.rcseng.ac.uk/client/en_GB/lives/search/detailnonmodal?qu=LIVES_OCCUPATION%3D%22Maxillofacial+surgeon%22&qf=LIVES_HONOURS%09Titles%2FQualifications%09MRCS+1920%09MRCS+1920&d=ent%3A%2F%2FSD_ASSET%2F0%2FSD_ASSET%3A378202~~0&ic=true, accessed 6 May 2021.

Phillips, H., *In a Time of Plague: Memories of the 'Spanish' Flu Epidemic of 1918 in South Africa*, Cape Town: Van Riebeeck Society, 2018.

– *Plague, Pox and Epidemics: A Jacana Pocket History*, Johannesburg, Jacana, 2012.

– *UCT under Apartheid: Part 1—From Onset to Sit-In, 1948–1968*, Sunnyside, Fanele (Jacana), 2019.

Pierce, G.W. and O'Connor, G.B., "The Tubed Pedicle Flap in Reconstruction Surgery", *California and Western Medicine*, 35, 2, August 1931, https://www.ncbi.nlm.nih.gov/pmc/articles/PMC1657906/?page=1, accessed 9 December 2020.

Plaatje, S., *Native Life in South Africa*, Northlands, Picador Africa, 2007.

Posel, D., "The Apartheid Project, 1948–1970" in *The Cambridge History of South Africa, Volume 2, 1885–1994*, Ross, R., Mager, A.K. and Nasson, B., eds, Cambridge University Press, 2012.

Pottinger, B., *The Imperial Presidency: P.W. Botha, the First 10 Years*, Johannesburg, Southern Book Publishers, 1988.

Ramaphosa, C., "Deputy President Cyril Ramaphosa: Unveiling of new wing at Cecilia Makiwane Hospital in Mdantsane", South African Government, https://www.gov.za/speeches/remarks-deputy-president-cyril-ramaphosa-during-unveiling-new-wing-cecilia-makiwane, accessed 28 March 2021.

"Rare Disease Database—Yaws", *National Organization for Rare Disorders*, https://rarediseases.org/rare-diseases/yaws/, accessed 8 January 2021.

Reader's Digest, Illustrated History of South Africa: The Real Story, Cape Town, Reader's Digest, 1992.

Reidy, J.P., "The Formation and Early History of the Stoke Mandeville Plastic Surgery Unit", *British Journal of Plastic Surgery*, 39, 1986.

"Robert Vansittart", *Spartacus Educational*, https://spartacus-educational.com/Robert_Vansittart.htm, accessed 3 February 2021.

Roberts, F.W., "Working with Albert Schweitzer", http://www.nigel-roberts.info/Working-with-Schweitzer.htm, accessed 5 August 2020.

Roi, M.L., "Sir Robert Vansittart, The Global Balance of Power and Nazi Germany, 1934–1937", Unpublished PhD dissertation, University of Toronto, 1996.

S2A3 Biographical Database of Southern African Science, http://www.s2a3.org.za/bio/Biograph_final.php?serial=344, accessed 14 August 2021.

"Saints and Sinners: Sir Harold Gillies", *The Royal College of Surgeons of England Bulletin*, 2013, https://publishing.rcseng.ac.uk/doi/pdf/https://doi.org/10.1308/003588413X13643054409063, accessed 9 December 2020.

"Schlesinger, Izidore Williem: Business Magnate and Property Mogul", Artefacts.co.za, https://www.artefacts.co.za/main/Buildings/archframes.php?archid=6355, accessed 16 April 2021.

Scotland, T. Heys, S., eds, *War Surgery, 1914–18*, Solihull, Helion and Company, 2012.

- Holmes, J.D., "Development of Plastic Surgery"
- MacDonald, A., "X-Rays during the Great War"
- Robertson, E.A., "Anaesthesia, Shock and Resuscitation"
- Scotland, T.R., "Evacuation Pathway for the Wounded"
- Scotland, T.R. and Heys, S.D., "Setting the Scene"

Scott, D.L., "Hypnosis in Pedicle Graft Surgery", *British Journal of Plastic Surgery*, 29, 1976.

Schweitzer, A., *My Life and Thought: An Autobiography*, CT Campion, C.T., translator, London, George Allen and Unwin Ltd, 1933, 1948.

- *The Philosophy of Civilization 1: The Decay and the Restoration of Civilization*, London, Adam and Charles Black, 1950.
- *The Teaching of Reverence for Life*, London, Peter Owen Limited, 1965, 1966.

Segev, T., *A State at Any Cost: The Life of David Ben-Gurion*, Watzman, H., translator, London, Head of Zeus Ltd, 2019.

Sewell, B., "Reconsidering the Modern in Japanese History: Modernity in the Service of the Prewar Japanese Empire", https://www.researchgate.net/publication/254167793, accessed 25 August 2020.

Shain, M., "Jewish Cultures, Identities and Contingencies: Reflections from the South African Experience", *European Review of History*, 18, 1, February 2011.

Shain, M., Mendelsohn., R. and Bickford-Smith, V., "Testing Cosmopolitan Tolerance: Port Jews in Cape Town During the Late Victorian and Edwardian Years", *Jewish Culture and History*, 7, 1–2, May 2012.

Shimoni, G., *Community and Conscience: The Jews in Apartheid South Africa*, Glosderry, David Philip Publishers, 2003.

Silverman, M.E., Hollman, A. and Krikler, D.M., "The Hammersmith Hospital and the Royal Postgraduate Medical School" in Silverman, M.E., Fleming, P.R., Hollman, A., Julian, D.G. and Krikler, D.M., eds, *British Cardiology in the 20th Century*, London, Springer, 2000.

Singh, M., Barrett Noone, M.R., Afolabi, H. and Caterson, E.J., "A Tribute to the Founding Figures of the American Board of Plastic Surgery", *Plastic and Reconstructive Surgery*, 135, 6 June 2015.

Sir Roy Welensky, https://www.oxfordreference.com/view/https://doi.org/10.1093/oi/authority.20110803121643788, accessed 14 February 2021.

Sir Roy Welensky, Transcript of talk given on 12 October 1963, NYPR Archive Collections, https://www.wnyc.org/story/sir-roy-welensky/, accessed 14 February 2021.

Snijman, C., "The History and Development of Our Society", http://www.drsnijman.co.za/association-plastic-reconstructive-aesthetic-surgeons-southern-africa/, accessed 20 April 2021.

"South Africa: His Father's Son", Time Magazine, 2 August 1963, http://www.time.com/time/magazine/article/0,9171,870366,00.html, accessed 15 April 2021.

South African Medical Journal, 16 December 1967.

Spinney, L., *Pale Rider: The Spanish Flu of 1918 and How it Changed the World*, New York, Public Affairs, 2017.

Stadler, J. and Dugmore, C., "'Honey, Milk and Bile': A Social History of Hillbrow", *BMC Public Health*, 17, Suppl 3, 444, 2017.

Stanger, C.D., "A Haunting Legacy: The Assassination of Count Bernadotte", The Middle East Journal, 42, 2, 260-272, 1988.

Starzl, T.E., "Peter Brian Medawar: Father of Transplantation", *Journal of the American College of Surgeons*, 180, 3, March 1995.

Stelnicki, E.J., Young, V.L., Francel, T. and Randall, P., "Vilray P. Blair, His Surgical Descendants, and Their Roles in Plastic Surgical Development", *Plastic and Reconstructive Surgery*, 103, 7, June 1999.

Styan, J., *Heartbreaker: Christiaan Barnard and the First Heart Transplant*, Johannesburg and Cape Town, Jonathan Ball Publishers, 2018.

Susman, D., *An African Shopkeeper: Memoirs of David Susman*, Martin, L., ed, Fernwood Press, 2004. Excerpt taken from http://www.machal.org.il/index.php?option=com_content&view=article&id=287%3Adavid-susman&catid=45%3APersonal+Stories+&Itemid=392&lang=en, accessed 29 August 2020.

"Susman's Woolworths a Legacy to be Proud Of", *Newswires*, 14 May 2010, https://insurancenewsnet.com/oarticle/Susmans-Woolworths-a-Legacy-to-Be-Proud-of-a-190373, accessed 16 March 2021.

Susser, M., "A South African Odyssey in Community Health: A Memoir of the Impact of the Teachings of Sidney Kark", *American Journal of Public Health*, 83, 7, July 1993.

Teller, E., *Energy from Heaven and Earth*, San Francisco: W.H. Freeman and Company, 1979.

– "Science and Morality", *Science*, Vol 280, 5367, American Association for the Advancement of Science, 22 May 1998.

Thompson, L., *The Political Mythology of Apartheid*, New Haven and London, Yale University Press, 1985.

"Trachoma", https://www.mayoclinic.org/diseases-conditions/trachoma/symptoms-causes/syc-20378505, accessed 21 March 2021.

Tong, D., Bamji, A., Brooking, T. and Love, R., "Plastic Kiwis—New Zealanders and the Development of a Specialty", *Journal of Military and Veterans' Health*, 17, 1, October 2008.

Van der Waag, I., *A Military History of Modern South Africa*, Johannesburg and Cape Town, Jonathan Ball Publishers, 2015.

– "The Union Defence Force between the Two World Wars, 1919–1940", *Scientia Militaria*, South African Journal of Military Studies, 30, 2, 2000, http://scientiamilitaria.journals.ac.za, accessed 26 November 2020.

Van De Laar, A., *Under the Knife: Remarkable Stories from the History of Surgery*, Brown, A., translator, London, John Murray, 2018.

Van Onselen, C., *New Babylon New Nineveh: Everyday Life on the Witwatersrand, 1886-1914*, Johannesburg and Cape Town, Jonathan Ball Publishers, 2001.

Van Zyl-Hermann, D., *Privileged Precariat: White Workers and South Africa's Long Transition to Majority Rule*, Cambridge, Cambridge University Press, 2021.

Wallace, M. with Kinahan, J., *A History of Namibia: From the Beginning to 1990*, New York, Columbia University Press, 2011.

Watson, D.M.S., "Robert Broom 1866–1951", *Biographical Memoirs of the Fellows of the Royal Society*, November 1952.

Wilson, L., *Steve Biko*, Johannesburg, Jacana Media, 2011.

Wobst, A.W.K., "Hypnosis and Surgery: Past, Present and Future", *Anesthesia and Analgesia*, International Anesthesia Research Society, 104, 5, May 2007.

Wood, C. and Bioy, A., “Hypnosis and Pain in Children”, *Journal of Pain and Symptom Management*, 35, 4, April 2008.

Worley, M., “Why Fascism? Sir Oswald Mosley and the Conception of the British Union of Fascists”, *History*, 96, 1, 321, January 2011.

Index

S. Chetty, *Reconstructive Surgery and Modernisation in Twentieth-Century South Africa*, Medicine and Biomedical Sciences in Modern History, https://doi.org/10.1007/978-3-031-38673-2

J

K

O

P

S

T

FSC
www.fsc.org
MIX
Papier | Fördert gute Waldnutzung
FSC® C083411

Kolibri 360 GmbH
Ferdinand-Jühlke-Straße 7
99095 Erfurt, Deutschland
produktsicherheit@kolibri360.de